THE NEW VET'S HANDBOOK

Information and advice for veterinary graduates

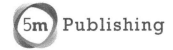

5m Publishing

To my son Guy, who was born with severe learning difficulties but who has taught me more about non-verbal communication than anyone could ever appreciate. Here he is with Spencer, our horse, with whom he has a special bond.

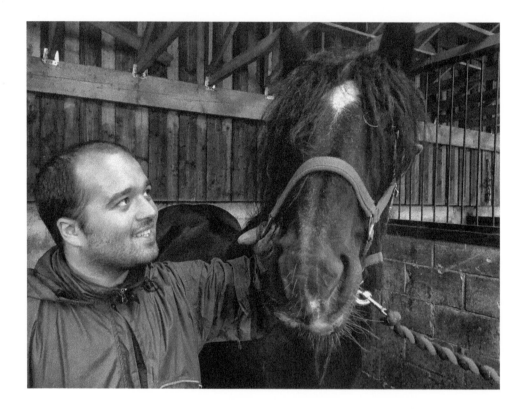

THE NEW VET'S HANDBOOK

Information and advice for veterinary graduates

Clare Tapsfield-Wright

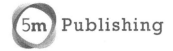

5m Publishing

First published 2018

Copyright © Clare Tapsfield-Wright 2018

Published by
5M Publishing Ltd,
Benchmark House,
8 Smithy Wood Drive,
Sheffield, S35 1QN, UK
Tel: +44 (0) 1234 81 81 80
www.5mpublishing.com

A catalogue record for this book is available from the British Library

ISBN 9781912178360

Book layout by
Keystroke, Neville Lodge, Tettenhall, Wolverhampton

Printed by CPI Anthony Rowe Ltd, UK

Photos by the author, Wendy Jones and Richard Tapsfield
Cartoons by Nigel Sutherland, www.nigelsutherland.co.uk

This book is intended to describe events that vets may typically encounter
during their careers and is based on the personal experience of the author.
It is not intended to replace formal advice and guidelines laid out by
veterinary regulatory authorities. Should occasions arise that require
additional input readers are advised to seek advice from their employer
or from experts including indemnity cover providers such as the VDS.
Any instances of veterinary procedures or encounters performed
sub-optimally have been included in the book for educational purposes
and are not intended to reflect on the character or competence of any individual.

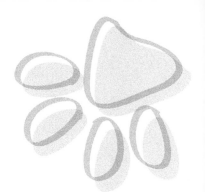

Contents

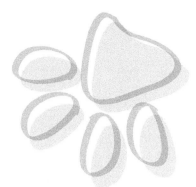

Introduction

I have written this book in the hope that it will act as a helping hand for veterinary students and newly qualified veterinary surgeons during the transition from student to working veterinary surgeon.

If you are a vet student reaching the end of your course and about to enter the world of work, you are a highly intelligent individual who has been through years of higher education both at school and at university to reach this point. This book is not a formal textbook or a manual, but a written mentor to help with some of the other stuff that comes with being a vet, and is not intended as a substitute for a human adviser but hopefully an additional useful resource to help you.

I hold my hands up and say unashamedly that this book is anecdote-based advice and comes from my years of experience of actually being a vet and from trial and error on a life-time scale. I have reached the stage of my professional life where I can freely admit to all my mistakes and I would like you to benefit from them and avoid making similar ones. I have been a vet for such a long time that much has changed in the veterinary world, but animals have not changed, and deep down their owners are very much the same too, even though their expectations and demands may be different.

Starting work as a qualified vet is a time of great transition when every day brings new experiences and challenges and you will frequently wonder if you are doing the right thing and how you should use all those skills you have acquired at vet school once you are out in practice. You have the attributes and knowledge to be an excellent veterinary surgeon and now you just need the experience to hone those skills and techniques in the reality of veterinary practice.

There will be times when you read something in this book and think that it is stating the obvious and you may wonder why I have included it at all, but I do hope you will also read about something you had not considered, and however insignificant or trivial it may seem, perhaps that small nugget of information could make your life as a vet just a little bit easier. There may be a few pointers which may throw light on something or prevent you from stumbling over a minor problem you didn't see coming.

We are all used to the perennial question of why we decided to choose this career and everyone has their own story. I am not from a farming-related background but decided at about the age of ten, having always been interested in animals and science, that I wanted to be a vet and from then on I worked through school with that aim in sight. I am sure many of you have experienced the same vocation and I hope that when you reach the same age as I am you will still be glad that you made that career choice. I often hear that many vets would choose a different career if they had their time again and that saddens me, because I can honestly say that I would do it all again and that training to be a vet has been one of the best decisions I ever made.

The life of a vet is not always sunshine and fluffy kittens, however, and I have had my ups and downs during my years in practice. I can still remember vividly how I felt when I first started out and how over the years, something always managed to pop up and surprise me, however well-prepared and experienced I was.

Like all vets, I have made mistakes over the years and I have included some of them here in the hope that I can help you avoid them, but also to illustrate that you can and will make mistakes and you will survive and can still be a good vet. Ours is a job which inevitably trips you up from time to time and I include the odd anecdote and tale of disaster because the unexpected happens all the time when animals are involved and it always will. This is what makes ours such an interesting and varied career and never boring, but there are times when it is difficult and demanding.

My career as a vet

I have been qualified as a vet for 38 years now and my first two jobs in practice were each of three years' duration and in mixed practice. I then decided my future lay in small animal practice and I was employed as an assistant for a further two years before being invited to become a partner and buying a 50 percent share in a small animal practice in West Yorkshire.

I was joint owner of an expanding practice for the next 28 years and over that time we employed many new and recently qualified graduates, some of whom stayed in the practice and some who moved on. It is a great privilege to see those new graduates transition through those first years in practice and to see what excellent vets they become. I still meet some of them from time to time and many have become more successful and much more highly qualified in various disciplines than I ever was. I have always been happy and proud to be a general practitioner and practice owner and it has been the right career choice for me.

The practice we owned is located in the north of England in Halifax and the surrounding Calder Valley and is typical of many small animal practices in the UK, being in an area where there is a wide range of client income. It has always covered its own out of hours work and is located in premises which are not purpose-built but converted from other uses and it employs a range of vets of differing ages and experience. There are many similar practices throughout the country which are neither state of the art nor minimal and basic and which provide good-quality, affordable veterinary care for the general public and their animals. The majority of vets start their careers in practices like this and the service these practices provide in nurturing newly qualified veterinary surgeons often goes unrecognised.

Veterinary practice has changed over the years and will continue to change with new medical advances and emerging diseases and other challenges such as antibiotic resistance and new technology, but the fundamentals remain the same and those are the needs of the animals, and the interactions with their owners and the colleagues you have to work with.

When I first graduated, female vets were very much in the minority and were a novelty for practices, farmers and pet owners. In the first two practices I worked in I was the first female vet the clients had ever seen and there were still a significant number of farming clients who thought women could not and should not do the job. I will always remember a sheep farmer insisting on carrying a bucket of water up the yard for me to a lambing and mumbling about this being no job for a lady.

The expectations of those who work as vets have altered and we should no longer allow the job to engulf our entire family life but quite rightly enjoy a healthy balance between work and other life interests. When I was first employed, a one in four rota was considered very generous and while my partner and I were building up the practice, we were working a one in two rota and I was paying 14 percent interest on a loan from the bank to buy my share of the partnership. When my veterinary partner was on holiday, I worked full-time all week and I was on call every night and all weekend. Some older vets look back and say that it was better being a vet back then, but in reality life in practice was often unhealthily all-consuming, and vets and their families suffered from the consequences of that, so I am glad things are changing for the better.

We now recognise the need for working reasonable hours and having a life outside work but the mental health of vets is still of great concern; it is not an easy life but it can be a rewarding and interesting career in the right circumstances. The nature of the pressures of veterinary work that we face nowadays have changed but they still exist for vets in practice particularly when we first start work and in the first few years after graduating. Thankfully, the recognition of the need for mentorship and support for young graduates and the will to provide it is increasing all the time although there is still much to be done. Support needs to be accessible to all vets throughout their lives because working as a vet is demanding and it takes its toll unless we improve the way we look after ourselves as a profession.

Writing this book

We sold our practice a few years ago and I am now a client and seeing veterinary practice and veterinary surgeons from a different viewpoint. It was attending veterinary practices and seeing the other side of practice with my two old dogs and a horse which prompted me to write this book. My dogs and horse were all in their last year of life and, like most clients with elderly animals, I was a frequent visitor for various reasons until their lives ended.

I now have a young Labrador bitch called Nelly who is also a patient of the small animal practice I used to own and I am a client of a local mixed practice with my new horse who is a sturdy cob called Spencer.

The experience of being a client as well as being a vet has been invaluable in writing this book as it has given me the perspective of being the end user of veterinary services and how it actually feels to consult the vet instead of being the vet.

I was also an elected member of the Royal College of Veterinary Surgeons Council for eight years from 2006 to 2014 and chaired the Standards Committee, and at the time of writing I am chair of the Primary Qualifications Subcommittee which advises on accreditation of vet schools in the UK and overseas.

I have written this book in an informal manner in the hope that you will find it useful and entertaining and feel able to pick it up and read a bit over a cup of tea or while you are waiting for a client. I hope you can read a section and find something which is relevant to you, wherever you are in your veterinary career and whatever type of work you may be doing at that moment. The thoughts expressed in it are my own and there will undoubtedly be vets who disagree with my opinions and the ways in which I approach being a vet but I hope you enjoy it, and if it provokes some thought and helps you in any small way at all then I will be happy to have been of help to another member of the profession I care about so very much.

CHAPTER 1

Becoming a vet

The beginning of your veterinary career

You may now be in your clinical years at vet school, or have just graduated and are about to embark on the start of the exciting life of a qualified veterinary surgeon. There are so many different career pathways for a vet but the majority of graduates will go into general practice which may be small animal, large animal, equine or mixed, and the aim of this book is to give you a helping hand as you navigate the first days, months and early years in practice.

Your weeks of extramural studies (EMS) will have given you the opportunity to have an insider view of veterinary practice and will have assisted you in making the decision as to what sort of veterinary work you would like to do. You have been trained to treat all species of animal to the level of the day one competencies but some vets will know from the outset that they only want to work in small animal practice whereas others have a special interest in equine or farm work. Whatever you decide to do, make the choice that you know is right for you, not because of anyone else's expectations or external pressures, or fear of making the wrong choice, but because you want to follow that path.

It is wise to think very carefully about the choices you make now because, even though it is entirely possible to change your mind in the light of experience, your first job is inevitably very influential in the direction your working life will take. Employment with a good practice with the right amount and quality of support will, however, provide the foundations for your future life in the profession and will be a springboard for your career and your happiness in your life as a vet.

What type of practice do you want to work in?

If you are convinced that you only want to work with companion animals, then your choices are clear when you look at the adverts and you will be considering all the ones which are small animal-orientated and disregarding any offering large animal work. If you are a little undecided, then you may find it a little easier to change to a small animal practice from a mixed practice rather than the other way around, and currently there is a reasonable variety of advertisements for new graduates for work both in mixed practice and small animal practice.

If you have always wanted to work in an equine practice, you may find the choice of positions available for a new graduate limited and there are likely to be many applicants for those that are advertised, but you may be able to find a mixed practice with a proportion of equine work in which you can gain valuable experience which will enable you to find an equine-only position in the future.

Mixed practices can offer you a broad range of experience in many species and a change in career path is always an option in the future once you know what you want to do. Be aware that if you are employed in a mixed practice where you are mainly performing small animal work in the daytime but are included in the out of hours rota for both large and small animals, then this can be quite a challenge as you have limited opportunity to learn the basics during the day. You only meet the farmers when faced with a large animal emergency, fire brigade work as we call it, and this can be daunting even with another vet on second call. If you are attracted to working with zoo animals or wildlife generally then a good grounding in a mixed practice will also give you valuable experience and transferable skills which will come in very useful in the future.

Some referral centre practices offer internships which might appeal to you, but they often require you to have some experience of working in first opinion practice beforehand, so that you become familiar with the common cases presented, and have the basic skills and ability to recognise what is normal and what is abnormal.

There are other options available to you such as staying in academia, and there is better advice on these options at the university where you are studying, but I will be concentrating in this book on aspects of working in general practice.

Many job adverts ask for a vet with some experience, but it is always worth considering sending a letter of application for such a position which you have found very appealing, if you feel you have something to offer despite being a new graduate. There are occasions when a practice asks for some experience but no suitable vets apply for the position, and an outstanding application from a new graduate might make a practice willing to invest the time and effort in bringing on a new graduate after all. Just make sure that they are able and willing to support a new graduate sufficiently and that you will not be asked to perform work beyond your capabilities.

If you had a good experience at a practice during EMS and you like the idea of working for that practice, then do write a letter to them even if they are not currently advertising. They may be prompted into considering you as an addition to their workforce and be glad to be approached, especially if you were a bright and willing student and they can see a role for you in the practice.

This is definitely the time to be proactive and go and look for the job that you want, using all your contacts and putting effort into your job search. If you know some recently qualified vets in practice then contact them and ask about any potential vacancies in the practices they are working in, especially if they have been treated well, because a word of mouth recommendation is invaluable.

Maternity cover positions may mean that the practice is going to ask you to fill a short-term vacancy rather than invest in you as a future member of the team, but this can also be a stepping stone to a permanent position, so do not discount them. Some vets do not choose to return to work after the end of their maternity leave so it may develop into a permanent position, but you still need to make sure it is a practice who is willing to give you good mentors and take time to integrate and support you as a new graduate.

When you are young, and you have a busy social life but few commitments, it may be tempting to work part-time with no evening or weekend work and to enjoy that precious work–life balance that everyone speaks of and treasures. The fact is, however, that if you take a part-time job at this stage of your career it will take you considerably longer to become experienced and confident, so I would advise you to take a full-time position as a new gradu-ate if at all possible. Working two days a week usually means that you have to hand over a complicated case to another vet and by the time you are back at work again the animal is either better or might even be dead! Learning case management by following cases through and assessing outcomes is so much easier if you are working full-time and can find out what happened and how accurate your diagnosis and treatment was. There are well-paid part-time positions in vaccine and neuter clinics but, if you restrict your exposure to more complex cases and sick and injured animals, you will limit your opportunity to become an experienced clinician so do not be tempted by pots of cash for uninspiring part-time work.

I believe that if you do not take a job which involves working out of hours in the first few years of your career then there is a strong likelihood that you never will, and some students have indeed told me that they never want to work in an on call rota. There is a great deal of discussion in the veterinary press about work–life balance and the stress of working out of hours but the fact remains that it presents a great opportunity to learn. Fear of not being able to cope with the pressure has been cited to me as a reason but in a moderately sized practice there are not as many dire emergencies out of hours as you may fear. Although we all fear the midnight GDV, these drastic emergencies are not nearly as frequent out of hours as less challenging but interesting cases such as acutely sick animals, cut paws, diarrhoea and collapsed, old dogs.

Out of hours work offers amazing opportunities to learn and can be exciting and interesting, offering you the time to work a case through from start to finish, and the chance to experience the responsibility of using your training and skills and seeing the results. You will really feel you are making a difference when you help a sick or injured animal out of hours and it is one of the many things which makes the job worthwhile. It is potentially easier to complete the requirements of the Professional Development Phase (PDP) if you work out of hours too, as during the day there may be fewer opportunities to perform more complicated procedures and surgeries.

It can help when searching for jobs to have criteria which exclude the practices which you would not consider but do not make those criteria too restrictive. Read every advert carefully so as not to waste your time applying for something unsuitable.

Look everywhere, in the *Vet Record* and the *Vet Times* and also online as increasingly this is where jobs are being advertised.

Some jobs advertised as farm animal positions may be primarily TB testing so make sure you read the advert carefully.

What area of the country do you want to work in?

It is not a good idea in a competitive job market to be too rigid about what geographical region of the country you are prepared to consider; if you are willing to work anywhere in the country then you are more likely to find the practice which offers what you seek.

I do understand that it can be attractive to be reasonably near family and friends as this is going to be a time where family support can be very helpful both emotionally and practically, but this will depend on your individual circumstances and your personality and needs. You have already been away from home studying and you know yourself best, and though some individuals thrive well without the support of family and friends, others do not and this will be a challenging year. You may feel that you need that level of proximity in your first year and would not be happy starting work in a completely new region of the country. It can make a big difference if you are near enough to drive home for some home-cooked food and a sympathetic ear from those who love you.

Do not limit your choices of job by imposing too many filtering criteria as it may be that the job market does not offer enough of exactly what you seek and you have to work in a slightly different type of practice or in a city environment when you would prefer a rural setting. You can always move practices in a few years' time. For a new graduate, choosing a good, supportive practice is far more important than the location.

What size of practice?

You will be faced with choices of a large practice with many vets, which may be part of a company or corporate organisation, or a medium-sized practice which may or may not have central management. There are still some small practices with one or two vets or nurses who are owners and who are planning on expanding and taking on a new graduate as their client numbers increase. Your employer may be working alongside you, or you may be supervised and managed by a clinical director who is also themselves an employee. Some practices, despite employing quite a large number of vets, are set up with multiple branches with one or two vets working at each branch, whereas a practice with one large building will have all the vets and nurses under the same roof. Practices come in all sizes and with multiple variations of management structures, with vets with different levels of expertise and the potential for expansion and opportunities for the vets they employ.

This can be a very important consideration and one you should look at carefully, so always search for the website of a practice and check how it is organised and who is working and where. In a large practice, the chances are that you will have vets of varying ages, some of whom will most likely have qualified relatively recently and with whom you will have much in common. This can also increase the opportunity for a good social life outside work which can be very important especially if you are of a sociable disposition and likely to enjoy the company of other young vets and support staff. Young, recently qualified vets will also remember what it is like to be a new graduate and may be more helpful, understanding and supportive, having experienced it themselves so recently.

I have been told by younger vets that in some large multi-vet practices, the more senior vets have a tendency to monopolise much of the interesting work and leave the younger graduates with a high proportion of the more mundane, routine work such as neutering and basic consulting. This is perhaps only to be expected in the first few months while you find your feet, but can become frustrating if you never get the opportunity to increase your experience as time goes by. Good management should prevent this happening but human nature being what it is, and a natural inclination by vets to look for the interesting surgical work, can make it more difficult for a recent graduate to get a look in with the exciting cases.

Some large practices can appear a little intimidating in size because they employ many vets, but the organisation of the premises may be that of several self-sufficient small branch surgeries which can mean that you are still working in a relatively small team. In some practices with small branch surgeries there may be just one vet at a branch, and I would suggest that it is preferable for a new graduate not to be expected to work completely on their own without the support of a more experienced colleague who is physically present and not just at the end of a phone.

In a small practice, there may not be the same number of complex medical and surgical cases as in a large practice and they may not have the top-of-the-range equipment that you have seen at vet school, but you may be more likely to get individual attention from an experienced vet who is highly motivated for you to succeed.

This is especially true if they are the owner or have a significant financial stake in the practice. They may be inclined to be more generous with their time than a fellow employee and may give you encouragement and the opportunities to gain experience in more complex procedures at an earlier stage.

You may be an individual who thrives better with this sort of personal, one-to-one mentoring by your employer or line manager, or you may prefer being part of a larger group, but it is useful to think about it in advance while you are looking at the jobs on offer.

Who will you be working for and who with?

Practices may be independent, small businesses owned by one or more vets or may be owned by a large company or a charity. Many investment companies buy independent practices and keep the practice more or less the same in terms of organisation and culture because this is the model which has made that particular practice successful. There may, as a result, be many different types of practices even within a group owned by the same larger company, and new graduates may have varying experiences despite being employed by the same company.

Some companies have their own internal new graduate support and mentoring programmes which are structured and consistent and this approach may appeal to you more than the informal mentoring which exists in some practices. As previously mentioned, you may prefer the personal approach from an independent practice owner who is mentoring you on a daily basis as well as employing you.

I recommend that you make some enquiries and see if you can get feedback from vets who work there such as graduates who qualified a year or two ago, or see if you can speak to the vets employed in a practice as this may be more revealing than the information you receive from the prospective employer. Vets are more willing to be frank with their views if you contact them by phone or private message rather than asking them to put anything in writing or in an open forum online.

When to start work?

After all that studying for your final exams you may have plans to go travelling after you qualify or you may be eager to use your skills right away and start applying for jobs. Once you are working in practice you will be highly unlikely to get more than two or three consecutive weeks of holiday unless you are between jobs, so if you are desperate to go to Thailand, now might be a good time.

At a recent congress for final year students, a panel of graduates qualified for one year said that they felt they needed a few weeks off to recover from the last six months of vet school because they were exhausted, but they also felt concerned that they would forget things if they took six months off to go travelling.

It is worth considering that practices looking for a new graduate may be targeting their advertising right now and there is competition for jobs out there. Starting work at the same time as your vet friends can also provide you with an unofficial support group because you can compare notes and keep in touch with people you know who are experiencing the same situations as you are in the same timeframe. The first few weeks and months are exciting but can also be bewildering, exhausting, wonderful and terrifying and speaking to people who are experiencing the same feelings can be very comforting and helpful.

Applying for a job in practice

I am sure you have had plenty of advice and instruction on the practicalities of applying for jobs and composing CVs, so I am not going to duplicate that here but instead explain just what I was looking for when I was advertising as a prospective employer of a recent graduate and of assistant vets generally.

Over the years, I must have read thousands of CVs and covering letters from new and recently qualified graduates. The advent of the computer has been both a blessing and a curse as in the past I have received handwritten letters of application which allowed for a certain amount of early filtering. Applications on lined notepaper with fluffy kittens and letters full of spelling mistakes, such as spelling veterinary as 'vetinary', and hastily dashed-off letters which were virtually illegible, went straight into the rejection pile. You may think this harsh, but if an applicant cannot be bothered to compose a good letter of application, then an employer may have less confidence in their potential to be a diligent and organised employee. Many applications are now online and you will have been told the importance of a good CV and covering letter.

Nowadays, every veterinary graduate can use spellcheck and will have received training in producing a professional-looking CV, which is good news for the applicant but means that it is also more difficult for you to make your application stand out from the others. Employers have to use other means to weed out the poor applications and other criteria are used to decide whose application goes into the 'maybe' file and who receives a polite rejection.

A good first impression with a well-written CV is the key to getting on that shortlist because time is very precious to a busy employer who may be confronted by a large number of applications for the position and may also be working as a vet at the same time with all the inevitable time pressures that presents. You may have just 30 seconds to impress a potential employer with your CV because they may be scanning a stack of applications at the end of a busy day and will be ruthless in culling badly written, waffly applications. It may seem unfair after all the effort you have put into composing your application and sending it in, but this is the harsh reality.

The good news is that when practices advertise they may well be on a tight timeframe to fill a position that has become vacant without much warning, so you are at a definite advantage as a new graduate who is available right now. You do not have to hand your notice in at a previous practice and work your notice, but can start work right away which might be just what the interviewer is looking for.

Apply as soon as possible after the advert appears because an employer in a hurry may employ someone as soon as they find a suitable candidate, even if this is in the first week of advertising. You do not have time to hang around so be prepared with your CV and covering letter composed and ready to go after minor adaptations to suit the position advertised and make sure that you have included information that demonstrates that you fulfill the criteria.

What to include in your application

As an employer, I am looking to recruit a vet who my clients will like, who I can work with and rely on and who will fit in with the rest of the team. I am not particularly bothered if you can play the violin or went to the Galapagos Islands on a research project, but I would like you to tell me you are keen and enthusiastic to work hard and learn and contribute to my practice. I want to know that you like people as well as animals and that you will be really keen to vaccinate all those puppies and discuss wormers with my clients time and time and time again. I expect you to care about and enjoy being with animals or you would not have chosen to be a vet, but I also want to see something which would make me want to meet you and warm to you as a person. If I like you and I like your attitude, then the chances are most of my clients will too.

I fully expect you to have the day one competencies and if you have come from abroad and taken the RCVS statutory exams then I am assuming your knowledge is up to the required standard. I may be impressed by any honours or awards you have won but I will be looking for other subtler abilities when choosing my successful applicant.

If you have had practical, hands-on experience, then that will impress me too as will enthusiastic references from places where you saw practice, especially if they are relevant to my practice. Make sure you inform the people you have asked to be referees so that they know that they might receive a phone call, and keep them up to date about which positions you have applied for so that they are ready to sing your praises when I contact them.

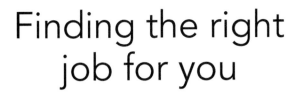

CHAPTER 2

Finding the right job for you

Interviews and finding the right job in the right practice

When you receive an invitation to come for an interview, pause for a moment and congratulate yourself, because this means that the practice thinks that you stand out above other applicants and your application has been proven to be effective. This should give you a big boost of confidence and, if you have been honest about your suitability, and the practice has been honest about what they are offering, you have matching expectations and a good chance of success.

Find out who owns the practice and their names by looking at the practice website and do some research which will also stand you in good stead when you come to the interview. It gives a good impression if you have some knowledge of the practice and are familiar with the information it provides to the general public. Make sure you make a note of the correct name of the person interviewing you and their title if possible.

Having received an invitation for an interview, it is not unreasonable to contact the practice and find out what form the interview process is likely to take. You should be given some idea of how long it is likely to be and what to expect on the day so that you can plan your travel and your time. Interviews vary greatly and might be composed of an informal chat after morning surgery, a meeting in a pub on a weekend or a full day at the practice with a formal interview panel of one or more people and a practical assessment of basic skills. If the invitation has not made it clear, then email the practice or phone up and ask how long you might be expected to stay and what the day will comprise.

It might also be possible at this time to enquire if interview expenses are paid although this will vary from practice to practice and might require tact at this stage. I was recently party to a discussion about this and there was considerable variation, with some practices always paying expenses whereas others felt that this was not reasonable. Use your own judgement about asking but our practice always used to pay travel expenses and it is worth making sure you keep your train ticket receipt or petrol receipts with you in case you are asked for them if you have travelled a long way.

Some practices may ask you to work a half day or more to give them and you the opportunity to assess how well-suited you are to the practice. Employment is a very important commitment both for you as the potential employee and for the practice employing you. The cost to the employer of advertising the job, reading and sifting the applications and interviewing is considerable and if an employee and a practice are incompatible it is an expensive procedure to go through again for all concerned. Working for a few hours or a day can give you the opportunity to experience what it is really like to work in that practice, which could be invaluable. You will have the chance to find out what the practice and personnel are like, even though it may seem daunting and you may feel it a little unreasonable not to be paid for your time and effort. Look on it as good experience and an opportunity to increase your chance of working for a good practice with high standards.

The formal interview will vary widely from practice to practice, but may include some form of personality assessment or psychometric testing to see how you might perform within the veterinary team. These tests have been designed to prevent an individual pretending to be something they are not, so answer the questions honestly and do not worry too much about them. There are no right and wrong answers and there is no one personality type who makes a good vet, but the practice may be looking for a certain personality type to complete their team. You are who you are and although you can modify your own behaviour to some extent, you will be happiest and most confident being yourself so do not try to double think the answers and pretend to be someone you are not.

First impressions

As an interviewer of a new graduate, I will be interested in your attitude and approach to working in veterinary practice and your interaction with me and with my staff. You do not have much time and opportunity to impress me, so make the most of it; you can give yourself a head start in many small ways even before the interview begins.

First, do not under any circumstances be late for your interview unless there has been a terrorist incident or a natural disaster outside your control, such as a hurricane or an unexpected outbreak of the black death. Plan your journey, leave a good margin for error and if it is not too far away then perform a dummy run the day before. This can also give you the opportunity to explore the area and surrounding countryside.

If you arrive early on the day, having found out exactly where the practice is you can park and go for a walk around, calming yourself and collecting your thoughts while getting a feel for the local area. You will be able to arrive at the practice several minutes early, calm and composed rather than falling in through the door spluttering apologies, all sweaty and dishevelled, having been stuck in traffic and having parked in the disabled parking bay.

We once invited a new graduate for interview and arranged to meet them in the local pub for lunch before taking them on a tour of the practice and progressing to a formal interview at the surgery. She arrived at the pub and said she had come for an interview and the manager of the pub assured her she was in the right place. She was taken into the pub kitchen and it was only after a few minutes of confusion that she realised the manager thought she had come to be interviewed for a bar staff position in the pub itself. Fortunately, the mistake was discovered before she had to demonstrate pulling a pint of bitter or making a cocktail.

The atmosphere in a practice when you walk in or while you are sitting in the waiting room is a strong indicator of how happy a practice this is going to be to work in. If the greeting you receive is warm and friendly and you see the same kindness and friendliness towards the clients and between the reception staff, then this is a good portent. Give yourself the time and opportunity to observe the area where the practice meets the general public and assess this first impression.

Appearances do matter

On our first meeting, as a prospective employer I would like you to be smart and clean and to look as if you have made an effort to look like a professional person who I would be happy to introduce to my clients.

You should be wearing shoes (not trainers), have clean hair and finger nails and should not be wearing jeans, because at this moment you do not know the sartorial preferences of the person who is about to interview you. It does not hurt to have gone to the trouble of being dressed in a slightly over-formal manner and, even if you are wearing a jacket and tie and your interviewer is not, this does not mean you are overdressed. It is you who are looking for a job and seeking to make a good impression and not the interviewer.

I once arrived for interview wearing the only respectable clothing I possessed which happened to be a wool jacket and trousers. This was in a July heatwave and the vet interviewing me was in a pair of shorts and a shirt; after the formal interview he took me to watch the vet nurse competing at a local horse show. I sweltered in scratchy wool all day long and was definitely overdressed for the local show but eventually I was offered the job.

Ladies, please wear something practical which covers your thighs and which you can reasonably wear for work as a vet, so no high heels or nail varnish thanks, and please do not subject me to a full montage of your tattooed cleavage.

I would prefer piercings to be left at home and although I don't mind you expressing your own style, I am also mindful of my more conservative clients so if you look as if you are on your way to a nightclub or a festival I might have some reservations. I prefer to be surprised and interested by body ornamentation when it appears at the Christmas party rather than during the interview process.

This may all sound very old-fashioned and there are vets who have made unconventional dress their trademark and become known as 'the vet who always wears leathers', or who has different coloured hair every time a client sees them. There are practices and practice owners who have no problem at all with informal or alternative appearance and once you are employed you will find out what is acceptable in that practice. Different can be good but it can also be a bit of a gamble and can backfire spectacularly if you are going for an interview at what turns out to be a very conventional practice with a strict dress code. An employer has to consider how their clients may feel if they are faced with you wearing thigh-length boots and a nose ring or dressed like Lady Gaga. Your expertise as a vet is the most important consideration of course, but when everything else is equal between applicants then appearances may determine which candidate is employed and you want it to be you.

Please turn your mobile phone off before you enter and do not look at it at all under any circumstances while you are in the building for the interview, or when being taken on a tour of the practice, not even for one second. This is not the time to be wondering who has sent you a text or phoned you and it will distract you even if it is on silent by vibrating in your pocket when your mother rings you every ten minutes to see how you are getting on.

You might think this is all very obvious advice and old-fashioned, but the chances are that the person interviewing you will be considerably older than you are. You would be amazed at the variation in interviewees even though they have been through the filter of the application selection process.

I have had vets arrive for an interview 40 minutes late without an explanation or an apology saying 'Oh, that's me, I'm always late for everything!'

I have interviewed vets in tee shirts and cycling shorts, jeans and dirty trainers, short skirts and high heels with eye wateringly low-cut tops and crimson talons for fingernails. I have been astounded that the applicant has not bothered to take the time and trouble to arrive at an interview looking clean and presentable.

I have listened to interviewees who have criticised my staff and told me of the shortcomings of the equipment and practice facilities compared to their EMS practice. Some have thought it reasonable to tell me that they are waiting for a reply from a practice they really would prefer to work for, but might just have to settle for mine instead. There have been candidates who have insisted quite aggressively that they will bring their dogs to work as a condition of employment, and others who have addressed me by the wrong name and not let me get a word in edgeways to ask them a question.

I have been asked about the amount of holiday on offer in the first minute of the interview and one who informed me that if they got the job it would just be a stopgap before they could get the job they really want in an equine practice.

I have had interviewees answering their mobile phones during the tour of the surgery, one who criticised the way a vet was suturing a wound, and one who stank of alcohol at ten o'clock in the morning.

When you first meet me, I am mindful that the first impression I receive within the first half hour will be the impression that my clients will most likely receive on meeting you for the first time. Please give me eye contact and smile and greet me speaking clearly. I understand that you may be nervous so I don't mind you speaking a bit rapidly or making a couple of garbled remarks until you settle down, but my initial assessment will be based on how my clients will take to you and be able to communicate with you. I will be asking myself if I will enjoy working with you and how you are going to get on with the rest of the veterinary team. Are you going to relate well to others or get right up the nose of my head nurse and are you speaking over me or not listening to me? The first few exchanges during an interview are intended to set you at your ease and give me the opportunity to see how you approach meeting new people, and during these moments I do not intend you to be imparting impressive knowledge or information. The interviewer will not usually start the formal interview until they have seen that you have relaxed a little and they want to give you the opportunity to present yourself at your best.

Once the interview starts in earnest, the format may be highly structured or remain more informal but, whatever the arrangement, this is your opportunity to sell yourself as a prospective employee.

During the interview I may appear to ask a fairly random assortment of questions and although I am interested in the detail of your responses I am also observing how comfortable you are when talking to people and considering whether I feel that you would fit in with the practice team. I will not be trying to catch you out at all and the questions are unlikely to be particularly intellectually challenging, so my advice is to be yourself and be as open, honest and sincere as you can be in answering my questions. I may be making notes – do not let this put you off or worry you about my reaction to an answer you have just given. It is important for me to make notes to jog my memory when I have interviewed several individuals so just continue to concentrate on your own answers, even if I am scribbling away.

This interview is your opportunity to convince me that you are the best person for the job so focus on imparting the positive factors which might make choosing you preferable to the other applicants. Expressing a willingness to work hard, appearing likeable and approachable and demonstrating an open mind and a keen interest in learning and contributing to the practice team will all be perceived as positive factors and carry more weight with me than any spectacular academic achievement.

This is not the time to be shy or overly modest and if you do have positive information to give, such as having won a prize or having worked in a neutering project spaying 20 cats a day, then make sure that I, the interviewer, knows about it.

Do not volunteer any criticism of the practices where you did your EMS as I will think you sound precocious and ungracious to the practice which hosted you and I will wonder if you will be equally indiscreet and critical of my practice sometime in the future. I might even know the practice owner because the veterinary profession is relatively small resulting in many vets knowing one another and meeting through various societies and functions, so always have this in the back of your mind.

The interview is a mutual process and you should be assessing me as an employer and deciding if you think you would be happy to be employed by me and would like to work in the practice. Observe the manner in which I speak to other members of staff such as the receptionists and other vets and nurses and how well organised the practice appears to be. If I am abrupt and offhand with the staff as I move around the practice, then however pleasant I am being towards you at the moment, it will reflect what sort of a person I am and what sort of an employer I would be.

Make some preparation before you come to the interview so that when I ask you about your positive attributes you have some means of illustrating that you have good communication skills, for example, or an interest in a certain species. Tell me about working in a coffee bar and how much you learned about customer service and bring your relevant experiences in where appropriate to differentiate you from other new graduates. You might be asked for examples which illustrate your approach to certain situations and it is worth thinking about an interesting case you were involved with at vet school to use as an example.

Many interviewers will ask each candidate the same questions so that they can compare their responses, perhaps on how you would approach a case commonly seen in practice. You cannot prepare for every single question that you might be asked. The important thing is to collect your thoughts and respond in a thoughtful and organised way, drawing on your existing knowledge and presenting it clearly. Do not rush into speech immediately but give yourself time to think and formulate a concise answer. I know this will seem to you like a long uncomfortable silence even though only seconds will be passing, but it is much better to say a few well-thought-out sentences than to gabble away like a turkey on speed, making no sense.

I am highly likely to ask you as the interview progresses if you have any questions for me and this is the time to ask those questions that you have prepared earlier but which I have not already given you the answers to. Take a list with you and do not hesitate to refer to it because it shows me that you have prepared in advance for the interview and are organised and methodical.

This is a good opportunity to ask about mentoring and support that you should expect as a new graduate; this can vary a great deal in different practices but is extremely important. If no mentor will be allocated and you will be expected to work on your own or with little support, then it is best to know now.

I am quite likely to ask you about your ambitions and which aspects of veterinary work you are particularly interested in and, although it is good to aim for the stars as far as your career is concerned, it might be better not to dwell on your ambition to be an equine vet in a small animal practice or to say that you want to work in a referral centre if you are at an interview for a very small mixed practice in the country. Most practices will be looking for vets who are interested in the type of work they are likely to be involved with, so an interest in canine and feline internal medicine and dentistry will be music to the ears of a small animal practitioner and an interest in mastering general practice and herd health in mixed practice will go down well. Employers like to hear that you are willing to work hard and are interested in general practice and doing the basic work well and that you like talking to people and improving their animals' overall health rather than your aspirations to be a supervet.

You might want to know more about the way the working day is structured and exactly where you would be working in the practice. If you are being interviewed in a different branch from the one in which you would actually be working, then you might receive a different impression of the job that is on offer. Working on your own in a branch surgery with minimal equipment is very different to being in hospital-status premises with digital X-ray, in-house laboratory facilities and ultrasound on hand. An employer should be honest and open about this, but it makes sense to be aware and ask the relevant questions and if you are going to be working at a different branch, then ask if you can see it.

By all means ask me what hours you will normally be working and what the usual rota is, but do not place undue emphasis on time off and the holidays too early in the interview. You do need to know this information and it is entirely reasonable to ask about it, but it is best if this does not appear to be your number one priority.

Ask about accommodation and if a practice vehicle will be provided although this is less common than it used to be partly because of the tax implications for you as an employee. If accommodation is provided, then ask if you can see it, and ask if there is an accommodation allowance allocated if you decide to move out of practice property.

Take notes of important things that are said so that you have a record of them and have the correct facts at hand when making further decisions if I offer you a job. If you are successful, a written job offer will usually fill in the gaps concerning the rota and what the conditions of work are; you can contact the practice to enquire if all is not completely clear and seems different to what was discussed at the interview.

Once you have had your initial interview, I would probably take you on a tour of the premises and introduce you to the other vets and the nursing staff. Beware the 'secondary interview' which takes place when I leave you alone with the other vets and nurses and you relax and think the interview is all over. These are the people who are going to be working with you and mentoring you, getting you out of difficulties and preventing you from making mistakes when you first start. If they later express a reluctance to the idea of working with you, this will carry weight with me because the happiness of my staff means a happy working life for me. Make no mistake, this is still very much a part of your interview and will influence my choice of successful candidate because after your interview I will definitely be asking them for their impressions. I have interviewed vets who I thought were very pleasant only to find that their attitude to the other vets and nurses when I left them alone to chat had resulted in impassioned pleas to not even consider employing them.

The staff of a practice are usually proud of the place they work and while they might choose to criticise some aspect of it, they certainly do not appreciate a new graduate interviewee making any negative observations.

Make your own assessment of what it might be like to work in the practice, gauge the atmosphere and observe the demeanour and interaction of the members of the veterinary team. A standard practice without state-of-the-art equipment but with an excellent, enthusiastic boss and a happy team of vets and nurses can offer a much better starting point for a new graduate than a fancy practice with cutting-edge gear but with unfriendly workmates. This is the time to trust your instincts as you are going to need friendly moral support and guidance far more than access to an MRI scanner.

Ask about the inpatients as you are shown round, because vets and nurses care about their patients and they are joined with you in a common bond of enjoying working with animals. They want to know you are also a kindred spirit who cares and if ever you are lost for words or there is an awkward silence, just ask them what animals they have at home. You will hear all their tales about the stray dogs and three-legged cats they have rescued, the conversation will flow and they will be able to imagine enjoying working with you.

As we move around the surgery I do not expect you to pat and fuss every cat and dog you see, but if you ignore every single animal that you come across, I will think you don't like animals. Some people will even bring their own dog into the room during the interview to see what your reaction is, so do not blank the dog even if he is slobbering on your best trousers. An affinity with animals is something intangible that may not be on a CV but is extremely important in a vet. Vets are just as besotted with their own animals as the clients, so if the vet has a boxer then find something positive but genuine to say about boxers and don't say you disapprove of owning brachycephalic breeds. Do not recoil from the greeting of a smelly old collie under the desk because it has no doubt been rescued and is treasured by the person interviewing you as much or more than they value their partner.

If you ask intelligent questions and listen attentively to my answers, I will be more impressed than if you hold forth about everything you have seen and done elsewhere. I am also most likely very proud of my practice and it may represent years of my hard work building it up, so it would not hurt to find something complimentary to say about it.

It is reasonable to ask details about how the practice is organised in a general way, concentrating on the day-to-day structure and timings. Looking at the appointment book and the op list will give you a good idea of the workload and the hours expected of you and will also demonstrate your interest in the way the practice is organised.

If you are offered contact details for a member of staff to phone later for information, then do take them and do phone them because they will give you an employee's personal perspective of the practice off the record. You can ask those questions which may have occurred to you since the interview and you may also be able to ask why a new post has arisen and get some inkling of why a previous incumbent has left the practice.

At the end of the interview, do make sure you thank everyone for their time and ask for some idea from them of when you might expect to hear if you have been successful and whether the communication is likely to be by email or telephone. You may receive more than one job offer and you do not want to be in the situation of being reluctant to accept one offer because you are waiting to hear from another practice and you do not know if that job has already gone.

If you would really like to be offered the job then say that you are very interested without sounding overconfident of being offered it. If the timeframe in giving you a decision overlaps with your attending another interview, then say so, because if you have just given a really good interview and a practice is keen to employ you, it might hasten their decision for fear of losing you.

If you receive an offer from your second choice, you can always contact your first choice to double check and let them know that you have received an offer. This means they know you might no longer be available and might even focus their minds on offering you a position if they really want to employ you.

Vets who are working hard at clinical work and managing a practice simultaneously are always short of time and dealing with unforeseen eventualities, so may be more likely to delay contacting you than a large organisation. If you really want to work there, then telephone and politely ask what is happening. There are practices who do not have the courtesy to inform unsuccessful applicants but if you have been told a likely timescale when you can expect to hear back and you hear nothing, then telephone and check that the decision has not been delayed for some reason.

The right fit

It is a nerve-wracking experience to undergo, but you have probably performed much better in the interview process than you think you did. When I interviewed young vets, I was usually very impressed by how enthusiastic, approachable and employable most of them were. Selecting the successful candidate was usually more about the right fit and the dynamics of the practice team than because a new graduate did not come up to the mark. It was usually a simple choice, between candidates of equal ability, of the one who I thought I and my team would like to work with, and who my clients were going to have confidence in and want to see.

An unsuccessful interview is not a criticism of you as a person so put it behind you and think about the next one without going over where you think things may have gone badly. It is unlikely to be down to any mistake you made and each interview gives you experience which will be useful as practice for the next one, increasing your chances of success.

If you have several interviews without being offered the job, then you could ask for constructive feedback to help you in future interviews but often there is a reluctance to be brutally honest and the practice may prefer to give some bland comments rather than hurt your feelings.

Deciding which job offer to accept

Be prepared that you may be offered a job on the spot at the interview so consider how you would respond. It may be that you are uncertain, in which case it is entirely reasonable to require thinking time and resist being pressured into answering there and then. If a practice really wants to employ you then they will be prepared to wait at least a few hours to give you time to think.

They might want you to start tomorrow but you need to know exactly what you are being offered and the full job description and financial package. In these circumstances, it is even more important to make contemporaneous notes so that you have a record of what has been offered and it is reasonable to make a provisional acceptance dependent on the fine detail of the job offer.

Trust your instincts and your own judgement because you know what will suit your personality and where you will be happy, so do not accept a job on the day of interview that does not really appeal to you just because you feel pressured or grateful that they actually want you. Ignore that niggling voice in the back of your mind wondering if you might not be offered another one, and if it does not feel right for you or you feel the support offered is not adequate, then do not accept it.

If, after several interviews, you are offered only one job but you really didn't like the practice or the prospective employer, then do not let fear and panic push you into accepting it. It is much more difficult to move once you are working and more advisable to keep on applying until you find the job which will suit you.

Taking the wrong job and then leaving after a couple of months will mean that not only have you had a really unpleasant experience but also you have an employment record of a short term of employment and potentially not a fantastic reference. It is better not to have started work at all than have your first experience as a vet in practice such a negative one, so be prepared to be patient and wait for a more suitable job to come along.

If you are not being asked for interviews at all then have another look at your application and CV and ask someone with experience of employing people, preferably a vet such as your EMS practice owner, to advise you on improvements.

If you receive more than one offer of employment then it may be that the attraction of living by the sea or a better rota or a higher salary tempts you to accept one practice over another, but I would urge you to choose the practice where you feel reassured that you will be mentored and looked after and allowed to gain experience in a supportive atmosphere. Do not opt for the practice which lures you in and pays a relatively big salary with lots of time off but in which a new graduate may be left to sink or swim without good mentoring and care. No amount of sandy beaches or cash in the bank can compensate for a really horrendous first year in practice and a potentially catastrophic loss of confidence as you navigate your first year without the necessary support.

The importance of a good mentor

If you speak to older vets, you will usually find that they will name a certain individual vet who they credit with having taught them the building blocks of how to be a success in practice and it is often in the first year that a really good mentor can help you to become a really good vet and to enjoy being a vet.

In my first job in practice there were two partners who were a little bit like the good cop and the bad cop. I learned a lot from both of them in terms of clinical work but I also learned just how important it is to support a new graduate for the graduate's benefit and that of the practice. From the good cop I learned that encouragement and advice with a nudge was enough to make me challenge myself though I always knew that he would come and help me out when I really needed it without begrudging his time. He did not nanny me but he supported me and bailed me out when I was out of my depth and was generous with his time and his patience. The other vet was rather less enlightened about helping a new graduate and embraced the view that there is no point having a dog and barking yourself so offered little help or advice but plenty of feedback, all of it negative, but I survived. I progressed over the next two years until I was eventually mentoring new graduates myself and I will always remember the good cop with warmth and appreciation and am still pleased to see him whenever I meet him now. My boss in my second job was also wonderfully supportive on occasions such as when I was unable to replace a prolapsed uterus in a cow or needed a second opinion on a horse with colic. When I look back, I realise I was lucky and that my mentors went out of their way to make sure that I did not have my confidence undermined and allowed me to gain experience with my head held high.

I was very fortunate in having good mentors throughout my early veterinary career and even when qualified for many years, I still appreciated those colleagues who looked out for me and gave their time and expertise willingly, despite sometimes inconveniencing themselves. There is a long history of mutual support in our profession and however long we have been qualified there is always someone somewhere who knows more than you do about something and if you ask them they will give their help and advice with generosity.

The employment package

Make sure you have all the facts about any job offers so that you are completely sure of your complete employment package which will include salary and all other additional benefits such as accommodation, car, payment of subscriptions, CPD allowance, registration fees for RCVS, indemnity insurance, health insurance for extended illness or incapacity, and so on. You should compare like with like and be careful to take everything into consideration including working out of hours, holiday pay, weekend work and the length of the normal working day. Some contracts will offer more generous sick pay provision whereas others will offer the basic statutory sick pay and this will influence the personal insurance you will need to take out to protect you in the event of illness or injury preventing you from being able to work for a significant length of time.

Always get a job offer in writing so you are absolutely sure of the details and print it out and keep it on file just in case there is some future disagreement as to what was in the offer at the time you agreed to accept. Keep a copy of the advert for the job and all your contemporaneous notes from your interview with the written job offer, job description and your contract. Make sure you have read everything thoroughly to avoid any misunderstandings and ask for clarification if there is any ambiguity.

I still hear of a gender pay gap between male and female vets even at the new graduate level and the reasons for it are frequently debated. It is said that men are more likely to ask for a higher salary, although in my experience the reasons are more complex and the level of salary we offered was always dependent on how much we wanted to employ that particular individual and certainly nothing to do with their gender. I have interviewed very confident and assertive vets of both sexes including male vets who undervalued themselves and women who overvalued their worth to my practice in terms of salary.

I had a salary figure in mind for a new graduate and although an outstanding, experienced vet may command a higher rate of pay than the one advertised, this is less likely to be the case when employing a new graduate. There is often a pay structure already in place with other vets and nurses and once you have proved yourself to be a good asset to the practice, then your position is much stronger when asking for a salary increase as they will want to keep you. Some practices review the pay of a new graduate after the first six months in practice when they have seen how they are progressing, so look to see if this is specified in the job offer.

The provision of a car or practice accommodation will usually be in the job advert itself but the precise figure for the salary on offer may not be. They may ask you at the interview how much you are expecting to be paid and this can catch you unawares if you are not prepared. It can be a difficult question to answer, especially if you do not know the other factors such as the workload, the length of the working day or emergency rota. It is reasonable to avoid answering directly but if you check the SPVS salary survey to see what the average rate of pay is in that particular geographical area, you will have an idea of the expected rate in that area for that type of practice. Also, ask your friends what the going rate seems to be.

There are still accounts of new graduates being paid a pittance, well under the going rate, and being asked to work extremely long hours and in poor conditions in practices where, after a year or so, the lucky ones escape and are replaced by another new graduate. I would recommend that you do not accept a job where your first experience of practice is going to be such a negative one.

As long as new graduates are willing to accept work in these practices then this abuse of young vets will continue and the 'new graduate sausage factory' practice will persist. Some new graduates do not fully realise what they are being asked to agree to until they start work when it is too late, so make sure you find out all the facts before you accept.

You can ask politely but assertively for a written job offer and careful reading of an employment contract can avoid the situation where you find yourself in a practice where you are sucked in, overworked, underpaid and lose your enthusiasm for the vocation you have worked so hard for. No job is worth that, however worried you are about finding a job and once you are in that job it is much harder to get out and look for another one.

Most practices are not like this at all but have employers who care about their employees, paying decent salaries with good working conditions, reasonable hours and good support. Choose your first job wisely and it should mean a win–win situation for both yourself and your employer.

Having carefully considered the job offer and accepted, ideally you should be offered a written contract which you should read carefully; ask an experienced friend or relative to read it too or ask a solicitor to check it over. Some practices are regrettably slow in issuing a written contract, but contracts can be verbal too, so make sure you take notes at the time which could be used as evidence if for some unlikely reason there was a dispute in the future. It is a legal requirement to give you a legal statement stating your employment rights and benefits.

Useful websites for employment issues are www.gov.uk and www.acas.org.uk.

CHAPTER 3

Preparing for work in practice

Before you start your new job

Congratulations! You have applied and been interviewed and offered that first job in practice which is a great achievement; you should be feeling optimistic and rightly pleased with your success. There are many new graduates out there looking for work and you have been selected ahead of other candidates so believe in yourself because you have so much to offer and your career as a veterinary surgeon is about to begin. You have agreed the terms and conditions of your job with your employer and decided on a starting date and I am sure you are really keen to start work at last after all these years of study and exams.

This move into your first job is a significant occasion and more complex than when you first left home to start at vet school because you are now an independent person entering the world of work rather than becoming a student with the support of university and the vet school pastoral care. At university, you worked for yourself to achieve your qualification but now you will be working for someone else and will be a financially independent individual and a professional.

It used to be fairly common for practices to provide transport and some sort of accommodation as part of the employment package but over the years, changes to the tax regulations mean that if a car and house or flat are provided, you will be taxed quite heavily on it as a benefit in kind. It is much more usual now to be paid a total salary package and to organise and pay for your own car and accommodation. A car may still be provided in mixed and large animal positions where perhaps a four-wheel drive vehicle may be necessary, but it is far less likely that you will have the use of a practice car in small animal practice. Transport and accommodation may need to be organised quite swiftly after accepting a job and in the few weeks before you start work, so do not delay. Your employer may be able to help you organise finance or a reference for a lease if you do not yet have a credit rating and may provide you with letters for letting agencies confirming your future income.

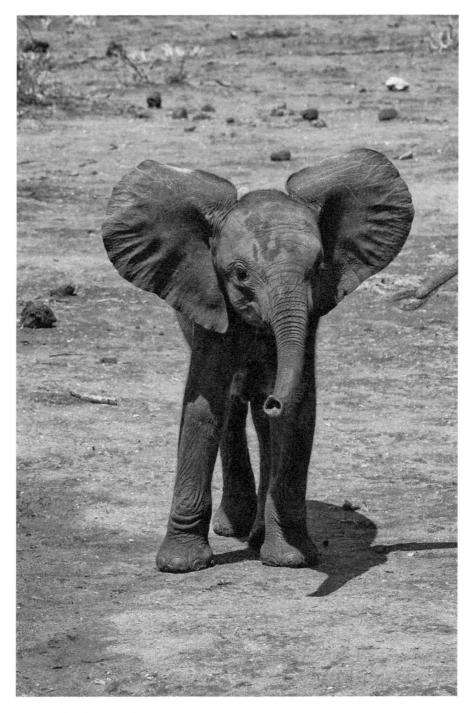

It is good to be confident; you do not want to charge in blowing your own trumpet and ill-prepared for what you may be facing. You are full of enthusiasm and fearless and whatever you may lack in wisdom you make up for with up-to-date knowledge and energy, but be prepared and give yourself a head start.

Practice accommodation, when it is offered, can be of varying quality and you may have been shown round the accommodation at the time of your interview. Some practices offer a flat or a house of a value far above that which you could afford to buy or rent on a new graduate's pay and in a first job this can present a considerable saving for you despite the tax implications. You will be responsible for keeping it clean and tidy, but not for the routine maintenance of the building and this can be a blessing.

Sharing accommodation, perhaps with another member of staff, needs careful consideration as your housemates may offer friendship and company but could also be loud, smelly and annoying, staying up until the small hours and with questionable personal hygiene. You most likely have had experience of this at university but, obviously, find out as much as you can before you commit to sharing with anyone. Falling out with a fellow student at college is much less of a problem than falling out with someone you have to work with and face over the operating table for the foreseeable future.

Transport

If you own a car which is unreliable and breaks down all the time on the way to work, you will not be popular with your employer. Choose a car which is going to start and get you to and from work without a problem and which is suitable for the area and your journey. Check to see if you will be expected to transport any animals for your work as you may need to notify your insurer. It does not usually cost much more, but they need to be informed.

Insurance

Check your other insurance requirements and look at the BVA website as you may be able to access favourable rates through them.

You should have indemnity insurance such as that provided by the Veterinary Defence Society (VDS); the practice may have enrolled you but check and make sure. The VDS is a non-profit-making company created by vets for vets and is the largest provider of indemnity insurance, although other companies are also available. Your indemnity insurer is there to support you when things go wrong, so make sure you have the phone number and your membership number handy just in case you need it.

I strongly recommend joining the BVA as, among many other excellent services, you will also pay a lower preferential rate for new and recent graduates and receive free legal assistance and discounts on various insurance products, which makes it worth the subscription from the outset.

Remember to arrange contents insurance for your property, car insurance and check out a sickness and accident policy to cover you if you are injured or ill and unable to work. You may be young and fit and feel invincible, but vets get ill and injured just like anyone else and you need to make sure that you are not worrying about money if the worst happens and you are out of action for weeks or months. The younger and fitter you are when you take out such a policy, the cheaper the premium. Read your contract about the arrangements for sick pay to ensure you get the correct cover.

Register with a doctor in the area and a dentist too while you have spare time before you start work and check all your vaccinations are up to date.

Clothing

Most small animal practices have some form of dress code so be prepared to follow it and have suitable clothing to wear. Many practices provide a uniform such as a scrub top, perhaps with a practice logo, while others just wear their own clothes, but usually there is a certain expectation so ask them what they would like you to wear. When you visit the practice, have a good look at what the other vets are wearing and wear something similar but possibly a little more formal when you first start work.

Looking smart and neat makes you look professional and capable and yes, it does matter to the clients, many of whom are older than you and may be more conservative. Vets who have been in a practice for several years often dress more casually and idiosyncratically than the more recent vets and I have seen vets working in their own practices in all manners of dress. They have already established their reputation in the practice and, unfair though it may seem, the clients will be more forgiving of them for wearing jeans or looking a bit scruffy than they will be of a wackily dressed new graduate.

Take at least one spare top to work with you and even a spare pair of trousers is a good idea for those little accidents, not yours of course, but those of your patients. It is highly likely that you will get something gross, colourful and probably very smelly on your clothing early on in the day and clients prefer their vets not to have the previous patient's bodily fluids adorning their chest.

Many a vet and nurse will have held a cat under their arm as a means of restraint and experienced the 'pocketful of cat diarrhoea' moment. It is not unusual to find that the terrible smell in the supermarket on the way home is in fact coming from you because you have accidentally knelt down in tom-cat urine or an anal gland has emptied over your sleeve.

I risk stating the blindingly obvious, but do make sure you have comfortable working shoes on as you will be on your feet for most of the day and at the end of a long week of walking round the practice and being constantly on the go, your feet will feel like a couple of tenderised fillet steaks. There was a whole thread on footwear recently on one of the veterinary forums with some

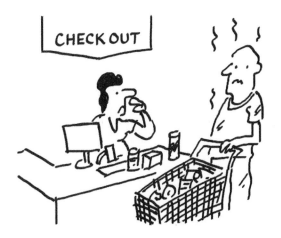

recommending walking shoes and others boots and specific brands of shoe. The length of the thread and the amount of passionate discussion reflected the importance of not having sore feet at the end of a long day.

Finally, do make sure your personal hygiene is impeccable as a long hot day in a veterinary practice is not helped at all by a colleague who suffers from body odour. Be generous with that deodorant and have a shower in the morning, even if you are exhausted from the day before. You will be working closely with other people and often in close proximity, holding a dog to examine it or taking a blood test and it is not unusual for someone to be restraining an animal close to someone else's armpit.

Planning for arriving for your first day

You do have a choice about the manner in which you arrive at the practice for your first day at work. Hopefully you will have contacted the practice well in advance of your start date and found out exactly what time you start work and where. Make allowances for the morning rush hour and make sure you know exactly how long it takes to get from your home to work at that time of day in case you get caught in the work and school traffic. It is a good idea to get there early to make sure you are calm and collected and to make a good impression, not just for your boss but also for the vets and nurses you work with. This is your chance to make an immediate good first impression and present yourself as calm and efficient, friendly and in control, and on time ready for work.

I would very much like your first few days in practice to be perfectly planned by your employers so that you would be allocated a more experienced vet as a mentor to ask questions of and who would nurture you in your first few days and weeks with patience and sympathy. The importance of a good mentor has been mentioned earlier and practices are becoming much more aware of the importance of mentorship for their new graduates. The BVA provides advice and support for mentors for practices and hopefully the practice you start in will have already allocated yours to you beforehand and that mentor would have been in touch before you start work.

Ideally, each member of staff would be introduced to you by name and role and they would have plenty of time to make you feel welcome. In the first week or so, it would be helpful if you could be allocated two or three times the normal amount of time for a consultation and that these cases would be simple and straightforward so that you could settle in without any time pressures. In an ideal world, everyone would be happy to take time to answer all your questions and show you where everything is and you would have ample time to read about the practice protocols on vaccination, neutering, laboratory testing, pre-med protocols, euthanasia protocols, admission forms, fluid therapy, coffee breaks, lunch times, uniform, expenses sheets, the ultrasound machine, and so on. The fact is that in the reality and unpredictability of general practice they may simply not have the time, so if you have been sent information beforehand then be prepared and take the time to read it in advance of starting work.

A well-run practice will usually give you plenty of written information before you start and it is worth asking for it in advance if they haven't volunteered it. There may be a practice handbook containing the answers to the many questions that you are likely to need to ask. Read as much as you can about how things work in the practice before your first day and look on this preparation as an investment in yourself, facilitating a calm introduction to being a working vet. Every practice is different and may not be organised in the same way as the one in which you did your EMS, so make no assumptions but do the research.

You will be faced with a tsunami of new information in your first few days at work and hopefully the vets and nurses in the practice have sympathy with how you are feeling and will be supportive. It is natural to feel that you are standing in the way as the team move around the practice and as soon as anyone tells you anything you forget it because there are 20 other things to remember. Do not worry about it, this is completely normal but help yourself by being prepared and by looking and listening.

It may help you if you take a small notebook in your pocket so that you can jot down important pieces of information and make a note of questions you may need answering later in the day when it is quieter.

Here are various random pieces of advice for you before you start work:

- Make sure you have some decent, easy to cook, healthy food in the fridge for when you arrive home exhausted so that you can whack it into the microwave and collapse. This is not the time for creating a culinary masterpiece involving fancy food preparation, nor should you resort to junk food.
- Try to be organised about your home even if that is not your usual approach to life, because you are going to be really busy and very tired at the end of the day. Fill your car with petrol, make sure you've done your laundry and you have enough food and toilet rolls, because once you start work that first week, your feet are not going to touch the ground.
- Read the RCVS Code of Conduct with which you should be familiar from your time as a vet student; it is a good idea to look at the code again before you start work and remind yourself of the guiding principles. There is supporting guidance about various topics to help you navigate the demands placed on you as a vet in practice, so do not forget about it and remember to consult it during your career whenever you are unsure if you are doing the right thing as a vet either ethically or morally, and you are likely to find the answer there.
- Add the phone numbers and contact details for people at work onto your mobile phone so that you have someone to call if you need assistance.
- Make a note of who people are and what their role is in the practice.
- Ensure you have the contact details of the practice manager in case you need to check anything to do with your employment or are ill.

Do not worry too much!

You might be anxious about starting work as a vet but be aware that, however confident everyone you meet appears to be, they all felt the same way that you do now when they first started work. In a busy practice in your first few days, expect to be surprised, nervous and excited and to feel a bit like the new kid at school. You want to join in but you're not sure who everyone is and what you are expected to do but if you are willing and helpful you will soon find your feet. Most vets and nurses are really good, caring people and are sympathetic towards you and want you to succeed and already consider you to be a part of their veterinary practice team.

Don't worry about proving your abilities right away

You have graduated as a veterinary surgeon and you have the training to do the job but no one is going to expect you to be a good vet straight away. You have the foundations of knowledge and you can and will make it, but it is going to take time so do not expect too much from yourself. You should feel nervous and have a heightened sense of awareness because excessive confidence and lack of awareness of your limitations is dangerous for a new graduate and can lead to avoidable errors.

Even the most confident, experienced and skilled veterinary surgeon in the practice still has the odd case where they do not know what the hell is going on and are completely baffled. They will use their knowledge and skills to take steps to find out, but they might not actually know right now. Animals do not read the textbooks and do not always present with every symptom of the disease they may be suffering from in a textbook manner.

Remember that every vet in the world had to do each procedure, however basic, for the first time and they needed help and support.

The art of being a veterinary surgeon is in using the skills we have to work through a case to a satisfactory conclusion and also in giving the clients confidence that, although we may not immediately make an accurate diagnosis, we know how to treat the patient and how to reach a diagnosis eventually. There are some cases which will resolve without a diagnosis having been made and the capacity for our patients to heal themselves is a continuous benefit to the practising veterinary surgeon.

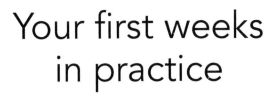

CHAPTER 4

Your first weeks in practice

Your first day in practice

It is your first day in practice and here you are, finally realising all the hopes and dreams of your ambition to be a vet. Your hard work over the years at vet college has paid off and your parents are incredibly proud of you and are telling everyone they know that you are now a real working vet! Excitement and apprehension combined is making you feel a bit sick and giddy as you wake up to face your first day. It has finally dawned on you that you are no longer a student but actually 'the vet'; you will not be a student but actually doing it and the buck now stops with you.

I hope you will feel confident and prepared because you have read the previous chapter and have had the common sense to get ready for this day as much as you can in advance.

You will have arrived at work at least half an hour early and found out where to put your coat and bag and where the toilet is. You have located the kettle and discovered where the tea and coffee are kept. You may even have earned the priceless approval of Chirpy Cheryl on reception who has been answering two phones both ringing simultaneously since she arrived at work an hour ago by bringing her a cup of tea. You have already contacted the practice a couple of days ago asking what you might be doing today and perhaps even called in to check out the practice management system and follow the on-screen tutorial so that you can at the very least access the histories of the inpatients.

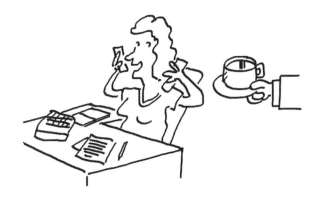

Every practice is different, but in many practices the very nature of the work means that although there was every intention of slowly and gently inducting you into the practice and concentrating on you, the reality is that if you arrive on a busy day you may feel like a spare part for the first day or so. It may feel a bit like seeing practice when you are always in the way and not sure what to do, despite being really eager to get in there and work. Just show an interest in everything and try to be as helpful and willing as you can and if there is anything that obviously needs doing, then offer to do it.

Although I would like your first day at work and induction to be perfect and the mentoring and support to be exactly as discussed previously, unfortunately this is not always the case. The reality of your first day may be that the practice is unexpectedly incredibly busy, or it may be that you have been employed because another vet has left or because the practice has expanded so rapidly that they desperately need another vet and are understaffed. The holiday rota will have had to be honoured so the practice may be a vet down already that week, and perhaps a second vet is off sick unexpectedly too. The carefully planned and well-intended induction plan goes out of the window in these circumstances and everyone is rushed off their feet, leaving you spinning around wondering what is going on and where everything is. The consulting session during which they had carefully allocated you extra time per client has been altered to squeeze in a few extra appointments and you have your first client facing you before you know it.

If this is your experience, then stay calm and do whatever you reasonably can, focusing on the job in hand, and usually the apparent mayhem will settle down. Many busy days in practice can seem unmanageable at times to the observer, but the team just steps up a gear and copes with the demand by prioritising and working harder. If you appear to have nothing to do, then be patient and helpful and wait for further instructions as your induction may not be an immediate priority just at that time.

It is inevitable that there will be practices which are better organised than others and larger organisations often have protocols in place for new members of staff, but the best-made plans can be affected by pressures of work. Do not be too quick to judge and assume that your induction plan is not being followed as it might just take a little while to get going.

First impressions are very important and if it feels as if everyone is weighing you up then that is because they probably are doing just that. They do not know if you are going to be the willing new graduate who hits the ground running with a smile or the pompous one who stands around aloof, without offering to mop up the wee in the corridor or help carry a fat, reluctant Labrador to the wards. They might refuse your help even if you do offer, but will certainly appreciate your willingness to be a worker and not an observer.

Induction

The induction period should give you the time to familiarise yourself with the work of the practice and should cover topics such as:

- ❧ the practice management system (PMS)
- ❧ the practice protocols for common treatments and procedures
- ❧ the pharmacy
- ❧ the equipment in the consulting room
- ❧ the equipment in the preparation and operating suites
- ❧ imaging equipment
- ❧ laboratory equipment and protocols
- ❧ rota and responsibilities
- ❧ recording data for the human resources department
- ❧ health and safety regulations and training
- ❧ in-house further education and clinical audit
- ❧ practice financial protocols
- ❧ practice social opportunities.

Ideally you will be given written resources for the induction period stating all the necessary information and the sooner you study all this information the better, as there is an incredible amount of new material to absorb in the first few days in a new practice. Read it as soon as you can and be prepared to read it more than once as it will help you to know what is expected of you.

The practice management system (PMS)

You may well be familiar with one or two practice management systems you have seen during your EMS and a familiarity with a system can be a great advantage to you in your first days at work. The important thing in your mind will be correctly performing your job as a veterinary surgeon, but do not underestimate how important the correct use of the practice management system is too. You may have had the chance to check it out before your first day at work but, if not, then the quicker you can use it effectively the better.

Be proactive about this and put some time and effort into learning how to use it because you need to master it quickly or it will slow you down in consultations and make you appear less competent to the clients. Being able to use the PMS efficiently will save you so much precious time in consultations that are better spent in examining the animal and talking to the client.

Most systems have a tutorial function and hopefully you will be given plenty of time to check this out. Most employers fully intend to give you plenty of time to get up to speed with the management system, but asking in advance might just prompt them to factor time into your induction process to do this. You may be given the assistance of a veterinary nurse or receptionist when you start consulting and they may also help you with the computer system at first, if you are lucky.

Recording information and treatment may not appear to you to be a high priority when you have so many other things to occupy you, but for maintaining the confidence of the client it is vitally important. Case notes must be accurate and easy to read for anyone following on with a case or in the rare case where there is a dispute. Do not sacrifice clarity and use too many obscure and unique personal acronyms and do not sacrifice spelling and grammar for speed as this can give a poor impression of your professional skills. Make it concise but comprehensive and understandable by any veterinary surgeon who may read it at a later date. Touch typing is a very helpful skill which you may have already mastered and which will save you valuable time. There are online courses available which are excellent.

It is most unfair, but the client may quite unreasonably judge your capability as a vet on producing the wrong invoice rather than the brilliant diagnosis you just made. Clients are also reluctant to accept being charged at a later date for something you forgot to enter at the time.

I once employed a new vet who decided that it would be a lot easier if she just concentrated on the consulting alone and wrote up all the history and differential diagnoses at the end of the two-hour consulting session. She wrote up the treatment she had given at the time so that the medicines were dispensed and the labels printed but decided it would take too much time to record the history and clinical findings.

It turned out to be a nightmare for her and us as she struggled to remember all the details of how big the lump was on the black Labrador and what the temperature was of the anorexic cat and who had what symptoms. Keep an accurate record at the time, as you cannot reasonably expect to remember everything during a busy surgery.

Pharmacy

Explore the pharmacy on your first day and find out by what Machiavellian system it has been organised so that you can easily find the most commonly used medicines such as ear drops, topical creams, antibiotics, nonsteroidal anti-inflammatories, and so on. Some practices stock items in alphabetical order and others in body systems and it helps to be able to find things quickly in the middle of a busy surgery if you need to. Most importantly, you need to know what they have in stock for you to prescribe when you are consulting.

Do not assume there is always logic applied to this, and never try to rearrange it in a way you consider more sensible or all the vets and nurses who have been there for years will go crazy. Practice pharmacies may appear bizarrely organised because the senior vet may be very reluctant to change a system which has been there for years. He or she likes everything to be kept where it has always been kept, however illogical that may seem, and maybe your first day is not the time to start suggesting changing things however helpful you may be feeling. Leave tactful suggestions for improvement until a later date.

The practice may use a different supplier of antibiotics and nonsteroidal anti-inflammatories from the brands you have seen before so make sure you can identify them and know what strength they stock and what the brand name is for the most commonly used injectables. Some large groups of practices buy medication in their own-brand outer wrappers and they may not look familiar to you at first.

Find out where the drugs are dispensed from and how they are packaged and labelled.

Take the opportunity to locate the usual disposables stocked by the practice, such as syringes and needles, bandages and dressings, and where and how the injectable drugs are stored including the ones which are refrigerated. Never leave the fridge open because there will be valuable vaccines stored in there and if the fridge temperature goes up they may have to be discarded. This is a very unpopular misdemeanour so make sure it doesn't happen to you.

Check where the prescription food is kept and the flea preparations for the different species and different weights, and who dispenses them and when. Some practices will have a member of the support staff to count out the tablets, label the ear drops and give them to the clients but you need to know how the system works as there may well be times when you need to do this yourself.

Be prepared for the most common consultations

The chances are you will see quite a lot of basic, routine consultations at first, so research the most likely information you are going to need. In an enlightened practice, easing you in gently, it is unlikely that you will be seeing many challenging cases or performing the more complex procedures straight away. You are much more likely to be seeing routine vaccinations, sore ears, lumps and bumps, diarrhoea and lame dogs. Lucky you, you will get all the puppies and kittens with their happy owners and all the healthy dogs and cats for their boosters.

These are the staple first opinion cases but though it is unlikely that you will be faced with a difficult diagnosis, you never know what underlying pathology an old dog who has come for a booster might have, so be vigilant and thorough and do not be afraid to ask if you are not sure about anything. Far better to ask a question and be reassured by a colleague than for a patient to go untreated for something like diabetes or a pyometra because you did not want to ask for help.

Make sure you have some idea of basic protocols, such as how to go about booking a case in for the next appointment or how to book a dental procedure in for the day. Find out the protocol for vaccination, the age at first vaccination, the time interval until the next dose and where the vaccination cards are kept. Do you fill in the vaccine record cards or does the nurse do that for you?

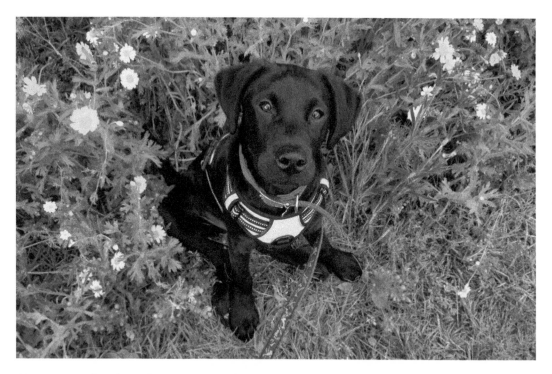

Always remember the end users in our work as veterinary surgeons: the animals in our care. Some are cute and appealing like this puppy and some are smelly, old and incontinent but still very special to their owners who love them.

Practice protocols

During the induction period, you should make yourself familiar with the protocols in place in the practice. There are so many different ways to approach the most common issues raised during a routine consultation such as parasite control, vaccination, neutering and diet and they vary from practice to practice more than you might think. The induction period is your chance to find out how this particular practice has agreed to treat certain conditions such as ear infections and diarrhoea cases. Protocols are reassuring for both vets and owners as it avoids a situation where the owner is being given different and sometimes conflicting advice each time they come in, and the vets know what advice the previous vet will most likely have given a client. Sometimes it is necessary for a vet to use their clinical judgement and go 'off piste', away from the usual protocols, but in this case it should be clearly recorded in the clinical records.

It is highly unlikely that any practice will stock all the different types of flea and worming products as this would not be cost effective because it would tie up too much money in stock on the shelves. Most practices come to a consensus about which anti flea products and worm control products they use and have client information leaflets explaining the recommended routine and product choice for parasite control in different species and ages.

Standard protocols for routine surgical procedures

There is a lot to learn about how the practice you are working in recommends routine procedures, but here are a few you might find useful to know:

- At what age do they usually recommend castration of dogs and cats?
- What age do they recommend spaying female cats and is it flank or midline approach? Some practices spay kittens at quite a young age, especially for cat rescue centres where they like to rehome them already neutered.
- What age and intervals between seasons does the practice recommend neutering bitches?

It is because the protocols for neutering vary so much between practices and also because of the different choices and recommendations of various vaccines and products that I am not going to state any recommended protocols here. You are now a qualified veterinary surgeon so will have your own ideas and use your own judgement, but most practices come to a consensus of opinion about the timing of these routine procedures. The receptionists and nurses need to know what to say when a client rings up asking for advice and it is disconcerting and unmanageable if every vet has a different personal regime which they recommend.

Equipment in the consulting and dispensing areas

Do investigate all the equipment in the consulting room such as the auroscope, ophthalmoscope, digital thermometer, and so on, and familiarise yourself with it before using it in front of a client. You know how to use many of these already, but find out the quirks of those provided for your use in this practice because there are subtle differences between makes of equipment.

Find out what the protocol is for cleaning the instruments between patients and if the table is hydraulic, then find out how to operate it and what to clean it with between clients. Clients love to see a clean consulting room table that has been freshly cleaned just before they come into the consulting room.

Find out where to dispose of sharps and clinical and other waste.

Find out where the suture and staple removal equipment is kept.

Equipment in the operation suite and prep room

There is a huge amount of equipment in the prep room and operating theatre and it is inevitable that you will need several weeks or months to discover where everything is and how it works, but it is worth having a good look during the induction period.

Whenever you have a chance, open the drawers and cupboards and see where everyday items such as curved scissors, cotton wool and syringes are stored. Find out where the stomach tubes and the urinary catheters are stored and keep looking and observing. You have an enquiring mind and if you do not recognise what a piece of equipment is used for, then choose the right moment and ask someone. Make sure that you take every opportunity to watch and learn and ask questions.

Imaging equipment

Find out where the X-ray machine is and over the next few days, have a look at the basics of how it works. It is highly unlikely that you will be using it without assistance, especially at first, but it is a good idea to know how to use it. It may be that the practice nursing staff usually take the X-rays, but you never know if a situation is going to arise in the future when you need to take one yourself.

Make sure you know and follow the safety procedures to ensure that neither you nor anyone else ever exposes themselves to radiation under any circumstances. The previous generation of vets had a far too relaxed attitude to exposure to radiation, and to health and safety generally, and you may still find practices where they are not careful enough to protect themselves and wear the right protective clothing and dosimeters. They are your precious gonads so look after them. Never hold an animal for an X-ray even if there are other vets in the practice who do, always close X-ray room doors and always assume that any female member of staff at any time could be pregnant.

Find out where the ultrasound scanner is and at the very least how to switch it on and where the gel is kept, but preferably how to use it. Not all practices have a scanner in every branch and not all vets are proficient in using one so you need to know who is the best practice ultrasonographer and what you should do if you see a case that needs scanning. Over time, you will of course be able to perform ultrasonography skilfully yourself and putting in the time to practise using it is the only way to improve, so grab those opportunities.

Laboratory

Most practices have an in-house lab of some sort and perform investigative work of varying complexity. Some will perform just basic biochemistry and blood testing with machines and routinely use an external laboratory as a backup, and for more complicated tests and for those that cannot be performed in-house such as examination of slides for histology.

If you are working at a branch surgery without its own lab facilities, find out how the transfer of samples to the lab is organised. As time goes on, you will become familiar with the different tests available but it is worth finding out the basics at this stage.

You need to know if it is usual to admit animals for blood sampling and how to generate an estimate for the costs. Admitting a complicated case for blood samples to be taken also offers a useful opportunity for a second opinion to be sought from a more experienced colleague.

Find out the usual turnround time for results so that when a client asks you when you will be phoning them back, you will have at least some idea of a timeline and know if it could be hours or days before the results can be expected.

Have a look at the in-house lab if there is one and ask those in charge for a tour and an explanation of what you are expected to do and how the results are reported back to the vets. Find out what to do with a sample you wish to have processed and where to look for the sample bottles and tubes and slides.

Look for where the prices for lab work are on the PMS so that you can give a quotation for the costs involved when you recommend them to an owner.

Rota and shifts

You should have been informed of your usual working hours but you may not be aware until you start how all the vets and nurses are organised to work the different sessions during the practice day. Most practices have a daily routine of when the reception staff and nurses start work and the phones go live and when the morning and afternoon consult sessions start.

There may be a set time for coffee breaks and lunch, but in many practices this is very flexible and can depend very much on the workload, with members of staff taking their breaks where they can.

You will find your first few days tiring because there is so much information to absorb even though you may not actually have been consulting or operating, and you will probably be on your feet for longer than you are used to. Make sure that you take the opportunity to have a break and to drink something and eat when it is offered as you may otherwise miss your chance. If everyone is busy then they will be following their own routines and may be snatching a chance for a bite to eat when they can and so might not actually prompt you to take a break. It will not benefit anyone if you pass out halfway through the afternoon because you have not had enough to eat or drink.

Find out where you are supposed to be and when and be there promptly without needing to be nagged or chased. You are part of the workforce now and much more will be expected of you than during your EMS. You are no longer a student and so your work should be for the benefit of the practice and not primarily a learning experience. It may be that the interesting and varied work that you used to observe when you were a student is happening, however you are not there to observe it but there to work.

When I was a new graduate I asked if I could watch my boss operate on a really interesting orthopaedic case one Monday morning and my boss gently reminded me that I was there to work not to further my education. Good employers are enlightened enough to realise the importance of continuous learning and to encourage this, but this has to be reasonable and fit in with the pressures of the working day. A change in attitude from being a vet student who is there to learn to being a working vet who has to share the workload is essential and the luxury of having the opportunity of watching really interesting operations for an hour or more or spending a whole morning on one case and looking up information at length is impractical on a busy day in practice.

You should expect to do the basic work such as vaccinations, suture removal, lumps, bumps and diarrhoea for quite some time as you become skilled and experienced in the consulting room. Opportunities to perform surgery, even such as a basic cat spay, will only be possible when there is enough time and supervision available to support you. It is natural to feel impatient and to want to get more involved with the exciting stuff but your time will come, so be patient and give each case your full attention.

Expect to feel the pressure and the uncertainty of being the new person in the practice and remember that everyone has been there and they all felt just the same. It will not be long before you are part of the team and no longer feel an outsider. People who are busy and focused can look bad-tempered or appear abrupt with you and even seem unfriendly but it is usually because they are concentrating on what they are doing and are distracted.

Practice days are often composed of frantically busy times interspersed with quiet times when nothing seems to be happening but there is always something to occupy you if you look around.

If you find yourself at a loose end at any time, go into the wards and read through the case records of the inpatients even if you have not been involved in that case. It is interesting and educational and gives you an idea of how they go about treating cases in this particular practice.

If, during your consulting session, you have seen a case which has since come back in for a re-examination by someone else, or has gone for surgery, then have a look on the case records and see what the outcome has been. This is feedback and reflective learning in action and you will learn from the case management of your more experienced colleagues. Seeing positive outcomes where you came to the correct diagnosis and seeing that you gave the right treatment and the patient recovered well, will encourage you and give you confidence that you are performing well.

Do not be tempted to rush off at the end of your shift but make sure you speak to your supervisor or fellow members of staff to ensure that you have done everything they expected of you and that it is all right to leave. They may want to have a quick chat with you and find out how your day has gone and it creates a better impression than running out of the building like a rat up a drainpipe the second your shift finishes.

If ever the staff are meeting up after work or there is a social function, then however tired you are, do make an effort to attend even if you leave early, because the team spirit that exists within the practice team will support you in the future. The members of staff will often make an effort when you first join the practice to welcome you and include you in social events and although you may be dreaming of collapsing into bed, accept the invitations whenever you can. It will give you the opportunity to receive positive feedback and reassurance; most members of staff in veterinary practice understand how hard it is when you first start and will offer you support and encouragement which is invaluable.

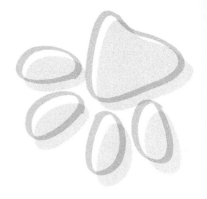

CHAPTER 5

Working with large animals

Starting work in a large animal or mixed practice

There is a huge amount of specific information which could be written about your first job in large animal practice but here I aim to illustrate just a few of the issues the new graduate may face in mixed practice. The information in the other chapters is just as pertinent to mixed practice as to small animal practice when it comes to communication skills, looking after yourself and working with others, but there are some special considerations when you work with large animals.

Working in a mixed or large animal practice brings its own unique challenges for the new veterinary surgeon. The day you start work in practice is very exciting and is the culmination of all you have worked so hard to achieve, whichever type of practice you find yourself in.

You should be proud of yourself for having come so far and the day you 'fly solo' is like no other. It is the start of a working life which will be incredibly interesting and mentally stimulating as you continue to learn every day and develop your skills as you go along. There have been so many advances in large animal veterinary practice over the years and these innovations and changes will continue throughout your career. There will never be a moment when you can sit back and think 'Right, that's it, I know it all' in any type of practice and good vets are always willing to progress and embrace innovation.

We have come a long way from the days of James Herriot driving round the Yorkshire Dales seeing one case of calf pneumonia followed by a cow with mastitis and stopping to admire the view with a tot of whisky in a hip flask. Many large dairy farms now do much of their own routine work that they used to call a vet for, such as calvings and treatment of hypocalcaemia, though there are still smaller farms where the vet may be called on to attend. Dairy farms are sophisticated businesses now and herd health visits are far more likely to be on your visit list than attending a milk fever.

Horse ownership for leisure is thriving and access to portable X-ray machines and the use of ultrasonography has hugely increased the accuracy of diagnosis in horse lameness and other conditions.

We are in danger now of losing some of the treatments we have been used to having freely available, such as a wide range of antibiotics, because of the development of antimicrobial resistance and there may be a risk of losing some of the freedom of the right to prescribe. We bear a responsibility to prescribe the drugs at our disposal wisely and on evidence-based decisions and must resist the overuse of antibiotics and anthelmintics, as has happened in the past.

Vets in practice have had to adapt to the changing times and you will find that there is still a large amount of variation between types of mixed practice and in practices in different geographical areas. You will need to be flexible and use the knowledge and skills you have and adapt them to the changing times and the work of the particular practice in which you find yourself.

You may have had experience of handling large animals before going to vet school, perhaps living on a farm or owning your own horse. You may have chosen mixed practice to work predominantly with horses or dairy cattle, but there are still many practices in rural areas where you will be seeing a wide range of domestic animals and will now be expected to handle species with which you are perhaps less familiar, such as llamas, alpacas and pet pigs. You have passed all your exams and are considered competent to treat all animals although it is inevitable that there will be some species you are more confident with and have more in-depth knowledge of than others.

You will have worked on farms and in mixed practice during your EMS but now you are working in practice and the responsibility for the animals you are asked to see is now yours. You are now 'The Vet' which can be very exciting, but also very daunting and in some ways this is more of a challenge for the new graduate in mixed practice than in small animal practice. There are some obvious differences, in that your patients are large and they have the potential to injure you unintentionally, and your clients are farmers and horse owners who know their animal husbandry and know what they want and expect from their vet. This can be quite intimidating to a new graduate and you have to maintain your authority as a professional, while also respecting the knowledge and experience of the animal owner.

With luck and having chosen your first job discerningly, you will be starting work with an enlightened employer who knows that you need good mentoring and support just as a small animal vet does. Every farmer and horse owner will be new to you and every farm gate and track is a voyage of discovery and is what I used to love about setting off on a round of large animal visits. Your boss will be aware that the first days and weeks in practice are exhausting and so should have organised your work sensitively and with a reasonable induction period to bring you up to speed. Routine work such as testing, if still performed by the practice, is a good way to introduce you to the farmers and hopefully you will be shielded for a little while from the really challenging work until you find your feet.

Just getting to know the local area at first is a challenge and even the organisation of the boot of your vehicle so that you know exactly where everything is, takes time before it becomes familiar. Every farm you visit for the first time, you need to know how to find the right building to meet the animal owner and how the gates open to even get to the animal you are meant to be treating. It's a steep learning curve and everything will take you twice as long at first, so most employers know you will be really slow getting around and will allocate your calls to take this into account.

There will be practices where there may have been delays in recruiting or a sudden loss of a vet due to illness or accident and the practice owner may find it more difficult to ease you in as gently as they would like. This can happen in any type of practice, but in a small animal practice at least you are likely to be under the same roof as another vet, whereas in large animal practice the other vets may be out on their rounds despite intending to be around to support you. If this happens to you, then do not panic but do the best you can and thank goodness for the advent of the mobile phone.

If you can maintain a can-do attitude and show willingness and a sunny disposition, it can be a real help when you are experiencing all the inevitable hiccups in your first few days in practice. People are much more likely to be sympathetic towards you and help you if you are friendly and approachable and demonstrate a sense of humour in the face of adversity. It does not help for a new vet to appear cold, aloof or pompous so although you should try to stay as calm and efficient as possible, you can still smile and ask for help.

> *Farmers tend to think new graduates look about 12 years old and they can be a bit resistant to accepting a new, young vet rather than the older vet that they may have been seeing for years. One farmer greeted me with the comment 'Is this the best they can send us?' in a disparaging manner when I got out of the car on his farm for the first time. I could have been defensive, but I smiled and said that I was the only available vet at the moment but that if I could not do the job then I would call someone else but would appreciate being given a chance. 'Fair enough,' he said, and we got on really well after that rather negative start.*

If unreasonable expectations are made of you on a farm visit, then make sure your personal safety is not compromised by your desire to comply in a dangerous situation. If you are struggling to cope with what is being asked of you, then stop and do not risk your safety or that of others under any circumstances. Contact your employer and explain what the problem is and ask for help if you need it. You will be expected to work hard and you might be fine going out and performing a procedure for the first time, but do not attempt anything that is way beyond your capabilities. Nothing is more important than your welfare and the welfare of other humans and that of the animals in your care. It is one thing being faced with a small animal case that you can admit for a second opinion but, as the only vet on the farm or at the stables, you may feel under pressure to act and it is at times like these that people get hurt.

My first morning in practice I was asked to go to a farm to clip a Jersey bull's feet. I arrived on the farm and calculated the dose of sedative under the dis-approving eyes of the farmer and his son, listening to sub-audible grumblings about 'was expecting one of the blokes' and 'looks like a school girl'. The bull was in a pen and I climbed in and whacked the sedative into his rump while he had his head through the bars of the hayrack. Pleased with my success, I clambered out and waited for the drug to take effect. 'Well lass, you're the first person who's been in wi' that bugger,' said the farmer as he smiled approvingly. It was my complete naivety which made me take such a stupid risk and, in retrospect, I don't know what I was thinking of. Fortunately, I survived and was able to trim the bull's feet which took me four times as long as anyone else with the result that my boss sent out a search party to find why I hadn't returned to the surgery by mid-afternoon.

If you cannot manage a case, be prepared to ask for help without fear of losing face and being judged. No one, including the farmer, wants you to struggle on failing to complete a task to the detriment of an animal when the best thing for your patient is to admit defeat and seek assistance. It takes courage to admit that you need help and reasonable owners will respect you for having the intelligence to realise your limitations; the worst thing to do is to carry on struggling and failing in order to protect your own pride. Make sure you know where and from whom you can seek help and what arrangements are in place before you start out.

Every single time I ask a vet what key advice they have for a new graduate, one of the first things they say is to ask for help if they need it and not to struggle on.

I went to see a cow with a prolapsed uterus quite early on in my first year in practice and I did my best to try to replace it, but it was like trying to squash a duvet cover into a pint pot. After struggling for a while and being covered from head to foot in lubricant and body fluids, I realised that it was beyond my capabilities and I reluctantly called my boss. I thought the farmer would be very critical of my failure but he was really understanding, and while we waited for the cavalry to arrive he said that he appreciated my seeking help rather than damaging his cow by trying and failing for too long. He said he had seen young vets who had put their own pride before the welfare of the cows with a diffi-cult calving and preferred a vet who accepted their limitations and accepted they had some learning to do and some experience to attain. This was from a Yorkshire farmer and believe me, if they think you are in the wrong, they show no mercy and they take no prisoners.
A year or two later, the same farmer and I were treating a horned suckler cow and her calf in a yard when she took umbrage at our presence and came for us at speed. We both managed to leap into the hayrack fixed to the wall and

while we were waiting to be rescued, the farmer chose to remind me about this failure, as farmers do. He then went on to tell me about another newly qualified assistant who had come to a calving and not asked for help, despite the farmer urging him to, until after the animal had been irreparably damaged and who he never allowed onto the farm again.

Horses

A considerable proportion of leisure horses are owned by individuals who may be working and unavailable to handle the horse or pony at the time when you are calling to vaccinate or examine them. In this situation, beware the inexperienced friend or parent of the horse owner who may not be able to handle the patient effectively and who has been left to hold the horse for your visit. Vaccinating a stroppy pony held by a mother in high heels with a handbag over one arm is not an experience I wish to repeat. Once I became more confident and aware of the potential risks, I would not have agreed to put myself or the owner in that situation and would have insisted on someone holding the horse who knew what they were doing. Always put your safety and also that of the person handling the horse first, as it is your responsibility to ensure that they are not injured during the consultation, and do wear a hard hat.

Take care of your vehicle

If you are working in large animal practice, you will most likely be given the use of a vehicle which you need to look after and keep clean and maintain the drugs and equipment in order and restocked. There is a unique smell to a vet's car, which is usually a mixture of manure, disinfectant and other unidentifiable aromas. This can cover the full spectrum from faintly veterinary to completely nauseating, so try to keep it as clean as you can. It helps to use washable covers, boot liners and storage boxes in your car and to clean it out regularly. It is important for hygiene and to show the animal owners that you take biosecurity seriously.

Biosecurity

Make sure you dress like a professional, even in large animal practice, and that you clean your hands and disinfect thoroughly between visits. Looking grubby and disorganised may not appear to be a problem as long as all goes well, but will become significant in a disease situation or if a case goes wrong. Clean your boots at the end of a visit and make sure the client actually sees you doing so, even if the postman is just as likely to carry disease on or off the farm. The hygiene routine of the veterinary professional must be above reproach as far as disease control is concerned.

You will smell at the end of a day working in farm practice and as you walk down the street you will find that dogs lunge towards you to check out the fascinating medley of aromas emanating from your clothing. I remember standing in a supermarket checkout on a warm day and being aware of a terrible aroma which I soon realised was coming from my own clothes which had become permeated with the heady smell of Essence de Pig Farm! People were backing away, and I was certainly served quickly just to ensure that I vacated the building.

You will learn that there are different standards of hygiene in different households and there are some farmhouses and small animal homes where it is not always wise to accept a cup of coffee. As your feet stick to the carpet and you see the quick rinse of a filthy mug, you may regret accepting that offer of a hot drink. There should always be washing facilities but do keep some antibacterial hand wipes and hand gel in the car for the situation where it is not easy to clean your hands properly.

If you are out on calls, do record exactly what you use and dispense on the farm at the time before you leave and start thinking about the next call. Most practices will have mobile devices to record any drugs injected and dispensed and the procedures you have carried out. Be disciplined and record everything as you go along or you will inevitably forget that box of medication.

One of the best things about working in large animal practice is that after a time, you can relax more because you know what to expect at each farm or premises. When you regularly go onto someone's farm, you will inevitably become closer to some clients and become involved in their lives and that is one of the charms about being a large animal vet, where getting to know your clients is one of the great rewards of mixed practice.

You may become quite close to people and in a small community, this can be very supportive and provide a social life such as Young Farmers' Clubs and other friendships. This can bring its own complications too, but as long as you ensure you maintain the usual safeguards of preserving confidentiality and your veterinary principles, then any other complications are your own business. Take care when going on to social media that in the course of chatting you are not indiscreet about a client's business and make sure you preserve your own privacy too. In small, farming communities it is even more likely that everyone knows someone so be careful never to comment about one client to another. The chances are that the word will get round and someone somewhere will take offence.

I have been invited to weddings and to join farming clients for Christmas day when I have been on call and a long way from home and have been welcomed into families and plied with drinks in the pub when off-duty. It is inevitable that you will make friendships in the course of your work and your time off and this is highly likely in a small community. It does make sense to tread carefully when crossing the line from a professional to a more personal relationship with someone who is a client or part of a client's family, and make sure you maintain confidentiality and discretion.

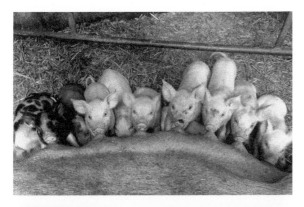

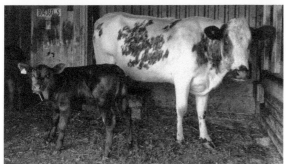

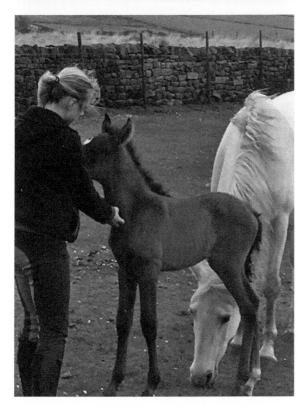

You never know what you are going to see as a large animal vet and although your work may involve complex herd health planning, there will still be occasions when you are in a less sophisticated environment with your patients. Smallholdings with a collection of different species and breeds are still relatively commonplace and you may need to compromise and adapt to conditions that are far from state of the art.

Large animal practice has changed over the years and continues to do so at a pace. Farmers are much more likely to be performing the routine tasks once performed by their vet and many are highly educated and know more than you do about the husbandry of their particular species and breeds, so we must treat them with respect. You will need to be robust in your role as the veterinary surgeon because diagnosis and prescription of drugs is your area of expertise and the decisions are your responsibility and yours alone. You will find that some large animal owners may try to pressurise you into doing exactly what they want you to do and coerce you into dispensing medication against your better judgement. Be polite, explain your reasoning and stay firm in the face of any pressure or manipulation by the owner because it is you who is the professional and who would face the music should there be any repercussions.

You are likely to meet a wide variety of sizes of farming enterprise and the hobby farmer can be a completely different challenge, as they may have little or no knowledge about their animals but hold some very strong views gleaned from a variety of sources both genuine and dubious. You may need to educate them as well as treat their animals, but these owners are often very interesting and great fun too.

There is never a dull moment when you are a vet in mixed practice and in my first six years, I thoroughly enjoyed the variety, working with all species, large and small, and the people I came into contact with. I would have continued to work in mixed practice but I developed an interest in small animals and soft tissue surgery and I found a small animal practice which fulfilled my dreams and aspirations. Many mixed practices are now structured into species subgroups with dedicated vets for each large animal species, but there are still practices where a true traditional mixed job remains and thrives.

Once I had to visit a disease-free pig farm because the extremely knowledgeable pig vet in the practice who usually attended was away from work unexpectedly. I arrived to find that biosecurity measures were in place and I was expected to enter the building, strip to the skin in the first changing room, pass through a shower and into a second changing room and then put on the clothes provided by the pig farm. They were obviously expecting my boss who was a middle-aged man of generous proportions and so I emerged on to the farm wearing a size 46 boiler suit and size ten boots under which I was wearing a string vest and a pair of Y fronts, which was all that had been available on the other side of the shower. While leaning forward trying to take a blood sample and trying to pre-serve my modesty, at least I had the comfort of knowing that I was not passing on any diseases and was also giving some free entertainment to the pig men who had all gathered round to have a good laugh at my expense.

I was asked to attend the local theme park which was owned by a farmer who was rather an entrepreneur and who had decided to build a visitor attrac-tion which consisted of a pig farm behind Perspex windows, open to the general public. It displayed all ages of pigs, including sows in farrowing pens, boars and piglets and the general public could look through the Perspex walls of the building to observe the pigs without having their delicate noses subjected to the smell of the pig muck. I was lying on the floor of the barn assisting a sow who was farrowing when I heard a child's voice saying, 'Mummy, why has that lady got her hand up the pig's bottom?' and I looked round to see the traumatised faces of a family of four watching through the window. I held up a piglet glistening in afterbirth and I don't think that really helped at all. The pig observation attraction was closed down shortly afterwards, and the farmer concentrated on other more aesthetic money-making schemes, such as a carvery and a garden centre!

Health and safety

The risk of injury is all too prevalent for large animal practice vets and, in my experience, it is during the first few months of practice that you are most likely to be injured by your patients. There is so much to learn and to concentrate on, and it is extremely tiring because everything is new and unfamiliar, and so a moment's lapse of concentration can have serious and painful consequences. As you gain experience and familiarity with the work, you will develop an awareness of the signals your patients display when they are becoming less passive and compliant. You will become much more adept at avoiding circumstances when you may be injured and it will become second nature to you with time, but it is very easy to get hurt when you are weary or distracted in a new and unfamiliar environment.

Large animals can cause severe injuries which can be life-changing and even life-threatening and you must ensure your own personal safety above all other considerations. The work itself can be very physical and every large animal vet over a certain age seems to have a bad back. Do look after your back and use the aids such as hoists and calving aids rather than demonstrating your strength and magnificent physique.

Make sure you take out insurance against sickness and personal injury before you start work in any type of practice because you do not want to have any financial concerns to worry about if you become injured and unable to work. It is easy to think it will never happen to you, but most vets will have a tale of doom and gloom where a colleague has been put out of action by an injury during the course of their work.

Euthanasia in large animals

There may be occasions where you will need to euthanise a larger animal such as a farm animal or an animal on a petting zoo. This is not a task to be approached lightly without being well-prepared and is one of the skills that you would be wise to go out of your way to learn from more experienced vets. If there is a chance that you will have to perform this task, then take the opportunity to learn how to do it before you need to do it in an emergency where an animal is suffering. This might mean observing or assisting another vet on your day off when an opportunity arises.

You will need to warn the owner what to expect when they have a large animal euthanised because they will most likely be extremely shocked, especially when seeing it for the first time.

Equine euthanasia

Equine euthanasia is a unique situation because the logistics can be more challenging and the attachment of an owner to their horse is usually strong and an emotional one. It is much easier to give a small animal such as a dog a gentle death in its owner's arms followed by a discreet and dignified disposal than it is with a horse.

Equine euthanasia is always a dramatic event and the size of the body and the moving of it afterwards for disposal is inevitably potentially shocking and traumatic for the owner. Careful planning is crucial, as is taking control of the situation firmly but kindly. Your first priority is your patient and if the emotional manifestations of the owner are distressing the horse then you need to deal with the situation with authority.

However many times you witness it, it is still a shock to see a horse drop and it is also a potentially dangerous situation, so make sure your willingness to ease the pain for the owner does not prevent you from ensuring everyone is safe, including yourself. I strongly believe that anyone dealing with a horse should be wearing protective headgear at all times and that includes veterinary surgeons. There is growing awareness of the need for this, but there is still some strange and illogical reluctance to do so from both veterinary surgeons and some horse owners. Ski helmets were a rarity a few years ago, but are now increasingly worn and wearing a hat should be a no-brainer for vets dealing with horses so that you protect the brain you were born with.

It is very tempting to try to make things as easy as possible for a distressed owner when you are putting a horse to sleep and a friend of mine went out of her way to do just that. She was asked to put an elderly horse to sleep for an old lady who was very attached to her ancient mare and wanted to bury her at home. Being a practical lady, she had arranged for her brother to bring down his digger and dig a suitably large hole because she wanted her to be buried in the paddock where she had enjoyed many a happy hour munching the grass. The brother had really taken the advice to dig deep to heart and had dug a hole of considerable depth and then gone home to await instructions to come back and bury her later.

The elderly mare was waiting patiently by the side of the grave when the vet arrived and was very quiet and easy to handle. After a catheter was put in easily, the owner said her goodbyes but was so upset that she was quick to take up the vet's offer to leave her to perform the final injection.

The injection was administered smoothly and there was a short pause as the drug took effect, whereupon the mare started to buckle at the knees and move inexorably towards the gaping grave, then went down and died on the edge of the hole. The body relaxed and started to gradually slide over the edge into the hole. Initially impressed by the efficiency with which the mare had interred herself, the vet then thought that she must check that she had actually died and was not just anaesthetised. She jumped down into the hole and reassured herself that there were no vital signs. Looking round, she then realised just how deep the hole was and looked for ways to get out. She tried everything, but all her attempts to climb out proved fruitless.

Visions of the old chap, possibly deaf, coming back with his digger and burying her alive with the body flooded into her mind and she desperately tried various options, even trying to climb out by standing on the body, but to no avail.

Eventually, she was rescued after shouting for help for what seemed like hours but was in fact only 20 minutes. Time passes slowly when you are in a very deep hole with a very dead horse.

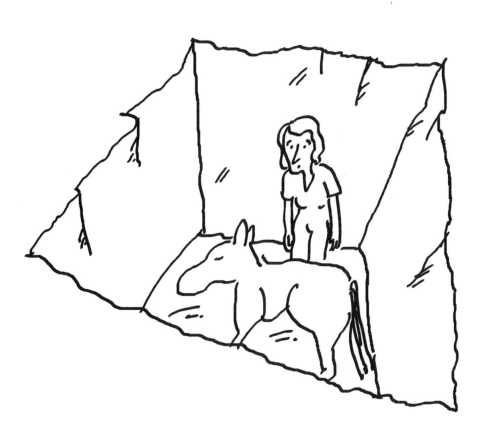

TIPS FROM VETS IN PRACTICE

I could never cover all the aspects of mixed practice even in a hundred books, but here is some miscellaneous advice from some mixed practice vets:

- Ask for advice sooner rather than later and learn the right way to do things by watching and asking advice from your more senior colleagues.
- Never assume anything when it comes to your safety in handling animals. Nothing is more important than the safety of the humans present, so do not take unnecessary risks.
- In all species of animals, do consider the common and the obvious before you start looking for obscure and rare conditions.
- Always make sure you hand over any swabs or blood samples for processing by the lab and that they are not left to fester in the recesses of your car.
- Phone the owners promptly with the results of any tests.
- Remember to inform the owner of any withdrawal times for drugs that you prescribe.
- If you perform a pregnancy diagnosis and you are uncertain, then do not inject the cow.
- If you calve a cow, always check for a twin still in the uterus. (I've made this mistake and the memory still makes me squirm.)
- Make sure you know exactly which address you are going to when you set out on a call and beware the same surname at different farms. (I have arrived at 3 a.m. to see a sick cow at the premises of the farmer's brother who shared the same name but whose farm was ten miles in the other direction.)
- Always keep your boot tidy and replenish stock efficiently, keeping an accurate record of what you have used and handed out so that you do not reach for something at two in the morning only to find it missing. Make sure you maintain stock control and book all the items used and dispensed to clients.
- Make sure your tablet and phone are charged at all times.
- Clean your scissors and keep your hoof knife and other equipment clean and sharp.
- Carry some drinking water, phone charger, spare shirt, wet wipes and plasters in the car.
- Carry heavy-duty barrier hand cream especially in winter, to save your hands getting chapped with being washed all the time.
- Use any quiet times when you are on call to catch up with all those routine tasks which need doing, such as organising your paperwork, filling in your mileage forms, phoning clients for updates and filling in your PDP online. If you do this while you are at work, then when you are off-duty you can enjoy yourself without all these minor housekeeping tasks hanging over you.

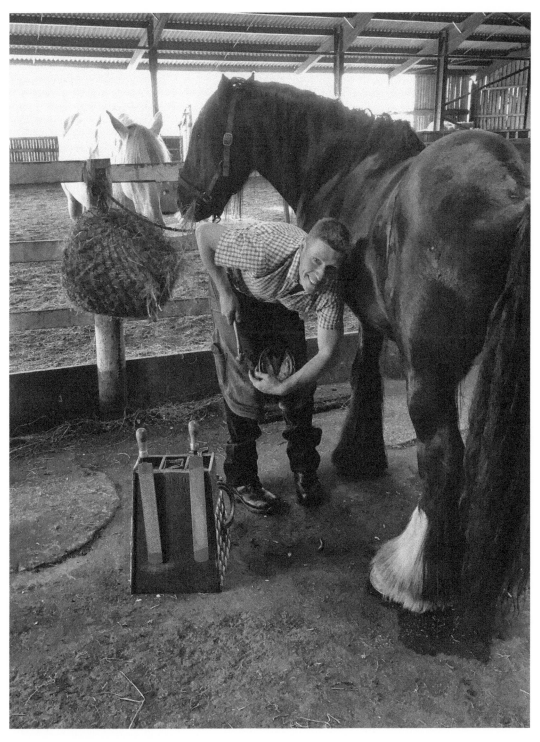

It is always a good idea to maintain good relationships with fellow professionals, such as farriers, as we can learn a great deal from them and our patients benefit by us working in partnership.

You will often be working alone so learn by following up cases and ringing to see how they are progressing. It gives you constructive feedback and the farmer will appreciate the fact that you are interested and care enough to lift the phone.

Many farmers will have a farm dog and quite often this is a Border collie, usually one or possibly more, and there are a few things to remember about these individuals. They will be highly valued by the farmer and his family, very protective of the property and usually they have a habit of nipping ankles and chasing cars. Take care not to run them over as you leave the yard and check that there is someone around to call the dog off before you get out of the car in the yard.

One of my bosses, who was a bit of a petrolhead, took delivery of a rather racy new car which he enjoyed positioning strategically in the farmer's yard for a quick and impressive getaway in a cloud of dust. One day as he was driving away, he and the Border collie tried to go through the farm gates at the same time and the Border collie came off worse and suffered a fractured pelvis. Not a word was spoken by the glowering farmer as the vet laid the casualty on the back seat of his car and assured him apologetically that he would be fixing him free of charge.

A vet told me the tale of how he attended a farm where the notoriously aggressive farm dog was always on a sturdy chain in the farmyard; when you arrived, the dog would hurtle towards you at throat height only to be arrested in flight by the chain. Considering himself to be safely further than the reach of the length of the chain, he left the car to treat a case of hypocalcaemia and was halfway across the yard with a bottle of calcium in his hand when he heard a clank and a twanging noise. He realised, in horror, that the chain had broken and the trajectory of the snarling Border collie was an airborne, vet-eating missile who was coming towards him at speed. An instinctive realisation of essential self-preservation and perfect timing resulted in him thwacking the dog across the head with the bottle and knocking it out cold. It possessed a good thickness of skull fortunately and lived to threaten subsequent vets who visited the farm with renewed vigour, although he always maintained a healthy respect for that vet.

Many vets move from mixed practice to small animal practice after a few years, as I did, but I have never regretted the six years I worked with large animals. I think I learned a great deal during that time which was useful in my work in small animal practice, especially the necessity to be resourceful and make necessary compromises in situations where the facilities were not perfect. There will be times during your career when you have to use your skills in the situation in which you find yourself and adapt, and large animal practice can train you to think laterally and use your initiative.

CHAPTER 6

How to look good
in the consulting room

You will have observed many different characters and personalities in the vets you have met during your weeks of EMS and it is likely that there are individuals whose style of consulting you admire and would aspire to. Most experienced vets make consulting look easy and enjoyable and watching them in action is like watching a skilled actor on the stage with each performance unique, entertaining and subtly different. A stage actor speaks the same lines in every performance, but no two performances are exactly the same and this is what it is like to be a really good vet who has perfected the art of consulting. Each consultation is indeed a unique occasion and the performance of it should be given your full attention and commitment. You would not want to pay to go to the theatre and see a careless, perfunctory effort by an actor who is having a bad day and your clients should always receive your best performance. There really is an element of getting into character and whatever may be going on in your private life needs to be left at the door with no negative influences on your delivery.

Being a chameleon in the consulting room

Not content with asking you to be an actor, I also expect you to impersonate an animal and to be a chameleon in the consulting room. Vets in practice are often presented with the same situation time and time again in consultations, but the really good vets deliver minute changes in their response to each person they meet. They become chameleon-like and subtly alter the way they extract and deliver the same information with different people. Consulting is indeed an art and though some people are by nature excellent communicators, others are not naturals but it is possible to learn techniques to improve your skills and you will become more proficient with practice.

You may be reserved by nature and given the choice, you might prefer to conduct a consultation in silence and in an analytical way, approaching each case scientifically and concentrating on making a diagnosis without indulging in any distracting discussion with

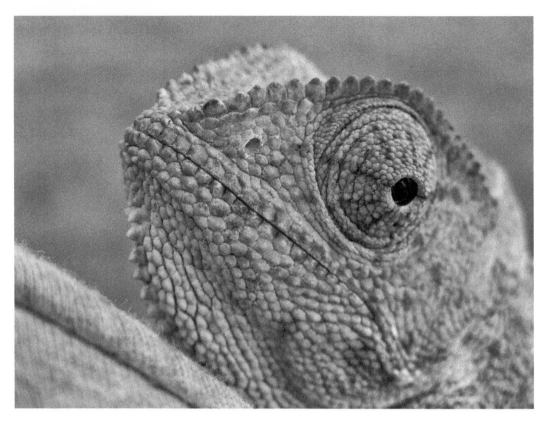

When we are in a consultation, our task is to help the client to tell us what they know about our patient and what they want from us for that animal. We then need to be able to communicate our recommendations back to the client in a manner which they will fully understand. To achieve optimum exchange of understanding, you need to able to change the way you interact and so become a chameleon by being sensitive to the situation your client is experiencing and responding accordingly. You may need to use different complexities of language and vary your consulting style to achieve this. Photo: Richard Tapsfield.

the owner or interaction with the animal other than examining it. In practice, however, in order to extract the information you need to be effective and to gain their agreement to necessary intervention, you will need to interact with your clients and you cannot simply be a silent but brilliant boffin. You may indeed be an absolute genius and a brilliant diagnostician, but you will not be successful as a veterinary surgeon in practice if you cannot conduct a consultation in which

a) you receive the correct information from the client,
b) the client hears and understands your opinion and advice, and
c) the client agrees to your treatment plan.

Clients tend to gravitate towards the vet whose consulting style they like and who they respond to, and they will give their appreciation of that vet's style and their own enjoyment of the consultation as much weight or more than they give to their appreciation of the vet's actual clinical skills. When you start your career, you will find it quite hard work because you have not yet perfected your own personal consulting technique and every consultation is a new and novel challenge. You do not yet have a familiar framework and a routine to your consultations, so nothing happens by automatic pilot and it requires effort, but there are techniques which you can use until you have developed your own unique way of communicating with your clients. If you are finding consulting difficult, go back to these basic principles and you may find your consultations more enjoyable and productive.

What clients really want is a vet who is friendly and who cares about their animal and they want them to listen and to explain what is happening in language which they can understand. They want their vet to be interested in all aspects of their pet's life and to acknowledge just how important that animal is to them and their family.

Clients are often worried when they come to the vet and they worry about many things which are nothing to do with their pet's current condition. They worry about where they should sit and stand and how much or how little information they should be giving to you. They worry about looking stupid in front of you and about how their pet will behave in the surgery and if their pet will be hurt during the consultation. They worry about how much it is going to cost and if they will be able to get tablets down their cat or be able to put ear drops in their ears. They worry about remembering everything you have said because they have to tell their partner what the vet said when they get home. They worry about all these things and more, and it is part of our job to ensure that they are reassured and relaxed as far as is possible, and that they get the best outcome from their visit to the practice. We want them to bond with our practice and trust us and want to come back to see us again.

I believe that sincerity is the key to success with all interactions with clients and that if you are sincere about what you do and say, you will not go far wrong. Although it is true that consulting techniques can be learned and communication skills acquired, genuine empathy and sincerity shine through and will be recognised by clients. They will forgive you for asking the same question twice or getting a bit flustered if they can see that you genuinely care about them and their animal.

Every interaction with every patient deserves your full attention and your best effort and will be appreciated by the owners. Every client, young or old, well dressed or shabby, should be treated with the utmost respect and you should do your best for each and every one of them.

I might consult in different styles with different people and may be more or less formal as appropriate, but I always give each one of them my full attention from the outset to ensure that the communication is at an optimum. I make sure that they have had their questions answered and their concerns addressed and that they know what I am going to do, and what they need to do, and when they have to come back to be seen again.

Most vets really enjoy being around animals and this is one of your greatest advantages when it comes to meeting your patients and their owners. Do talk to the owner, of course, but never forget to acknowledge the presence of the pet with word or touch as this will instantly bond you with the client as it shows you care about his or her companion as an individual.

Companion animals arrive in all variations, young and cute, old and doddery, scared and confident, with soulful eyes and beautiful coat colours, but even if they are carried in growling, hissing and smelling to high heaven, always find something positive to say about them. The owner is probably slightly nervous that you will not see how special their pet is, despite the bad behaviour and the smell, and if they immediately recognise that you see their pet as a valued individual and that you care, they will immediately relax and become more receptive.

You will meet people with all different levels of education, of all ages and abilities, and from varying economic circumstances who are far more diverse than you would ever meet in your social circle. Humans tend to socialise with those who have things in common, but in the veterinary practice waiting room you will see a kaleidoscope of the human race come and go with their animals.

Forget any preconception that you are superior to any of your clients and reach out and try your best to work with them for the benefit of their animal, putting aside your prejudices. You only have to spend the duration of a consultation with them, not become best friends, and at the end of the day they are paying your wages. They are paying for your time and undivided attention and should never be shortchanged in your attention or hurried or ignored.

I had a relatively sheltered life as a child and attended an all-girls grammar school before going to Glasgow University and enjoying my student years with my fellow students. My first job on graduation was in Rotherham, a gritty, industrial town, and was at the time of the miners' strike against pit closures in the 1970s. I had never seen real poverty before and had my eyes opened to reality when I went on a house call to a street on a housing estate in an economically deprived area of the city. On arrival, I thought I must have been given the wrong address because all the houses in the street appeared to be derelict and boarded-up but as I reached the house at the address I had been given I saw that it was still inhabited. I was admitted by a young woman and entered to see a small dog lying on the floor having a fit, with the classic symptoms of terminal distemper. There were small children in nappies and wearing filthy clothing walking round the stricken dog and the soles of my shoes were sticking to the carpet as I walked into the room. There were dirty nappies on the floor and dog excrement, the walls were covered in newspaper instead of wallpaper or paint and the smell was indescribable. I examined the dog and told the woman it needed putting to sleep and she told me that she did not care how much it cost, but to get it out of the house as it was upsetting to see it fitting. I asked her to sign the consent form and told her how much the cost would be, and she laughed in my face and told me to leave using a few four-letter words to drive her message home. I decided discretion was the better part of valour and took the dog away for euthanasia. I look back now and think what a shock that was to me as a naive, sheltered young person. I just did not realise that people lived in such conditions and I did not realise until that moment just how fortunate I was never to have experienced such deprivation. My years of being a vet have educated me and the years in practice have also broadened my mind and my perspective. I am sure many people go through life and never see how others have to live their lives, but as a vet working in practice I have met all kinds of people, and seen slums and stately homes and treated animals in both environments and everything in between.

I have learned that some relatively wealthy people can be ignorant, cruel and unwilling to spend any money on their animals. I have learned that someone who appears to have nothing will prioritise their animals' welfare over their own comfort and pay a vet bill by sacrificing their own needs. I have seen old people on a pension save a small sum every week to pay for their dog's treatment and turn on the heating for their cat, when they would economise and not put it on for themselves. I have known misguided owners pay hundreds of pounds for a puppy only to say they have not got the money to protect it by having it vaccinated.

I have met seemingly intelligent, well-educated clients who genuinely believe in homeopathy and those who will not vaccinate because they think it 'weakens the immune system' and have done my best to educate them and change their views for the good of their animals.

Seeing how other people live and hearing many different viewpoints from my own have made my work as a general practitioner immensely interesting and thought-provoking and I am sure you will find the same.

How I perform a small animal consultation

The process starts well before the client comes into the consulting room with their pet; I make sure I have looked through the appointment list before starting the session so that there are no surprises. I like to have a printed list of all the appointments for that session and I look through the list before consulting starts, looking up relevant history and patient details.

This means that you are aware of previous events in that animal's life and gives the client confidence that you have some knowledge of their pet, which might have been in two weeks ago with a cut paw or a bout of diarrhoea. Checking the vaccination and neutering status can prevent you from advising neutering an already neutered dog and asking questions which the client quite reasonably expects you to know already. You can check if they are already on medication which might be relevant to any treatment you prescribe, and if they are allergic to anything, which may prevent you from making the mistake of prescribing corticosteroids to a dog already on nonsteroidal anti-inflammatories.

Before the client comes in you should:

- ❖ Have noted the name of your patient and its sex and age
- ❖ Be aware if neutered and vaccinated
- ❖ Have read the clinical history as far as is possible
- ❖ Be aware of current medication and allergies and noted any warnings about temperament
- ❖ Have noted the reason for attending the current appointment.

Consultations of 10 or 15 minutes are a very short time to achieve everything you need to do, especially when the patient and the client are new to you. In that short space of time you need to:

- ❖ Call the client in
- ❖ Greet them and their pet
- ❖ Ask how you can help them today
- ❖ Listen to the history from the owner
- ❖ Ask necessary questions to clarify the history and ensure you have all the facts
- ❖ Record the history on the system
- ❖ Assess the dog or cat for general demeanour before laying a hand on it
- ❖ Assess dog for safe handling on the floor before lifting onto the examination table, or extract cat from cat basket
- ❖ Perform a full clinical examination
- ❖ Inform client of significant findings and explain possible differential diagnoses
- ❖ Suggest treatment plan and possible further investigations
- ❖ Administer any treatments such as injections
- ❖ Wrap up the consultation and check the client is happy
- ❖ Thank the client for attending
- ❖ Usher the client out of the consulting room.

Phew, it looks an impossible task but it is achievable and vets manage this every day and so can you. One of the most common problems facing a new graduate is keeping to time during a consulting session. If you have ever attended an outpatient clinic or a doctor's surgery and had to wait a long time to be seen, then you will know that time passes incredibly slowly when you are waiting long past your appointment time. Waiting makes you very irritable as you think of all the things you could be doing rather than sitting on a very uncomfortable plastic chair surrounded by other grumpy strangers coughing and spluttering.

If you are lucky and logistics in the practice allow, then you may be given extra time per consultation when you first start, but there will come a day when you are expected to keep to the same time schedule as every other vet and become more efficient at keeping to appointment schedules.

Some vets always allow their surgeries to run late and, while in some instances it is inevitable, it does show a lack of consideration for both the clients and the people you work with. When the surgery is running late, the reception and nursing staff have to deal with the clients who are being kept waiting and it can also mean that they do not get home on time because once the consulting finishes, they still have to tidy and clean the surgery. It annoys the clients and the staff and makes your life more difficult; being persistently late is a choice and not a personality trait.

There are ways in which you can help yourself keep to the appointment times while still being thorough and not making the clients feel rushed. It becomes easier with practice and sometimes an emergency will come in or an unexpected event take place but try to resist becoming a serial offender for over-running surgery times. Do not look at the clock or your watch or phone in front of a client during a consult but have your watch face up on the work surface where you can glance at it discreetly to keep the consults to time.

I like to keep the printed list of the appointments for that consulting session in front of me so that I can swiftly check at a glance to see if I am on time for each appointment without having to open and close windows on the computer. It may be necessary to check for last minute changes on the day book but it is usually quicker and is not affected by the computer crashing, and means you do not have to open up different screens or windows on the system. Also, I find crossing off the names of the completed consults weirdly satisfying, but that's just me.

If you are ready to start and your first client is already there in the waiting room, then do start your consulting session early because if an unavoidable delay does occur, you are already slightly ahead and have some precious minutes in hand. Do not be a jobsworth who starts on the dot and has been lurking behind the reception desk waiting for the clock to strike four even though people are waiting.

I prefer to go out into the waiting room to call each client in rather than hiding in the consulting room and being a disembodied voice calling the next client's name or 'next' which can sound unwelcoming and can result in people not being sure whose name has been called, followed by awkward shuffling and whispering.

When I go out into the waiting room I smile at everyone, make some casual comment about the weather or a cute puppy and maybe say 'not your turn yet' to the dog who leaps to greet me. I try to create a friendly, informal and relaxed atmosphere as some clients can feel quite nervous when they are waiting, especially if they have not been before.

If you greet the waiting clients warmly with a smile, then they will already have a first impression of you as a friendly face and anticipate a pleasant consultation. They are much more likely to relax and if you have instigated a topic of conversation even as mundane as the weather, then this often triggers further exchanges between the other clients and the nurses which makes the time pass and makes the whole experience more interesting for them.

Smile, and look approachable but do not become involved in whatever else is happening out there unless someone is dying or being assaulted. The receptionist will look after everyone and it is easy to find yourself waylaid by an assertive client who has come in to collect some pet food or a prescription and who tries to start an informal consultation in the waiting room.

The only time to really engage with the waiting room may be when you are running late by a considerable margin. This is the time to address the waiting room collectively and apologise for the late running of the surgery. If there has been an emergency, then explain that this is why appointments are running late as most clients will understand this and sympathise with the sick or injured animal. They may start to chat to one another and this really helps the receptionist by breaking the frosty silence which is pervasive in a waiting room of clients whose appointment times have long passed. Your receptionist or veterinary nurse will really appreciate this as they are usually the ones on the receiving end of the sighs and the raised eyebrows as clients ostentatiously look at their watches.

When you call in a client you haven't met before it can be tactful to use the name and surname of the pet as in 'Fluffy Jones' as this avoids the Mr or Mrs or Ms conundrum. The potential for embarrassment is considerable, as you wonder if you have actually identified the correct sex of the client. Are they father and daughter or husband and wife, and if you saw them two days ago then they might expect you to remember their title. Calling the pet's name and the surname can help avoid the whole question of names and titles and also reinforces the fact that the animal is your patient. It also obscures the fact that they may have asked you to use their first name which you have subsequently forgotten.

Unless you are certain you have accurately identified what the breed of dog or cat actually is, do not compliment them on their choice of a Poodle only to be told in outrage that she is a Bichon frise. Many clients expect vets to be able to identify every breed under the sun simply because they have been educated at a vet school. I think they believe that vet students are set numerous examinations for five years simply on breed identification of all dogs, cats, rabbits and reptiles. Hopefully, the nurse will have filled in all the details of the animal on the computer system and they will be forgiven for not being aware that the puppy is a Bouvier des Flandres much more readily than you will be. In the case of a puppy, ask for the vaccination record card because this has the breed written in and you can nod sagely and say how much you like Patterdale terriers. The advent of Cockerpoos and Labradoodles has just made everything even more complicated, but most clients will announce the breed with pride and you can relax.

First impressions

First impressions of hygiene are very important to clients and although we know that some dog and cat hair on the table is inevitable, I always spray and clean the table just before the client comes in so that they know it is clean. I also wash my hands and am demonstrably drying them as I enter the waiting room to call in the next patient, so they are reassured that hygiene is a priority.

I hold the door open and, if appropriate, help them by carrying the cat basket in or closing the door after them so that they know I am there to provide a service for them and not there as a lofty, intimidating medical expert. Many clients are worried about being made to feel stupid or insignificant so the more we do to help them feel relaxed and to feel we are on their side, the better. Helping them by indicating where they might like to stand and possibly offering a place to put their coat if it is very warm, can make the client feel you care about their comfort. Some elderly or infirm clients may need to sit down, so be observant about how they look and be considerate.

I always greet the patient and say something complimentary however bald, smelly or snappy he or she might be. There is always something positive that you can say that shows the client that you appreciate their pet, whether it be referring to a snarling cat in a basket as a 'feisty little person' or expressing sympathy for a 'brave old soldier' when an elderly, wheezing, fat Labrador comes staggering in. If you say anything remotely derogatory it is just like going up to a mother of a newborn baby in a pram and saying she has an ugly baby that looks like a potato. It is easy with puppies and kittens, but you might need to be more creative with a toothless, drooling Yorkshire terrier covered in eczema. Watch and listen to your colleagues and shamelessly steal all their best lines.

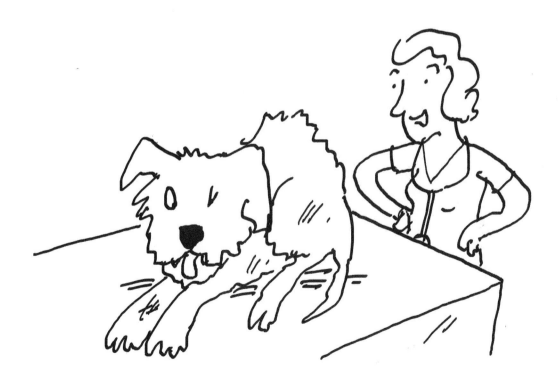

Dealing with dogs

In your enthusiasm, try to resist rushing in and starting to handle a dog straight away. They may need a moment or two to settle into their surroundings and calm down while you talk with the owner. Don't ignore them if they rush up to you, but just let them sniff or greet at their own pace; delay lifting them onto the consult table and do not stand looming over them as this can be challenging. If the dog is obviously friendly, then you can let them greet you and if they are over exuberant and jump up at you, then turn away and with luck the client will restrain them appropriately. If not, then you might have to help them and I am sure you know how to handle the average friendly dog by now. It is important to show the owner that while you appreciate their beautiful dog, you also show the dog that you are neither a threat nor a pushover. There are times when a dog remains very exuberant and the owner is struggling to listen to you, in which case the sooner the dog is on the table, the better, as they will usually feel less confident and will usually calm down.

With small dogs, ask the owner to lift them onto the table, but if it is a bigger dog then offer to help and confirm with the owner that they are happy to lift and handle their own dog. Watch out for asking pregnant women to lift up their dogs, although never assume a woman with a large stomach is pregnant!

Some owners have bad backs or other infirmities so you may have to ask a nurse to help you or, if appropriate, examine the patient on the floor. You need to look after the owner's welfare when they are in your consulting room, so if they are not able to lift or restrain their own animal then you have to find another way. Look after your own back too, as a substantial dog which shifts its weight about as you lift it can put quite a considerable strain on your back over the years. If you are examining a big dog on the floor, then be aware that your face might be quite close to the teeth and it can be harder to get out of the way. Many dogs do not like you bending over above them and prefer you to crouch down at their level.

Some practices use small, edible treats as a reward for the dog and to make them happier about coming to see the vet, but do always check with the owner before giving them any as a dog may have a food allergy or the owner may not appreciate your feeding them anything.

My own personal style is to chat to the patient with a sore paw or a cut ear and commiserate with them on their discomfort, and I also sympathise with the owner if they have had to clean up after a night of their dog's vomiting and diarrhoea. It just shows that you actually care and that you understand what it is like being a pet owner with a sick dog. I confirm that they have done the right thing by bringing their pet in to be examined, because some clients worry that they are overreacting or wasting your time. They transfer that reluctance to waste a doctor's time with wasting our time even though they are paying for the privilege of a consultation with us.

Talking to dogs

Personally, I am a great believer in talking to animals and over the years I have burbled and babbled away to many a dog or cat while I have been examining them. For one thing, chatting to them illustrates to the owner that you perceive them as an individual personality and not just another dog or cat. I find that the dog or cat will pick up on the comforting tone of your voice and often become more relaxed and compliant, making the experience of being examined so much more pleasant for everyone in the consulting room.

Companion animals are spoken to all the time in the homes of our clients and respond to human tone of voice, and soothing words are very effective with many patients. The byproduct of this is that the more relaxed your patient is, then the more relaxed the owner will be. You cannot announce to the client that you really like animals without sounding like some sort of a kitten-hugging loony, but you can demonstrate it in your manner and approach in interacting with the animal. After nearly 40 years as a vet, when I meet an old client it is rarely my surgical skills they mention, even if I saved their dog's life, but they will comment on how Dennis used to love me because I talked to him when he was scared.

I do not advocate going over the top and cooing like a soppy teenager over a puppy or a kitten, using nauseating baby talk, because you are there as a veterinary surgeon to perform a professional service and it is possible to go too far. There are some clients with whom you may need to maintain a much more reserved and scientific approach and who prefer a more formal consultation style; this is all part of the art of consulting and taking notice of your client and assessing their preferred approach to communication. My partner and colleague has a different approach and says he rarely talks to the animals but always keeps a physical reassuring contact with the dog or cat where reasonable to do so, and some of our clients preferred his style of consulting and some preferred mine. I seem to remember he used to get bitten every so often whereas I did not, but you must make up your own mind as you develop your own unique style.

The reluctant patient

Always look at the messages that your patient is giving you when you are examining them and if you feel uncertain of the way they are going to react, then do trust your instincts. The more time you spend around animals, the better you become at reading all the small signals of changes in body language and demeanour, and you develop a far better understanding of those signals than the owner of just one or two dogs or cats.

We put a great deal of trust in owners of animals to restrain them for us to examine and treat them without anyone getting hurt. The owner's knowledge of their animal's behaviour does not typically extend to how they will behave at the vets when being injected or examined. Do not feel you always have to believe an owner when they assure you that their pet will not bite. They may express amazement when he launches over the table to sink his teeth into you, but then the dog may never have had a thermometer inserted in his anus before so it can be surprises all round. Some owners can hold their dogs properly and some cannot and it is not always the strong man who you can trust to hang on to a difficult patient. Some clients at the first movement from their beloved pooch will just let go and allow them to bite you, and then probably blame you for hurting them to boot.

Controlling and handling dogs

There may be occasions when it is necessary to use a more direct tone to ensure compliance if a dog is resisting examination and squirming, but compliance should be rewarded by vocal praise. Most dogs know the instructions 'sit' and 'stay' and it is much easier to examine a dog who is cooperative. Ask the client to help you by holding the dog and reassuring him or her; this also makes the client involved and they feel useful. Some clients do not know what you want them to do and think that once they are in the consulting room, their role is redundant so you may need to give clear instructions.

For some bizarre reason, it is not unusual for some clients to take the lead off their dogs when they enter the consulting room as if to say, 'here you are, he's all yours', so if you see them about to do this then gently stop them before the dog is charging round your feet off the lead and jumping up at you. It will only take up valuable consulting time getting him back under control and back on the lead.

Ask the owner to get their dog to sit and hold them gently with their heads resting against their shoulder, reassuring them without restraining them too hard unless or until it is necessary. If they are held in a vice-like grip by a worried owner from the moment they are on the consulting room table, they will become tense and will resent the restraint and start to struggle before you have had a chance to examine them. Once on the table, I let the patient sniff me and I stroke their head or shoulders and touch them confidently, depending on their demeanour and the signals they are giving me. This is a skill that you will learn with time and experience and when you first qualify, do take care because in my experience you are more likely to be bitten in the first year or two of practice before you have acquired that second sense and honed your skill at interpreting the subtleties of animal behaviour. Remember that your face is close to their teeth when they are being examined, so try to keep a reasonable distance away so that you can take evasive action. No one wants their face washed by the tongue of a halitotic old spaniel or a French kiss from a vomiting Labrador.

The average dog:

- Usually behaves better when on the lead.
- Likes being spoken to and reassured.
- Usually knows the words 'no' and 'sit'.
- Does not like humans looming over them in a dominant way.
- May protect the owner and be more defensive if the owner is distressed.
- Is easier to examine on a consulting room table.
- Is sensitive about their eyes, ears, underbelly and orifices.

- Usually enjoys edible treats (depends on the breed and always ask owner's permission in case of food allergy).
- Will often look less ill when they get to the vet than they did at home. The journey there will have been stimulating and animals instinctively hide physical vulnerability, such as illness, in a stressful situation such as the vet's surgery.

There are still animals who give no apparent warning before launching an attack but these are few and far between, and you will develop an awareness of the signals given by the dog who bites because of fear.

> *I have had a German shepherd dog clear the consulting table in one bound and become airborne, heading straight for my face, and I managed to turn away just in time to avoid my face being bitten. He gave me a bruising bite on my shoulder but fortunately I had enough layers of clothing on to prevent the skin being punctured. Those were the days where we wore white coats when consulting and some intelligent dogs do remember a previous unpleasant experience from an individual in a white coat or someone who smells of surgical scrub and perceive you as a threat from the outset.*

Dogs can behave very unpredictably in the surgery and your safety and that of the owner are vital. If in any doubt at the start about the signals a dog is giving you, ask the owner how Fluffy usually behaves in the vet's, as in, 'is he happy being at the vets'?' and 'will he mind me examining him?' Over the years you will hear countless tales of vets who have been bitten by a dog and heard the client say afterwards, 'Oh, he hates the vet, he tried to bite the last one too.' Clients often think that we will know telepathically that their dog is likely to bite because we are meant to be pet whisperers and being bitten is 'part of the job'. Some obnoxious clients are almost proud of their dog exerting its authority over you, so do ask the question and look after your safety. If you are in any doubt about being bitten, then discuss other options with the owner, such as muzzles and sedation. With a really good owner it may be possible to practice examination from the blunt end if you are sure they are going to hang on, but a nasty bite can put you out of action for weeks, so never try to be a hero.

Muzzles

If you cannot examine or treat a dog safely, then do not just baldly announce that you are unilaterally making the decision to put a muzzle on. Discuss the situation with the client and explain that it is entirely understandable that Fang might want to defend himself, but that to examine him thoroughly you need to make sure that neither you nor the owner is going to get hurt, putting a muzzle on will then be perceived as a joint decision and necessary with Fang's best interests at heart. It may help if you point out that once a muzzle has been put on, many dogs accept that they are disarmed and become more submissive and cooperative and hence they are less stressed about the whole examination.

If you do not feel that you and the owner are safe, then do not proceed with the consultation. There will be a way to solve the situation without risking injury, so never feel you have to take the risk.

If a muzzle is not an option, you may need to organise sedation of the patient and it may be necessary to defer the examination and treatment. If you think you need to sedate and admit a case, then make that decision and do not be persuaded otherwise because this is your responsibility and the health and safety of everyone involved is at stake.

Clients are often unhappy with this decision at the time because it makes their lives more difficult. They may have to come back at another time and it will probably involve more expense for them. This is a clinical judgement that has to be made in each individual case, depending on the individual and the urgency of the case, but asking them to take their dog home and come back again may be a much better option. It may be preferable to let the dog calm down rather than struggling to inject an agitated patient and reinforcing their fear of vets so causing even more problems down the line.

Cats

Cat baskets and carriers and cages come in numerous designs and fastenings and the beginning of a cat consult usually follows the same course. The vet asks the client to place the basket on the table and get the patient out. The client will open the door of the carrier expecting the cat to walk out and will start patting the table in front of the opening saying, 'come on, Tiddles' for what seems like eternity. The cat has probably been fighting to get out of the carrier all the way in the car and was a hissing, scratching ball of fury when getting it in in the first place, so the client expects it to come out voluntarily. Some do choose to stroll out, but many decide that now they are at the vets they much prefer the safety of the cat basket and there is no way they are going to come out. Top-opening cat baskets are very easy, but with a front-opening basket I ask the client to place the basket on the table at the

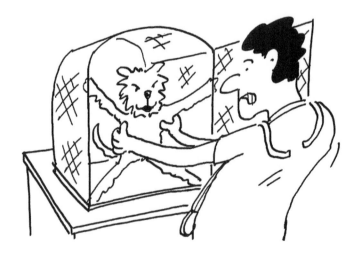

start of the consultation and leave the door open while we chat about the reason they are attending. Sometimes the cat will become bored or curious and venture out after a moment or two, but if the cat is still in the basket then I gently but firmly help them out myself.

Clients usually have no experience of extracting cats from baskets and will try to pull them out by their front legs, whereupon the cat braces its back legs against the inside of the aperture and hangs on with great tenacity. The most effective way to avoid an uncomfortable tug of war for the cat that is not aggressive but simply resisting, is to put a hand under the chest or gently grasp the scruff if necessary, place a hand round the rear end and help them out. You may need to grasp both front paws in one hand to prevent them clinging to the bedding with their claws and a hand under the sternum with the other. Gentle restraint of the odd stroppy cat by grasping the scruff does mimic the way kittens are carried by their mothers and they will instinctively cooperate for a time and you are in control of the teeth.

Restrain the cat on the table while you examine it by holding them facing away from you and towards the owner, with one hand under the sternum. They will try to move forward but they cannot go anywhere and you can tickle them under the ears or under the chin in a conciliatory manner while talking to the owner.

This sounds fine with a cooperative cat, but there are times when a cat violently objects to a hand coming into the basket and will attack, so then it may be necessary to tip the box up allowing gravity to assist. Feral and wild cats are a completely different matter of course, and should not be allowed out of the basket or handled without appropriate restraint such as gauntlets, sedation in crush cages and suitable assistance. Every vet has experienced releasing the cat from hell in the consulting room and watching it traverse the walls eight feet up for several circuits without touching the floor. Vet nurses are usually brilliant at handling cats and new graduates can learn a great deal about animal handling from experienced nursing staff, so watch and learn from the experts.

Cat scratches can be really painful and potentially dangerous, so always follow BVA or VDS guidelines if either you or an owner gets bitten or scratched. These may be more comprehensive than the advice given by doctors, so consider taking a copy with you to the surgery if you do get bitten and need medical attention.

Other animals such as rabbits, small furries and birds

Beware the client who opens a container and releases a bird into the consulting room before you can stop them, especially if there is any means of escape through a partially open aperture. You may note that extractor fans have a cover over them to avoid unfortunate accidents with free-flying budgies . . .

Clients seem to think you have mystical powers to control flying creatures or escaped small furries such as chipmunks, and it can take a long time and a bitten finger to recapture the patient in this instance. Children coming into the room in charge of the pet carrier should set off alarm bells and their parents may not predict the imminent release of the door catch by their little darling before the patient is ricocheting round the room.

Look for online resources about the recommended techniques in the manual handling of small furry animals and exotics and refresh your memory before you examine a rabbit or gerbil. It is a terrible experience for all concerned if an animal is injured while being examined by the vet, so make sure you know what you are doing. If in any doubt with an unusual animal, then try to avoid holding it on your own while you are examining it but ask the owner to hold it if appropriate, or ask a nurse for assistance.

There will be occasions when you are bitten by a small rodent. Do not instinctively flick the offender off your finger and across the consulting room risking death or a broken leg. This has happened to vets in the past and will no doubt happen again, and I know from experience that a hamster or a squirrel bite is extremely painful and your instinct is to immediately remove the source of the pain.

There is no owner, however understanding, who will think your instinctive reaction in hurling their pet across the room is reasonable. Grit your teeth, keep your hand still and extricate yourself, preferably without swearing profusely. Easier said than done, I know!

Beware of picking up hamsters by the scruff of the neck too, as they can still have enough loose skin to turn round and bite you, but beware that if you take up too much scruff, their eyes can be in danger of prolapsing from the sockets. Find out how much the hamster is usually handled at home and assess the best approach, but in my experience the fat, golden Syrian hamsters are more cooperative and less ferocious than the grey Russian variety. Good luck!

I saw a squirrel who had been brought in unconscious but who miraculously came to life in my hands just as I tenderly lifted it out of a cardboard box and it immediately sank its teeth into my index finger. I had to grit my teeth, control my language and transfer it hanging off my finger into a cat basket while stifling any four-letter words I desperately wished to utter. It was really painful for days.

Rabbits are prey animals and are notorious for sitting very quietly and apparently calmly and then making a massive leap for freedom. This may be from the consulting table or the owner's arms or even worse, while the vet is holding them or transferring them to their carrier. Most practices will have experience of a rabbit damaging its spine by diving off the table or out of someone's grasp, so always keep it in mind and never let them sit on the table without someone holding them.

Parrots and other exotic birds can inflict a very painful bite, and even a budgie bite can hurt so much that it tests your self-control and temptation to use foul language and flip the offender across the room. Take care with budgies not to hold them too tightly, as they are very talented in keeling over in your hand and expiring.

There are far too many practical considerations with all the different species of animal you may meet to cover them comprehensively here, but usually the less common they are, then the more likely it is that the owner will know how to handle their iguana or pygmy hedgehog. Use every opportunity that arises to learn about them if the practice has a client who keeps more unusual pets such as a ferret lover or a rat fan.

Taking a history

Always read the clinical records in advance and try to have a brief scan through them before you call the patient in. You may be in a tearing hurry but blundering into a consultation without reading the history is the quickest way to lose the confidence of a client. You need to know if they are in the middle of a course of treatment or were in last week. Addressing a female patient as 'he' instead of 'she' and discussing a possible pyometra in a neutered bitch, or not being aware of a drug intolerance or an existing condition such as epilepsy, can make you look careless, ignorant and incompetent.

The first question you ask should be on the lines of, 'How can we help Gnasher today?' If you ask the client, 'What is wrong with Gnasher today?' they will invariably say, 'You tell me, you're the vet!', which they think is an original and witty remark but gets remarkably tedious over the years.

Listen carefully while the client tells you why they have decided to come for a consultation and let them talk without interrupting for a minute or more so that they have the chance to tell you everything that they are concerned about. They will have prepared for this prior to coming into the room and will feel better if they have been given the opportunity to say everything that is in the front of their mind. Try to ascertain if they have given you the full picture as clients have a habit of introducing new symptoms or problems halfway into the consultation or even as they are just about to leave the consulting room. You do not want to produce a differential diagnosis or a treatment plan only to be told at the last minute that the patient might be pregnant or has had a nasty discharge from some orifice or other.

You might want to take down a few notes but give the client as much eye contact as possible and do avoid standing at the computer screen with your back to the client as you take the history. If you think you won't be able to remember details, then make some notes on paper. Clarify the history you have been given and repeat a summary back to them of what you have understood and this will help ensure that you have all the relevant history.

You will have had training and experience in taking histories as part of your vet school education but in practice you will usually have much less time at your disposal and some clients can find communicating a history accurately and concisely to a professional quite challenging. If you have ever been to the doctor, you may have experienced this yourself and found yourself babbling trivia and forgetting something important. You know what it is you wanted to say before you went into the consulting room but you may not be able to relate it succinctly without rambling and missing things out.

Putting your client at ease and giving them your undivided attention will give them the confidence to compose and relate their thoughts, helping you to take an accurate history. Do not let your mind wander to what might be happening in the waiting room or what you are going to prescribe, even if they seem to be rambling on telling you inconsequential rubbish, as you might miss a vital piece of information. Your client may be nervous and distracted by their pet's behaviour or worried about what dreadful disease you might diagnose and the potential cost of tests, treatment and operations.

If you have two or more owners in a consultation you may receive a different history from each one and they will sometimes even start bickering about it. You need to bring them back to the question in hand, ask them to clarify their answers and use your own judgement as to who is giving you the correct information. This is especially true when you ask about the animal's diet where treats and titbits are conveniently forgotten by one owner, who is embarrassed about being the soft touch who always gives in to the pleading puppy eyes. Rather than come clean and face the wrath of their partner, they neglect to tell you about the sausages they gave to their dachshund with the pancreatitis. One of the skills you need to acquire is fostering trust between you and the client so that they feel that they can be completely honest with you even if they have done something stupid, and not be judged, and that your interest is wholly in the well-being of their pet.

It is always a good idea to make sure that you gauge the level of knowledge that a client possesses early in the consultation as you do not want to be talking about 'upset tummies' to a gastroenterologist. On the other hand, if you talk about defaecation to some clients, they will not know what you mean, so assess your client's understanding and also their sensibilities. Some clients will happily use the word faeces in a consultation, while others speak of number twos and doing a pooh. If you say the word 'shit' to some clients, they will be appalled so you do have to use clear terminology that is also acceptable from a professional, but which the listening client can understand.

There is great opportunity for confusion, incomprehension and hilarious occasions of malapropism when consulting.

Some clients have a stab at saying the correct anatomical word but get it just slightly wrong, so that when they want a female cat spayed they ask for it to be sprayed, splayed, spaded or neutralised. They will ask for their dog to have a vasectomy when they mean castration and if you are really very unlucky, will describe their own vasectomy operation in graphic detail. They will say they have used Doc Martens flea products and tell you that they have had their animals microwaved instead of microchipped.

Some clients will say anything to avoid the words penis or vulva. They talk about 'front bottoms', 'down below', 'frou-frous', 'fanny', his 'old man', 'dipstick'. One elderly client with apparent nautical experience referred to the vulva of his bitch in season as her 'rubber dinghy' which was a very descriptive use of language I thought, but took some working out.

You may have to temper your use of medical terminology in order to maximise understanding and with some clients, use layman's terms such as runny eyes instead of ocular discharge. It may be pointless asking about borborygmi or flatulence when passing wind, or even farting, will be better understood.

You can go too far, however, with the earthy language and in my first job a client complained to my employer because I had used the term 'snotty nose' to his wife instead of nasal discharge, even though she had looked completely blankly at me when I initially used the medical term.

A client once came to see me in the evening surgery having seen a different vet in the morning, and when I asked why he had come back again with his lame dog he said the other vet had used such big medical words that he didn't understand what he was being told. He did not want to offend the other vet or look a fool so came back to see me in the evening. As he explained:

'Ee were a nice bloke and I didn't want to offend him but he din't speak Yorkshire. He told me my dog had a Slim Panetella in its knee!'

I had to explain that his dog had a slipping kneecap, as I deduced that calling it a luxating patella was definitely not going to cross the language divide.

It is startling just how little some people understand the workings of the body and that includes their own bodies and not just that of an animal. Nothing should be taken for granted when it comes to knowledge of basic biology and physiology.

I told a client that their dog had a liver problem and she informed me that I must be right because the dog had been 'bringing up bits of his liver onto the bedroom carpet all night'. She clearly thought that the abdomen was like a large cauldron in which the organs and food churned round and it was possible to vomit up the internal organs when things went wrong.

Clients who are well educated in other subjects may well not be aware of the different breeding cycles of animals and not know that cats ovulate when they are mated, or that bitches come into season every six months, even though they have a female dog.

They may not realise that neutered male dogs have no testicles and therefore cannot and do not desire to mate a bitch, even if they are exhibiting mounting behaviour.

They may imagine the effects of castration to be the same as that of a vasectomy and be outraged that their dog has no testicles when they come home after the operation.

They will ring you up at three in the morning because their young female cat is crying out in pain and rolling round on the floor in agony, not realising that they have come into heat and are calling for the tomcat.

They may think that a male and female litter mate will not mate because they are brother and sister and that their well-behaved and discerning pedigree bitch will not mate with that rough-looking crossbred dog from down the road because they are not the same breed. Assume nothing at the onset of a discussion and ascertain tactfully just how much they know.

One of our clients assured my colleague that her dogs who were siblings would not mate with each other because she always left the light on at night!

Smart Alec

There will always be clients who give you the impression that they are questioning and disbelieving everything you say, and those who have already made a diagnosis and come up with a treatment plan all on their own before they arrived. They are very keen to impress you with their knowledge and may require tactful handling as they tell you their diagnosis and demand that you prescribe their choice of treatment. Be careful to listen to them in the first instance, because there are occasions when they actually do know as much or more than you. Tempting though it may be to stifle their enthusiasm with a knee-jerk denial, you may later find that they actually know what they are talking about.

With chronic illnesses, a client will often become extremely knowledgeable about that particular condition and you should appreciate and acknowledge that. As an example, when a pet becomes diabetic then an intelligent owner may well have amassed a great deal of information about the disease and will certainly know what is normal for their individual animal.

Some breeders are knowledgeable about the idiosyncrasies of their breed though many just believe that they are, when in fact they have accumulated a great deal of false information from various sources. For some reason, clients have a habit of contacting their breeder when a puppy they have bought becomes ill and, even more irritatingly, they will often prefer the breeder's opinion to the one they are asking you to give.

Clients may come in armed with a sheaf of notes, having spent the previous evening on the Internet googling all the symptoms that their pet is presenting and printing out the most lurid and bizarre information they can find. A small proportion of clients have potentially dangerous views sometimes based on ludicrous information and they can be quite forceful in trying to coerce you into providing treatment that you do not agree with. They need gentle reminding that they have attended for your opinion and that you are willing to listen to them but you will not be dictated to when it comes to doing your job, as the responsibility rests with you when it comes to prescribing medicines and performing procedures.

It is a fact that almost every longstanding owner is an expert in one thing and that is the normal appearance and behaviour of their own pet. If they say their animal is doing something weird and out of character, then do not dismiss it out of hand but listen, record it and think about what it might mean.

Clients can find it difficult to describe a petit mal or differentiate between a faint and a fit or an episode of collapse and can send you up the wrong diagnostic alley. They may not know the difference and you may need to ascertain if the animal was actually unconscious or if its jaw was chattering. It can be very helpful if they can show you a video on a mobile phone, so it is worth asking them to do so next time it occurs.

You need to get a client to be specific and if they say a cat has been 'vomiting all day', do they mean 3 times, 10 times or 20?

'It has been like that for ages' can mean two days or three weeks to different clients.

Beware asking a leading question such as 'is he drinking a lot?' because some clients love to tell you what they think you want to hear. Ask roughly how much and how often their pet drinks and make sure they include the water their dog may be drinking when out on a walk or in the garden, as they sometimes seem to think this doesn't count!

Find out how long the owner thinks a normal dog walk is, as one person will think it is ten minutes round the block but another may be expecting an elderly, arthritic dog to still walk ten miles a day because they themselves are keen hikers.

The patient may have been brought to the vet by someone other than the owner who does not live with the animal or who is out all day at work, and this can make it very difficult to obtain an accurate history.

When consulting, you do want the client to have had the opportunity to express everything that they are worried about, but you also need to stay in control of the consultation. With a voluble client in full voice you will run out of time while you are listening to them reminiscing about the dog they owned before this one or their latest cycling holiday in France. I find that saying 'that is very interesting, but I think I'm going to have to stop you there to get back to Hagar's problem' works well without causing offence.

These are situations which make consulting very frustrating, but usually the majority of clients really are lovely and a pleasure to meet and you need to remember the nice ones outnumber the not so nice.

Examination

You have been trained in examination of the different species of animal and the importance of a full and thorough physical examination of a patient should not be underestimated despite all the advances in investigative technology, such as imaging and laboratory testing.

Palpation is still a really useful and cheap diagnostic tool and the more you practise it the better you get at it. It is possible to feel a foreign body in a small intestine and even identify what the object is on occasion. It is possible to positively diagnose pregnancy in a bitch if you palpate between 21 and 28 days with the optimum time being 24 days, that is, three weeks and three days. If you palpate every normal abdomen, then when you do palpate one with an enlarged spleen or kidney it will jump out at you and you might save the life of an old dog who has just come in for a booster injection and has a huge splenic mass just waiting to rupture.

If you always perform a full examination, it is surprising how often you will pick something up that is entirely unconnected to the reason for which the animal was presented. If you miss a lump when examining a dog for diarrhoea, it will be considered your oversight by the owner if they find that lump a week later. If you can be confident that you perform a full exam every time you will reassure yourself that you have not missed anything and will avoid any surprises later. For every problem you miss diagnosing because you do not possess the knowledge, there will be ten things that you miss simply because you do not fully examine and look properly.

Puppies and kittens should always have a full examination before vaccination, not just of their hearts but also of their mouths to check for a cleft palate or abnormal dentition and of their ears, eyes, limbs and abdomens.

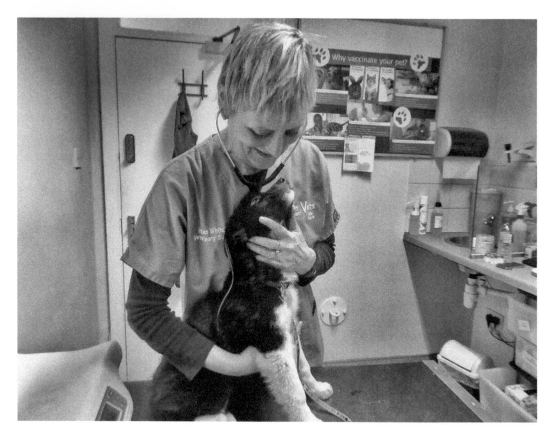

The first puppy or kitten consultation is a most important occasion for a client and the vet and one I never tired of in all my time as a clinician. Always give these consultations your full attention and never rush them or curtail the time because 'it is just a follow-up vaccination'. This is a golden opportunity to educate the client and also to make it a pleasurable experience for them and their pet. It is also a really happy occasion and a reaffirmation of what a great job we have being in the company of young, healthy animals as part of our working lives.

I always check male puppies and kittens for the presence of two testicles and if I cannot feel them on the first examination, I make a note to remind me to check the next time I see them.

The same is true of preoperative checks for routine procedures such as neutering, when it is not unheard of to find something of significance.

As you proceed with the examination, I find it helps to explain exactly what you are doing step by step as you work so that clients are aware that you are performing a full clinical examination. I use phrases such as, 'OK, let's listen to your heart' and 'let's look at your teeth' and I tell them when I am about to give an injection too so that the client is aware of what I am doing. Talking aloud while you work through the body systems in a regular sequence can also help you remember significant findings and inform the owner when findings are normal. It can prevent the client from distracting you with conversation while you are concentrating and thinking; I sometimes put the stethoscope on the chest and ask a talkative client for silence if I need valuable thinking time.

Thinking time can be quite limited in a consultation, especially if the patient and the owner require a lot of your attention and are demanding. When you have examined the patient, try to make a note on the screen of the key findings such as temperature, heart rate, and so on, and also significant abnormalities, before you forget. You may wish to add to the clinical notes later when the client has gone but it is all too easy to forget what the patient's temperature was, which leg it was lame on, or to notice an abnormality and fail to add it later. Write up each case as you go along and never at the end of a three-hour consulting session, even if you are running a bit late, as you may forget to record a vital piece of information.

Making a diagnosis (or maybe not)

Once you have thoroughly examined your patient you may be able to come to a diagnosis and be able to tell the client what conclusion you have reached, but in many cases you will not be able to reach a definitive diagnosis. You will have a list of differential diagnoses of varying likelihood and this is true for all vets, however experienced they are, who will always see cases where a diagnosis cannot be made, especially on first presentation.

This does not mean you are not a good vet and it is much better not to pronounce a firm diagnosis which might later be proven wrong, but to say it could be one of a number of conditions. It is acceptable to treat a baffling case that is not in a critical condition symptomatically and it is often the case on the follow-up examination a day or two later that it becomes clear what is actually going on.

If you are unsure, then do not feel pressurised into making a pronouncement but use phrases such as 'it appears to be' or 'the current symptoms suggest' because the progression of a case can change within a relatively short space of time. Clients will always remember if they heard you say, 'it isn't broken' or 'it's just gastritis', when a case later proves to have a fracture or a foreign body.

Do not try to do too much within one consultation session because you will be more likely to do something hurriedly and badly or miss something important, just increasing your stress levels. Focus on the main presenting problem and do not get sidetracked by other possibly unrelated symptoms or history which may be significant but may be clearly not. If a dog has come in for vomiting and diarrhoea, do not be distracted by the owner telling you it coughed once three weeks ago or that it had been limping six months before. You may need to address these problems at a later date so perhaps make a note of them on the clinical records, but there is only so much that you can do in one consultation and it is the current problem that should be focused on rather than problems which have resolved. Schedule a follow-up appointment and concentrate on the urgent problem first.

You may have seen other vets take blood samples and change dressings on the spot during a consultation, but it takes time, confidence and experience to be able to do that and as a new or recent graduate you may be asking too much of yourself. It is entirely reasonable to ask a client with a non-urgent case to come back in the morning for a blood sample or to organise for a case requiring a bandage changed to be admitted. Trying to perform complex dressing changes or fine needle aspirates in the middle of a busy surgery will cause your surgery to run late and you will potentially rush things for the rest of the session. It may be that you just need to ask a client to leave their pet with you for an hour or two so that you can make sure you have ample time and also a nurse to help you.

The client may well seem disappointed at the prospect of having to come back, but they usually agree readily when you explain that this is the best option for their pet. If you need to ask a client to come back for a consultation that is likely to be longer than the allocated time, then inform the receptionist and ask them to schedule a double appointment; if it is justified then charge for that double appointment too. Redresses often take longer than you think and it is always better to take time to do a good job than do a rushed job.

In many practices, the nursing staff do the dressing changes but it is a good idea to become proficient in bandaging for the occasions when you have to do it yourself.

There will be cases when you are faced with a really sick animal and you really cannot work out what could be causing the symptoms presented. You may have collected a full history and examined the case thoroughly, but do not understand what is going on and you are faced with a client who wants answers. Admitting a case for observation is the best action to take when you need time to collect your thoughts and perhaps ask another vet in the practice for their advice or opinion. Clients will usually be happy with this and observation is a phrase which they are likely to be familiar with. It reinforces the fact that you care about their pet and it is a far better option than appearing indecisive or sending a sick animal away without the correct treatment plan. It actually becomes much easier to say, 'I don't know' as the clients get to know you and as you grow in confidence and there will continue to be cases like this all your days in practice. It is far better to say, 'I do not know but I will take the necessary steps to find out' than to risk the animal's health for the sake of your ego, and rush into a wrong diagnosis.

Treatment plans

When proposing a treatment plan, it is important that you have the support of the client because treatment costs money and it is important for the sake of your patient that they agree to comply with the treatment or investigation you are suggesting. I make sure that the client has understood my explanation of my findings and proposals and I prioritise the pet's comfort and well-being in my explanation.

Laboratory tests, scans and X-rays should be used to confirm a diagnosis and not as a costly screening process to make sure you have not missed anything. A client can lose faith in veterinary practice if their trust is abused by untargeted, fruitless, blanket investigations that accumulate an enormous bill and nothing for the benefit of their pet and they may not readily agree to a subsequent essential work-up.

I make sure they know why I want to give them the treatment and I emphasise the importance of pain relief for arthritis for example, and clearly explain just how agonising a sore, infected ear can be. I ask clients with a pet with a skin disease to imagine how uncomfortable or itchy they themselves would be with similar lesions or how sore an arthritic joint can be. Some clients think that because their old dog or cat does not cry out aloud, then they are not feeling pain and it makes you wince to see the animal struggling to its feet. You may need to explain how animals in pain may present and that they may still ask to go for a walk but may be accepting their discomfort and suffering in silence.

I do warn them when conditions are likely to need more than one follow-up visit so that they are prepared from the outset and I emphasise that the reason I want to see them again is to make sure that they are responding well and so that I can change the treatment if necessary. As an example, I might say, 'This ear is so sore that I am not going to dispense ear drops today, but am going to take a swab and put some ear drops in for him now and give him pain relief by injection and ask you to bring him again in 24 hours so that he is more comfortable with me examining the ear canal. Is that all right with you?'

In cases of chronic skin disease, warn them that some skin conditions can require long-term management and they will probably need to come several times before the condition is controlled, and that there is a likelihood of recurrence.

When I give a client my opinion on the treatment their pet actually requires, I tell them with authority that we *need* to give a certain course of treatment. I do not say hesitantly, 'Well, we could always . . .' or 'I suppose we could take an X-ray.' If the patient needs an X-ray, then the client should be in no doubt that this is the course of action which they should take. If you sound uncertain, then the client will be uncertain too and wonder if her dog does really need that scan or blood test. Give your opinion and advice confidently because this is why the owner has consulted you. It is then the client's decision whether or not to take your advice and the responsibility for not taking that advice also rests with them.

When you discuss any suggested tests and investigations and develop a treatment plan, make sure you record this in the clinical notes. It is very important for any vet who sees the patient after you to know what has been discussed and planned for and it is also important to record what has been offered to the client but was refused or deferred, possibly on grounds of cost or for some other reason. Selective amnesia is very common in clients in my experience, and they can forget that you offered blood tests or X-rays earlier in the course of a disease and they refused!

Explaining costs of treatment

When you are proposing a treatment plan, try to make sure that as far as possible the client is aware of the likely costs. Veterinary surgeons are expected to offer the full range of treatments that are necessary and available and the client then decides what to opt for based on discussions with you. Do not quote for an initial treatment without mentioning the need for further treatment if it is obviously going to be needed. It is only fair to your clients to be open and up front about the likely costs for them to decide whether to proceed or not.

Many vets find discussing the cost of treatment really difficult and clients find it equally difficult making the decision to spend the money unless they are convinced the need is genuine. The media have not helped in this respect because they love to print articles about money-grabbing vets making outrageous profits from the pet-owning public. You cannot take on the moral responsibility for your client's financial position and you should not feel apologetic for a client incurring the expense of the necessary treatment of the animal they have chosen to own. You recommend the procedures and treatments that are essential and those which are advisable and the client makes their own decisions; they may decide they want optimum treatment and investigation or to treat the symptoms and wait and see.

I usually found it helpful for the client if I proposed three levels of plan: the treatment plan in a perfect world where cost was no object at all, the option which covered just the basics of what was necessary for the welfare of the patient and a middle path which would be what most reasonable people would opt for. Too many choices and the client may be overloaded with information and too many variables, but the three options can at least form a framework for discussion.

Some old dogs come in with multiple pathologies, such as osteoarthritis, lumps and bumps and bad teeth, and priorities and treatment plans need to be made clear for the owner. If budgets are tight, then different treatments may have different priorities and need to be discussed.

Do give a client time to think about the costs if the case is not urgent as they may need to consider their options for finance and their apparent unwillingness to agree immediately does not necessarily mean they disagree with your suggestions or are unwilling or unable to afford it. Veterinary fees are unforeseen costs which owners have rarely anticipated or budgeted for, and they may need to borrow from family or speak to a partner, so may not be able to give you an answer there and then.

Beware asking 'is he insured?' at the beginning of discussions of a treatment plan. Insurance cover or lack of it should have no bearing whatsoever on the treatment plan that you are proposing. The client has the right to spend money as he or she wishes and should be made aware of the treatment options irrespective of their insurance status. If you help-fully imply that insurance means that they do not have to worry about the cost, then the client may feel that you are looking on them as a cash cow and have less confidence that everything you are suggesting is in their pet's best interests.

You should explain and state the costs to an insured client just as fully and in the same detail as to an uninsured client, and insured pets should, of course, never have more investigation proposed purely because they are insured.

It is very easy to be tempted to keep costs down for the client by trying to avoid the need for a further consultation fee. If we see a case and then dispense a full, long course of treatment with the instruction to the client to come back if it is no better, then we are putting the onus on the client to assess responses to treatment and they are not trained to do so. The clients are rarely grateful for this approach as it leaves them without the reassurance of a professional telling them that there has been a good response to treatment, and often the cost of the full treatment plus a consultation fee for one visit is a relatively large sum which can actually deter them from returning if their animal is not improving. If they decide they definitely do not need to return, then they can make the decision and cancel the appointment.

Compliance

When you have decided on a course of treatment, do not assume that the client has the same level of knowledge and skill as you for the practicalities of administering it. Ask if they have ever put ear drops in a cat's ears or used a spot-on flea treatment before and if they have not, then be prepared to show them how to do it. Owner compliance has a major influence on treatment outcomes and we should take care to help the client actually get those ear drops down the ear canal or give the whole course of tablets to the cat. If not, then everyone loses out because the patient remains untreated, the client has spent money to no avail and the vet cannot understand why the patient is no better.

Clients can be very reluctant to admit to failure of compliance as it makes them feel incompetent and they are embarrassed. It is much easier to blame the treatment plan than admit to having plastered the ear drops everywhere but down the ear canal. Ask if they anticipate a problem with a treatment that you are suggesting, then consider alternatives if they are available, such as long-acting antibiotic injections instead of a course of tablets for an elderly lady with a grumpy cat. The optimum treatment does no good if it does not go down the patient but stays in the kitchen drawer.

One of my dogs was extremely good at avoiding tablets and I have had to devise all sorts of sneaky techniques with sausages, banana and bread and dripping to get a course of tablets down her. A discussion of ways to dose the patient with minimal resistance can make such a difference to a client and make much more of an impact on their opinion of you as a vet than your skill with an ophthalmoscope or an ultrasound scanner. This may seem unfair, but this is the reality and joy of the vet–client interface.

- Warn them that giving medication to a pet is usually a job for two people and it can be really difficult to do anything to an uncooperative patient on your own. Advise them that it may help if they lift the animal onto a surface such as a kitchen table, perhaps with a bath towel on it to stop them sliding around. This can bring the patient up to eye level, just as they would be on the consulting table at the vet's, in order to apply topical treatments.
- Flea preparations: show them how to part the hair to get to the skin so that it doesn't run off the hair and how to open the fiddly vial itself in the case of topical applicators.
- Creams and ointments: tell them how much to apply, for example a pea-size blob, or two massive squeezes and the tube will be finished in two days. Tell the owner to distract

the dog with a meal or a walk after application to allow some time for it to be absorbed rather than being immediately licked off.

- Ear drops: explain that the ear has a horizontal canal and a vertical canal and how to administer them to ensure that the drops hit the spot. Draw a quick diagram or show them a model so that they understand the anatomy of the ear, so that the ear drops do not end up in the hair around the ear flap rather than down the canal. If you instil the first dose, then the ear will hopefully be a bit less painful when an inexperienced owner repeats it at home. Tell them they need to get someone else to hold the dog so that they have a hand to hold the ear and a hand to squeeze the bottle. Cold ear drops are resented more than drops which have been brought up to room temperature beforehand.

- Tablets: just because you find it easy to give a tablet to a cat or a dog does not mean the owners will. Ask them how easy they find it and offer advice and a demonstration if they say they struggle. Smuggling medication in food is always easier if this is possible, because they do not experience a negative reaction from their pet when they approach with the tablet to administer it. It is all too easy for us vets to underestimate how tricky it can be to give a full course of treatment to an uncooperative patient. There must be many drawers in kitchens containing half a packet of the course of antibiotics we think has been completed when the client actually gave up after three days as the patient appeared to have recovered.

- Anti-lick collars and other protective measures: clients feel very sorry for their pets when they have to wear a lampshade and they often underestimate how quickly they can damage an area by licking or how speedily they can remove stitches or staples. Warn them that they should leave them on all the time and their pet will get used to it quickly, but never to leave them unattended even for ten minutes if they take them off.

- If you advise a client to purchase diet food for their animal, tell them exactly how much to feed per day, preferably with an easy measuring cup. If the cup holds more than the amount they are meant to feed, then they will sneak up the quantity, so advise a container such as a teacup or a mug which will hold the right amount and no more. If the practice offers a dietary advice service, then refer them to a veterinary nurse to help them be completely clear and label the food with the daily amount as you would with medication. Clients forget what has been said as soon as they leave, and the tendency is always to overindulge their beloved companion. Tell them clearly that the diet is not in addition to the ten treats the dog receives during the course of each day.

Wrapping up the consultation

This can be quite a challenge if you have a voluble client who enjoys your company. You have charmed her and her puppy and the relief that the clinical bit is over can result in a very happy, chatty client who wants to tell you all about her puppy and also about every dog she has owned in the past 40 years. Try to conclude the consultation a good couple of minutes early so that you can make sure the client has some time to confirm that they have told you everything they wanted to tell you and to say thank you and goodbye. It can be infuriating if they remember a wart on the dog's head just as you are saying farewell, but at least you have a spare minute left.

It can save time if you replace a cat into a cat basket yourself and fasten the door, checking thoroughly that it is indeed secure before they leave the room.

A helpful tip can be to stroll with the client towards the exit door and out into the waiting room chatting and usually they will follow you out. If they have a cat basket then pick it up and carry it out to the reception desk for them. Once you and the client have emerged into the waiting room you can hand over the client and the cat to the care of the receptionist, ask them to make the follow-up appointment and then nip back smartly into the consulting room. Performed efficiently, this can be more tactful than bluntly asking them to leave so that you can see the next client.

Sometimes, in the middle of a consultation, you may need thinking time with a complex case and especially one with a chatty owner who is preventing you from concentrating. You might need to check some facts online or in a book and rather than do so in front of the client, just say you want to check on something in the dispensary and this will give you a chance to review your findings and think calmly about a diagnosis and a treatment plan. You might also be able to check with another member of staff about an action you are planning to take that you are unsure about.

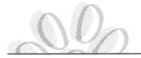

TOP TIPS

There are many sources of tips for new graduates, such as the handbook sold by the BVA for the Vetlife charity. Every vet you meet is a source of useful information, ideas and techniques they have found useful in practice. Watch and observe your more experienced colleagues and ask your recent graduate friends which tips they have received from another vet that they appreciate the most.

Miscellaneous advice from my colleagues

- Always start on time or early.
- Have a printed list of the appointments with times so that you know if you are running late.
- Cross off the list as clients arrive – it is motivating to see the list shorten.
- Write up cases as you go along wherever possible.
- Make notes and don't rely on your memory because there is too much going on to keep it all in your head.

- Pay attention to the time but without making it too obvious to the clients. Try to keep on time, otherwise your clients will be annoyed and may start to arrive later and later if you always run late.
- Don't rush the other clients when you are running late. It is not their fault and they should not be penalised. You might be able to catch up some time if it is a case of simply removing sutures, but do not make it obvious and cut people short.
- Always tell the client that if they are at all concerned about their pet they must feel free to contact the surgery and bring them in again, even if this is before the date of the scheduled appointment. This gives the client the confidence to make their own assessment and not to sit at home watching their animal's condition deteriorate, thinking everything must be OK because the vet didn't say to come back till Monday. A case can take an unexpected turn for the worse and you want to empower the client to use their own judgement.
- This applies to enquiries over the phone or out of hours. Always make them feel they can ring you back and that they own responsibility for a decision to present the case again. It prevents any accusation of 'I rang yesterday but the vet said it had to wait until morning'.
- Do not promise a particular brand of ear drop or cream because there will be the odd occasion when it is out of stock in the dispensary and you will have to convince the client of the benefits of an alternative, which they will think is not as good as your first choice.
- If you are giving an injection, warn the owner that it might sting a bit. If the animal yelps, the owner is prepared and if it doesn't, then they will think you are brilliant. (Some clients will still insist on telling you that their pet never cries for the other vet, Penelope Perfect. Smile sweetly even though it grates.)
- If you have offered the client several choices of treatment plan and they are dithering and unable to make a decision, then it is reasonable to tell them what you would do if the pet were your own.
- Be kind and non-judgemental. Help the client by being honest, but do not imply that you disapprove and think them unreasonable if they decide not to opt for the most expensive, top-of-the-range treatment. A vet is obliged to offer the range of treatments available but while protecting animal welfare as much as possible, we have to respect the choices and abilities of the clients to choose the treatment plan that fits in with their personal wishes and circumstances.
- Look in the mirror before you start the consulting session. Blood spatters on your face and a bloodstained, hairy top do not make for a good impression. Bring a spare top to work to change into in case you pick up a cat and it empties liquid faeces all down your front.
- Never forget that the client pays your salary. They are not the enemy, even if they sometimes behave outrageously.
- Laugh at adversity and remember you are part of a team and can lift the morale of

the rest of the team by the way you respond when things are hard going on a difficult day. A sense of humour and a generosity of spirit makes everyone feel we are all in this together. This sometimes includes the clients who will often be on your side when a client gives you a hard time or is rude.

🐾 Never criticise one client to another as they will wonder if you would discuss them behind their back too.

🐾 At the end of the day, try not to focus on the one case which you could not diagnose or the grumpy client who was having a bad day and complained, but remember all the small triumphs and the things which went well. Think about the happy and appreciative clients and the cat spay which went well, and not the one negative in a sea of positives.

Children in the consulting room

You will have learned all about techniques of animal handling during your training and may have owned your own dog or cat as a child, but the chances are you do not have one of the most challenging small animals of your own, the small human being!

I have written further of the delights of children in the veterinary practice in Chapter 9, 'Clients: the good, the bad and the ugly', and to be honest, they could feature in every one of those categories. Actors used to say never work with children or animals for a very good reason. They do unexpected things and they can make it a lot harder for you to maintain a cool, calm and professional demeanour.

When children are in your consulting room, you have a responsibility to keep them safe. This might seem unfair, but you really cannot always rely on their parent or carer to anticipate them picking up a syringe which you have left on the side or going into the bin for a bloodstained piece of cotton wool. Most parents will look after their own children, but they may be distracted by their animal during the consultation and some children are simply raised free-range and are completely out of control, especially in a new and exciting place. If something unfortunate happens to them, you will get the blame from the parents, so have a quick scan round your consulting room for any potential hazards and make sure they are not near the biting end when you inject their slavering, nervous Rottweiler.

Enjoy the experience

When you tenderly pick up a cat and it empties the contents of its diarrhoea-filled rectum over your shoes, then the only thing that you can do is laugh and metaphorically take it on the chin. There will be occasions when you are sprayed with bodily fluids and a golden rule is to keep your mouth closed when expressing an abscess or an anal sac. You will be anointed with unpleasant, smelly fluids and your friends and family will recoil from you when you come home until you have changed and had a shower.

Do not let all this detract from the enjoyment of consulting, because if you like animals and people it can be a pleasure to do a good consulting session. There are difficult experiences and very sad consultations where bad news has to be given or an animal has to be put to sleep, but you will also have the chance to meet some interesting and appreciative people and their animals in all shapes and sizes. It is a unique opportunity to use so many different skills and to improve the lives of animals, so can be extremely rewarding in a way in which someone who is not a vet themselves cannot truly appreciate.

You will do many consultations which are similar and talk about fleas and vaccinations time after time, but each consultation is also different and novel and if approached with enthusiasm and an enquiring mind you will enjoy it all the more.

CHAPTER 7

How to be a good vet in the back

Different vets gravitate towards and enjoy different aspects of general practice with some preferring to be in the operating theatre while others enjoy consulting. There are vets who complain all the time about having to see those pesky human beings when they would rather be operating and some who avoid operating and have to be encouraged to pick up a scalpel.

Working in the operating theatre and with inpatients can be very enjoyable because you are working within a team which is sociable, whereas when you are consulting you are on your own with the client. I believe that it is often a lack of confidence which can make a new graduate hang back and not volunteer to operate, and there are all too many keen surgeons who will be more than happy to hog all the operating and leave the new graduate to do all the consulting. If operating was always performed by the most experienced veterinary surgeons, then young vets would never become proficient, so a good practice should make sure you have the opportunity to gain experience and confidence in the theatre.

When you first join a practice as a new graduate, it is highly likely that you will be doing quite a lot of consulting as you get used to working in practice and finding your feet, but after a short time a good practice will look out for suitable, simple surgical cases for you to start with. They will understandably be more willing to supervise you in your first surgical procedures on a quiet day rather than in the middle of a busy day with a hectic operating list. Meanwhile, expressing an interest in scrubbing in to assist with operations or being willing to hold an animal while another vet is performing an ultrasound scan can be really helpful and you will learn a great deal. Be patient but be visible and even if you are nervous, do not skulk out of the way and become easily overlooked, but seize every opportunity to ask if you can help with an op or do some cat neutering or a stitch up where appropriate.

You have been given the latest surgical training while at vet school, so the following advice is simply my own personal and practical advice from over 30 years in general practice. Some of it will appear blindingly obvious but each piece of advice is here because over the years I have seen many a vet make a rudimentary mistake over what should be a routine procedure. Some examples come from my own personal bloopers and some from mistakes I have observed other vets make.

I would very much like to help you avoid making some of them yourself and the most likely time for something to go wrong is when you first start work. Everyone makes mistakes, no matter what they say, and this adds to your stress levels, so the following tips and hints may just help you on your way.

Cat spays and castrates

The chances are that, as a recent graduate, you will be doing a large number of cat spays and dog and cat castrates; this is why I have focused on them here. The more you do, the easier you will find them, and you will also find it easier to progress to other more complicated surgery. You might already have been performing plenty of neutering already, in which case you can skim over this.

Tips and tricks for neutering cats

Attempting to perform a cat spay on a male cat should simply never happen and it is your responsibility as the surgeon to make sure of the sex of the patient before it undergoes surgery. Many a Susie has come in for spaying and has turned out to be a Norman and you cannot always trust the owner to know. A neutered tom cat will not have testicles but is not a female, so look at the genitalia and do not just feel for some testes. Some clients will be very understanding as they may feel they should have known themselves, but the mistake is yours. Do not blame the nurse, as apportioning blame after the event helps no one, and although protocols should be in place, you should double check. Always examine and ensure that not one but two testicles are present, as you will find the odd cryptorchid individual presented and you will need to discuss this with the owner before the tomcat is anaesthetised.

The correct site of the incision makes all the difference to how easy performing a cat spay can be, so make sure of your landmarks before you make an incision. I incised approximately one centimetre anterior and ventral to the anterior of the wing of the ilium and I used the centre of the hinge of the artery forceps as a reference point, but this obviously depends on the size of instruments you are using. Ask other vets how they locate the right site and choose the rule of thumb that works best for you.

In a flank cat spay, an experienced nurse will most likely have shaved the correct area, but if you are working with a less experienced nurse this may not be the case and if the cat is under the drapes you can find yourself significantly off course if you incise in the middle of the shaved area. Check before the cat is under the drape and double check the landmarks of the pelvis before you start, because it is much more difficult to spay a cat when the incision is in the wrong place. I preferred the hind legs to be in extension and tied back so that the thigh muscle is out of the way and the flank extended.

When you first spay a cat, your incision will inevitably be bigger than many other more experienced vets' incisions. A relatively larger, clean cut with minimal blunt trauma which helps you perform the procedure quickly and cleanly results in less bruising and discomfort for the cat and a shorter duration of anaesthetic. Bigger can indeed be better for the patient when you are inexperienced rather than fiddling around through a tiny hole, bruising everything and prolonging the procedure. Your wounds will soon become smaller as you perfect your technique, but it can be less traumatic for the patient to make a decent-sized incision rather than making a small one when you first start.

This also applies to bitch spays and in gaining exposure for performing other surgical procedures where you need to have all the advantages of being able to see what you are doing.

Once you have opened into the abdominal cavity in a cat spay, there is usually a pad of sub lumbar fat at the dorsal aspect of the incision under which the uterus will be lying. If you locate this fat and locate the uterine horn underneath, it is much easier than repeatedly delving into the abdomen picking up random pieces of intestine and bruising everything until you get lucky.

Most cats do have two uterine horns so be very, very sure before you pronounce a cat to be abnormal and close up, diagnosing it as only having one uterine horn. Strangely, they often seem to grow another horn full of kittens later that year.

Cats in whose abdomen you do not find a uterus and who you decide have already been spayed also have a nasty habit of producing a litter of kittens six months later. Take a great deal of care when you discharge the apparently pre-neutered cat to make sure you stress to the owner that it is very difficult to be 100 percent certain that something is not there. You can say that you have explored it surgically very thoroughly, and have been unable to identify a uterus.

A lady once came in to the surgery saying that I had not spayed her cat and that six months after the operation her cat had had kittens. I explained to her that there was no way that I would say that I had performed a spay and closed up, leaving any ovary or uterus still present, without telling her. It then transpired that her cat had gone missing but she had gone to the RSPCA and there it was! She had recognised it because of its 'unique colour' which was so unusual. I had quite a job convincing her that tortoiseshell cats were not as rare as she thought they were and asked her if she had a photo of her cat before it was lost. Sure enough, the difference in markings proved that the cat in front of us was not her cat but an unconvincing doppelgänger.

When you ligate the ovarian ligament and the uterus, make sure that you have enough tissue on the distal side of the ligature to stop it slipping off. Try not to ligate where the tissue is too flattened by the forceps, because you will be ligating flattened tissue rather than spherical tissue and it does change shape. Once the forceps are removed, the ligature is more likely to slip off as the tissue returns to the unflattened state.

Do not let go of a ligated stump and allow it to go twanging back into the abdomen just hoping for the best, but instead hold on to it and be certain it is secure. Be sure in your own mind that you have ligated it securely and, if in doubt, put another ligature on but don't go mad and put seven on as this will just make things too friable and even more likely to slip off. Let it retract gently into the abdomen using the artery forceps to gently hold the stump and don't let it retract in like a piece of overstretched knicker elastic as this is the most likely time for a fragment of tissue to snag onto the ligature and pull the ligature off.

Never ignore blood that is steadily welling up from the depths of the abdomen after you have let the stumps go. There is a difference between seepage of a very small amount of blood, which is completely normal, and haemorrhage, and if one small dab of a swab does not easily staunch the blood then you may have a bleeding blood vessel; if so, you need to find it and ligate it. Some vets maintain that even if the ligatures have come off it is very unusual or even impossible for a cat to bleed to death, but I do not share their confidence.

Do not make your skin sutures too tight. They are not there to prevent bleeding but to appose the tissue to enable healing. Stitches that are too tight are uncomfortable for the cat and there is usually postoperative swelling which then makes them even tighter. Cats tend to leave a wound alone if it is comfortable but if there is a lot of bruising or excessively tight sutures, then they will lick excessively and are more likely to remove the sutures.

As time goes by, your surgery will be neater and your incisions smaller, and you will be able to complete the procedure much more quickly.

Bitch spays

This is rarely an easy operation to perform but with practice it becomes easier and so should not be disproportionately feared. It might be quite a while before you get to do one on your own – do not let the thought of them become a source of stress but concentrate on improving your general surgical technique.

Ligatures that are placed correctly using good ligating techniques are highly unlikely to come off and cause postoperative haemorrhage, but the blood supply to the ovary and uterine body in a bitch can be considerable. Some bitch spays are easier than others, but in a deep-chested, overweight bitch this can be a challenging procedure however long you have been in practice. Do not be concerned about needing help and support and always ask if you need that help because the patient is the priority and the potential risk is relatively high. Even if you do complete several uneventfully on your own, it is very helpful at first to have a more experienced colleague on the premises to help you if you run into difficulties.

There are many different techniques advocated by vets for bitch spays, but my opinion is that you should ensure you have adequate exposure to be able to see what you are doing and that tearing (not cutting) the ovarian ligament enables secure placement of the ligatures on the ovarian stump. It can actually be easier to operate on a pyometra than perform a spay on a young, healthy bitch because the incision is larger, exposure is greater and the broad ligaments are already stretched, aiding ligation.

Ensure that pain is effectively controlled in the postoperative period as there can be significant discomfort, especially if you are not experienced and have taken a long time and handled the tissues a lot so pain scoring is advisable. It is never acceptable to leave an animal in pain and this is not the fault of the inexperienced surgeon because we all have to learn, but it can be addressed with adequate analgesia. An animal in pain should not be discharged to the owner's care, so if in doubt and if it is possible, then keep the patient in. The observation of a bitch spay in the 24 hours after surgery is an interesting and revealing experience and one which I advise you to actively seek, as it will give you an understanding of what an owner has to deal with.

The death of a bitch spay during or after surgery is harrowing and one that I sincerely hope you never get to experience. It is an elective procedure on a healthy dog and is inevitably a young dog who is the pride and joy of the owner, who has bonded with her over the puppy months and who will be understandably devastated. Complications do arise from time to time which can include postoperative haemorrhage and anaesthetic death and, very occasionally and horrifically, the dehiscence of the wound which in the worst cases can mean the patient eating their own intestines. I am not including this here to scare you, but to ensure that you always take this major surgery very seriously, even though it is a relatively common procedure in practice. As the owner of a relatively large practice, I have seen the aftermath of things going wrong with bitch spays over the years and it is one of the most painful incidents to deal with.

Always ask for help if you need it, never close up hoping for the best when you know in your heart that you have not done a good job, and insist that someone comes and helps you if you need it. In very rare cases, I have heard of a vet leave the surgery with the bitch still open on the operating table because they have panicked and been unable to face the consequences, which is completely unacceptable. Take a few deep breaths, do not panic, ask for help, stay calm, stop the bleeding and remember that nothing else matters at that moment because you may be the only person on site who can save that life and you do have the training to do so.

Dog castrates

Always check that there are two testicles in the scrotum before you start.

Make sure that you clip or shave the area very gently. Clipper rash and harsh treatment of the scrotum causes postoperative discomfort, causing dogs to lick excessively; some vets leave the scrotum completely unshaved.

Some practices always give an anti-lick collar postoperatively, some use local as pain relief. Find out what your practice protocols are concerning postoperative analgesia. Protocols vary from practice to practice so discuss it with your colleagues.

If you feel your patient needs additional pain relief after a routine castration that you have performed, then make a clinical decision to give some because you may have caused slightly more trauma than usual through no fault of your own but simply inexperience. Pain relief can prevent self-trauma leading to complications, which are much more difficult to sort out after the event than it is to prevent them in the first place.

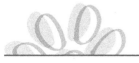

TOP TIPS FOR SOFT TISSUE SURGERY

- It is a false economy to staple a wound without an anaesthetic and without proper cleaning if it is contaminated, and there is a strong possibility that the wound will break down and need stitching again with all the possible complications. Cutting corners may save time and money but can cost more in the long run to both your patient in terms of pain and discomfort, and their owner in terms of money for further treatment.

- Take care when shaving an area prior to surgery; if you catch the skin in blunt clippers this can cause great irritation and inflammation postoperatively and the patient will lick the incision excessively. Blunt clippers can do a lot of damage to the skin if wielded carelessly, especially in rabbits or when shaving cats with matted fur when large skin wounds can be inflicted unintentionally.

- Tissue which is next to a traumatic wound may not be as healthy as it appears to be, so do not commence the bite of the suture too close to the edge of the wound as it may pull through.

- Take pride in your work and suture carefully but remember you are not performing fine needlework for decorative and aesthetic purposes, but putting tissues in a reasonable situation where they will heal. If it takes you three times as long fiddling about to make a wound look immaculate and perfect then you have probably done your patient a disservice by extending the time anaesthetised and will also have increased the likelihood of infection. As my old boss used to say, get in, do it and get out without messing around doing fancy needlework.

- Do trim the ends of the sutures to the same length and try to make the space between sutures the same, because it looks neater. If the ends are too long then it is easier for the teeth of the patient to get hold of them, but if they are too short then they are more likely to come undone.

- It may seem unfair, but clients can only judge the standard of your surgical prowess by the size and neatness of a suture line. You may have performed the most intricate and mind-blowingly difficult surgery inside the abdomen, but they cannot see it and will comment on the incision. They will not necessarily be impressed by a tiny wound with three sutures when you have spent ages searching for a retained testicle, but actually prefer to boast to their friends that Fang had to have 20 stitches and even assume the more stitches they had, the better value for money they have received. Owners judge you using different criteria than another vet would use.

- Cut pads heal much better if you take a deep bite of the pad tissue either side of the wound and appose the edges, but not too tightly. If there is too much strain on the suture then it will tear through or cut off the blood supply, preventing healing. I have often found that staples are too superficial and do not hold the deeper tissues of the pad together creating dead space which fills with fluid and often leads to wound breakdown and failure to heal.

* I prefer suture material to staples where a wound is mobile and under tension or swollen and bruised, as it is more pliable to movement and swelling.

Bandaging

You may have been given good training in bandaging different areas of the body at vet school, but this might have been minimal and theoretical – you may have only bandaged a real animal a few times. It is increasingly common in vet schools to train using models rather than live animals and this is understandably less stressful for the animals. It is, however, very different banadaging a model to bandaging a live patient, which is a skill you will need to perfect. In many practices, the nurses are responsible for this task and not the vets, but there will still be times when you need to apply a bandage effectively so make sure you know what the different dressings are used for and where the bandages are stored before you have a haemorrhaging dog to deal with or even a haemorrhaging human.

Good bandaging techniques take practice to perfect and poorly applied bandages can cause real problems in practice, with the most common error with the worst repercussions being a bandage on a limb which is applied too tightly. Elastic bandages should not be applied under tension for longer than is necessary to stop bleeding, as this creates continuous pressure and compromises blood supply. Tension should not be used as a means of keeping the bandage on at the expense of the circulation and adhesive bandage should not be applied directly to the skin as this causes great irritation for the animal who will chew at it, remove it and possibly inflict self-trauma.

Bandages applied to a limb which is bent at the joints tends to stay on much better than on a straight leg, so bandage above the elbow on a front leg or over the knee or hock on a back leg, depending on where the wound is.

Always tell the client to come back to the surgery even if it is before the arranged date of the appointment if the patient seems unhappy with a bandage. If an animal starts chewing or stops bearing weight on a bandaged leg, this can be a sign that the wound is infected or the bandage is too tight.

An animal with a bandage which is too tight will initially chew at it and be very uncomfortable and distressed, but it may then become pain-free as the blood and nerve supply is cut off and the animal may just become unwilling to bear weight. The observant owner might report a bad smell coming from the bandage, but it may be too late by that stage. It is a sad but true fact that bandages have been removed from animals containing the necrotic limb still in the bandage. Do not let this happen to you.

More helpful tips for general anaesthesia and surgery

There is a big difference between

a) flying by the seat of your pants and recklessly performing surgery which you have never done before and are not competent to do, and

b) finally flying solo and performing surgery for the first time having had the appropriate training and general experience.

I have no intention of duplicating all the training in surgical techniques which you have received at vet school, but there are certain simple guidelines which you should follow as an inexperienced surgeon and which you may find useful.

- Prepare well and make sure you have everything you are likely to need ready and sterile before you start.
- Weigh animals to ensure accurate doses for premeds and induction agents – never 'guesstimate' the weight.
- Old and sick animals may need less than the calculated dose of anaesthetic drugs so use your clinical judgement and continually assess their response to the initial dose.
- Do not cut anything unless you are absolutely sure of what it is.
- Do not remove anything if you are not sure you have correctly identified it. (More than one vet has removed a prostate gland mistaking it for a retained testicle.)
- Do not faff about when making an incision. Incisions heal across, not lengthways, so make a big enough incision when you first start, and with time you will be able to make them smaller as you become more proficient.
- If a piece of suture material touches a non-sterile surface it is still unsterile even if no one else saw it touch the table!
- If something starts to bleed, stay calm, apply pressure, think about what to do and do not panic.
- If something is bleeding deep down in an abdomen, then do what you have to do to locate it. This may include making a larger incision and getting everything in there out of the body cavity so that you can see exactly where the bleeding is coming from.
- If you perform a caesarian, always check the pelvis for a sneaky little puppy or kitten lurking in the body of the uterus.
- If you decide to operate on a cryptorchid dog, palpate the inguinal canal for the errant testicle before surgery and definitely before opening the abdomen and playing hunt the ball.
- Be organised with your surgical instruments and put them back on the instrument tray methodically and not balanced on the drapes as they will slide off and drop on the floor when you move something.
- Double check before you leave the abdomen and suture the abdominal wall that everything in the abdominal cavity is part of the animal and not a pair of forceps or a swab.

The abdomen becomes like the Tardis in Doctor Who and can conceal items in the hidden depths even in a relatively small patient. The nurses should count the forceps but you should also take care. Believe me, that is an X-ray you do not want to see!

> *I have closed an abdomen of a Labrador after a splenectomy and as I moved the dog, I felt a pair of artery forceps through the abdominal wall; I had to quickly resume anaesthesia and go in and open up again to retrieve them. Thank goodness that for some reason I ballotted the abdomen; I have no idea why I did but at least he did not go home with them still inside. Perhaps you are thinking that this would never happen to you but over 30 years, the opportunities for making mistakes are numerous so learn from mine here in black and white to help you.*

❧ Be aware of the breathing of your patient and the level of anaesthesia, because unless another veterinary surgeon is administering the anaesthetic then currently the responsibility is yours and not the nurse's. If you think an animal has stopped breathing, then speak up straight away and raise the alarm and do not keep quiet until it is too late, assuming that the nurse or anyone else is monitoring the breathing.

❧ Animals recovering from anaesthesia or sedated are unpredictable. They can lie motionless and apparently still unconscious and then come round quickly and lurch off the table.

> *My partner was just checking the tension in the jaw of a Rottweiler who was apparently unconscious when the dog clamped his incisors down on his fingertip, trapping it very painfully between his jaws. The treatment of his bitten finger demonstrated another salutary lesson in radiography of always taking two planes when X-raying; the first X-ray of his finger showed no fracture but the second set repeated several days later revealed that he had in fact got a chip fracture on the dorsal aspect where Nero had trapped it.*

❧ Never leave an animal unattended in the recovery phase until you are sure they are swallowing and have the endotracheal tube removed. Dogs have swallowed parts of tracheal tube before now when they have been left unobserved in a kennel.

❧ Be gentle with postural changes such as putting an animal which has been on its back suddenly onto its sternum.

Admitting animals for surgery or hospitalisation

I have owned dogs and cats all my adult life and as a small animal vet I have often operated on my own pets. There have been occasions when I have asked others more qualified than myself to attend to them but I always knew the vets and nurses looking after my animals personally and I knew they would do their best.

> *It was only when I took my young son into hospital for an anaesthetic and had to hand him over in the preparation room to a complete stranger who I did not know, that I really understood what it was like to entrust someone you really love into the hands of an unfamiliar medical professional. What an eye opener that was! It was not that I doubted their competence but the raw emotion that I felt seeing him go under the anaesthetic and having to leave him as he went into the theatre took my breath away. I look back at the times when I was working in practice on a busy day and admitting cases and I think I could have been a lot more sympathetic in the way I admitted a pet for a procedure under anaesthetic.*

How many times have I said to a client, 'oh, we'll just give him an anaesthetic and do x or y', and then blithely taken the pet away to perform an X-ray or dental without realising the emotions that client may have been experiencing? We are concentrating on our job and it is a procedure we do every day, but it is certainly not an everyday occurrence for that owner.

In addition to being calm and professional and explaining exactly what we are going to do and why, we should always remain sensitive to the feelings of a client and not be impatient with their need for reassurance or for that extra ten seconds to fuss Fluffy before we take him down the corridor to the kennel. They are probably a long way out of their comfort zone and possibly feeling guilty because they haven't come to the vet sooner, or because they are opting for elective surgery on a healthy animal for their own reasons, such as with neutering.

They may be thinking of the very worst-case scenario of anaesthetic death because we have quite rightly mentioned possible complications when they signed the consent form. People in this situation who are worried will often behave slightly erratically and dither, or appear not to be listening, or repeat themselves looking for reassurance as they ask the same questions that you have already answered.

In trying to reassure a worried owner, it is very tempting to say that there is nothing to worry about at all and that everything is going to be fine, despite having just explained that every general anaesthetic bears a risk. Choose your words carefully and express sympathy for the way the owner is feeling; acknowledge their concern but try not to promise them a positive outcome just to make them feel better.

The client often has no concept of where their pet is actually kept when they are admitted, and if we take the time to tell them that we are going to make Gnasher comfortable in a kennel with a comfy bed and look after him while he is in our care, this can go a long way to reassure.

As you admit a dog, the last thing the owner wants to see is their beloved pet putting the brakes on as they are dragged down the corridor and away from them. It is often more helpful to ask the client to leave the consulting room while you remain with the dog and you can gently close the door behind them. The patient will now most likely be happy to accompany you to the kennels rather than your trying to take them from their owner and have them struggling to get back to them as if they are fighting for their lives.

If they are coming in for more than one day and will need feeding, then make sure you ask simple questions such as what type of food they usually have, because a change in diet is best avoided. Sick animals may need tempting to eat and if they have a particular love of tuna or chicken then it is helpful to know this and have it in the records. Record any food intolerances, because even if you do not think them genuine the owner will latch on to a report of the feeding of a food that they consider their animal is intolerant to and blame the food rather than the medical condition for their pet's deterioration. It also makes the client feel that you care about their pet's happiness and well-being and reassures them that you will be treating their pet as an individual.

Always label dog leads, collars and cat baskets so that they can be returned to the correct owner when they go home. Avoid leaving dog leads hanging on cages to be chewed by the bored inhabitant of the cage. The nursing staff will be looking out for this, but it helps if you are vigilant too.

A colleague of mine told me their nurse once appeared ashen-faced with a chewed dog lead with no metal catch that had been found in the cage of a Labrador who had come in for elbow and hip scoring. Abdominal X-rays revealed the metal catch to be in the dog's stomach and, although the owner was very understanding and eventually nature took its course with the dog duly depositing it in a large pile of faeces, the protocol at the surgery was changed to prevent it ever happening again.

Looking after inpatients

As a veterinary surgeon you will have had training in animal handling and during hospital rotations and EMS you will have had to care for animals when they have been hospitalised.

I believe that one of the most important skills of the veterinary team is in the way we look after the animals our clients have entrusted to us. I frequently use the term 'entrusted to our care' because it encapsulates how our clients feel when they leave their pets with us to look after. They trust us to actually care for and about their animal, not just focusing on the clinical problems that their pets face, but also looking after their general well-being which encompasses their physical comfort and their freedom from distress.

We are so privileged in being allowed by virtue of our qualifications to be recognised as having the right to treat animals and I have been very lucky in working with so many nurses and vets who make such a difference to animal welfare every day of their working

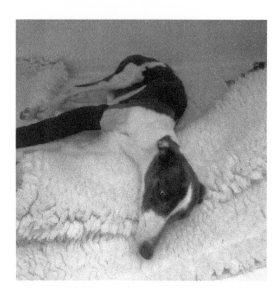
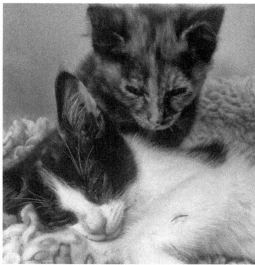

When you walk past a kennel with a dog or a cat, always make a point of observing the condition of the animal and the surroundings. The nursing staff may be responsible for their care but that does not mean that you should not be aware of the collective responsibility towards animals entrusted to our care. We should do our best to minimise fear and discomfort where we can, so never walk past a dog lying in a soiled kennel or with an empty water bowl without considering if you might need to do something to help.

lives. I believe the role and responsibility of attending to the nursing of sick animals should be shared by all members of the veterinary team and not confined to the veterinary nursing and support staff. If any vet sees a frightened dog or an animal lying in a soiled kennel, then they should not just walk by and assume that it is not their problem. They should make sure that they find an appropriate member of staff to attend to it or deal with it themselves and ignoring it should not be an option, however busy you are.

Companion animals who are sick or injured respond to stimulation, attention and human company and good nursing. Our pets do not usually live outside in a kennel as they used to do but are used to living closely with humans and being in the middle of the family, sitting with them while their family eat their meals and watch television. When they are in the surgery recovering from illness or injury, they are often left alone in a kennel surrounded by other animals and scents unfamiliar to them, scared and probably lonely and missing the human contact and reassurance that they are used to.

The skill of nursing and emotional support for injured animals is sometimes undervalued and overlooked in veterinary practices because the working day is so busy and these skills are not considered as being as important as those required in putting in an intravenous line or monitoring blood gas levels. I believe this is wrong both in the human medical and care fields and in veterinary practice.

Old cats with poor appetites will often eat if someone is willing to sit quietly with them, stroke them and hand feed them with tasty food. Warming the food can help and I always appreciated the really good veterinary nurses who would go out of their way to spend time with an inpatient, encouraging them to eat. Even though we had several expensive convalescent diets available on the shelves, there is still the odd patient who likes a bit of cheddar or a prawn, especially if offered by a kind and friendly individual who sees them as a patient rather than 'the renal failure cat' or 'the pelvic fracture'. There is more to the healing process than medicine and surgery and it is not just the nurses who can offer that care but the whole of the veterinary team as they go about their work.

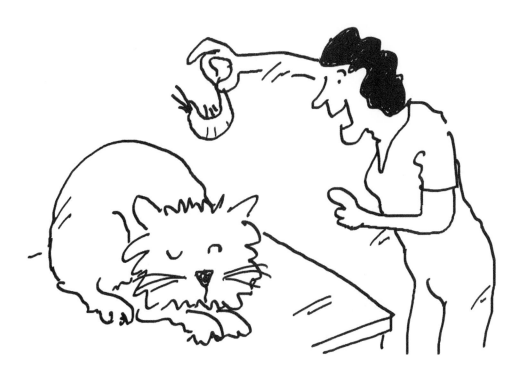

Forming a close bond with a recovering patient can be very rewarding and is one of the things which I believe makes the job worthwhile and gives our work meaning. Some may say that they always need to be detached and dispassionate about the cases they are treating and I am not recommending becoming over-sentimental or emotionally involved with all our patients, but I do think you have to be prepared to give a little of yourself. We have to be able to maintain a degree of perspective because some cases do not end well, and we have to protect ourselves from emotional damage and compassion overload, but being able to make a difference to the experience of an animal in our care and feel compassion is very special. When a client sees their pet being made a fuss of by the vet, and being really pleased to see the nurse who looked after them as an inpatient, it gives the client confidence in the practice and makes the experience much better for the animals, their owners and the veterinary team.

I will always remember a number of my patients, the ones that 'got to me' and who had that certain something that got under my guard. It is not possible to feel and grieve for all our patients as if they were our own but there will always be special memories of some of them, whether because of their personality or their acceptance of my administrations, however uncomfortable, without retaliation.

I remember Polly Collie, who was a great dog who chased aeroplanes when they flew over the garden and Siouxsie, a wonderful Siamese cat who used to walk across the car park to the surgery from her Bentley following her owner to attend her appointment. I have cried when a patient who has been for repeated chemotherapy treatments has finally succumbed and I think this is just a part of being a vet. You cannot let them all get to you, but you ought to care and we would not be human if we did not grieve for a patient once in a while.

CHAPTER 8

Working out of hours

Until relatively recently, most vets in practice worked nights and weekends and every practice provided its own emergency service that the clients could call upon when the surgery was closed. There were no dedicated emergency service providers and no referral practices other than the five university vet schools to whom you could refer very complex cases during term time only. Vets in first opinion practice had to deal with everything that was presented to them and the number of vets in the practice dictated how frequently each of them was on call overnight and at the weekends. This is still the case in many practices, particularly those mixed practices which provide farm animal and equine services, but also in some small animal practices.

An increasing number of small animal practices now refer a client who contacts them out of hours to a dedicated emergency centre and restrict their opening times to the daytime only, although the length of the working day varies from practice to practice. It is also increasingly common to refer a higher proportion of complex and challenging medical and surgical cases to specialist centres for treatment by a vet with greater experience and higher qualifications in a particular discipline, rather than attending to such cases in-house. There have been major advances in fields such as orthopaedics, cardiology and soft tissue surgery and there is no doubt that animals that would have died or been euthanised in the past have a much better chance of survival thanks to the advances in treatment available.

There are practices who choose to provide a complete service 24/7 for their clients because it suits their business plan and is perceived as a personal service and a positive in marketing the practice. Some practices have no choice, because their geographical location means that they cannot outsource their emergency work for logistical reasons, there being insufficient demand locally for an emergency centre. If you start work in a practice like this as a new graduate, you may be faced with some complex and challenging emergency cases where you are the best and only option available for that patient and in the majority of cases, you will be able to do a good job.

Large and mixed practices sometimes agree to share the burden of the out of hours rota with a neighbouring practice so that they can collectively reduce the number of nights and weekends that each individual vet is on call. This collaboration between practices necessitates excellent communication between neighbouring practices and great care is taken to ensure that all clients are looked after well and their routine custom is not subsequently appropriated by the practice dealing with an emergency call.

Outsourcing cases that occur out of hours has undoubtedly made a massive difference to the quality of life of a large number of vets who can now get an uninterrupted night's sleep, every single night. They usually have more time off than vets had previously and can enjoy more quality time with their friends and families at weekends. In the past, some vets would work incredibly long hours and their work became their life, often to the detriment of their family life, their relationships and their health.

Increasingly, the veterinary surgeons of today do not accept this way of life and working conditions for many vets in practice have markedly improved. Some vets today have never worked out of hours since the day they graduated and increasingly will not consider taking a job which includes an out of hours rota. I know that I may be looking back through rose-tinted spectacles, and it is a long time since I answered a call at three in the morning, but many of my most interesting and rewarding cases that happened years ago, but which I still remember vividly, occurred out of hours. I think working in the out of hours rota made me a better vet more quickly and increased my confidence and my job satisfaction.

Emergency medicine and surgery centres

Some vets thrive in well-equipped, dedicated emergency centres and relish the opportunity to deal with complex cases, and they may choose to make their career in emergency medicine and surgery. Some individuals adjust well to the working patterns of night and weekend shifts with all the pressures of changing sleep patterns, and tolerance of this varies between individuals. Many emergency service providers employ their vets on a pattern of a week of nights on duty followed by a week or two weeks off and the relative remuneration for working antisocial hours is usually significantly higher than in traditional daytime practice.

Vets studying for further qualifications such as certificates, or who have outside interests such as in competitive sport for which they wish to train and which may not fit with a traditional job, are also often drawn to this work as it frees up blocks of time while still enabling them to earn a decent income. It can also be very attractive for a vet with a young family when the cost of childcare and the demands of working full-time in a traditional practice are considered. Evening surgery times usually coincide with the busiest family time when children need collecting from school and with careful planning it can mean that a vet with a young family can participate in the usual activities such as collecting them from school and being there in the late afternoons and early evenings.

Several out of hours providers provide specific training in emergency work and this may offer the opportunity to become highly skilled in the treatment of a significant number of complex emergency cases which you might not have the chance to see in a smaller first opinion practice during daytime hours.

Having considered all these benefits and the potential opportunity of higher earnings you may be very interested in working for a dedicated emergency service provider, but I would strongly suggest that you initially gain some experience in a first opinion practice. There may be little or no support for you as a relatively new graduate in the middle of the night with a difficult case and your confidence could take a real battering, so make sure you are ready for it before embarking on this demanding but rewarding work.

At the time of writing, Vets Now does not employ newly qualified graduates straight from vet school but requires that recruits have done at least six months in first opinion practice, after which the company provides their own intensive training course in emergency medicine and surgery. The more experience you have of routine treatment in first opinion practice and basic surgery, the easier it will be to manage emergency cases and I would recommend that you get a good grounding of at least 18 months or more in first opinion practice before considering working in an emergency clinic.

Support when working out of hours

A good practice will initially offer considerable support and backup for you as a new graduate during the day, and also on the on call rota for a reasonable length of time while you gain experience and become proficient. This will vary from practice to practice and will also be dependent on how well a new graduate is performing. Some graduates need more practical support and continue to need it for a longer period than others and the time you take to become completely independent is not necessarily a predictor of how good a vet you will become. Experience gained before graduation varies a great deal between individuals and some graduates will have been neutering cats every day in their EMS practices while others have done very few. Some individuals may have more confidence than others from the outset and thrive under the pressure and excitement, while others take a bit longer to find their feet and will turn out to be just as good after being given enough time and support.

The BVA are currently very actively promoting mentoring of new graduates by their employers and recognise that employers need to be nudged, encouraged and supported to fulfil their obligations to their new graduate employees. There are still all too frequently horror stories of new graduates being insufficiently supported in their first months in practice and thrown in at the deep end to sink or swim. This is just simply not acceptable any more and a good employer will recognise this, giving you sufficient backup and providing you with a mentor.

The positives of working out of hours in general practice

Think twice before you say that you never want to work out of hours. Many new graduates express reluctance and sometimes fear about working out of hours but there are many positive aspects and advantages to gaining experience in this type of work, even if you decide at a later date that you do not want to continue in such a practice. If you do avoid it as a new graduate, then it can become a more frightening prospect as the years go by and a challenge that you may avoid for the rest of your working life as a vet, which could reduce your options to achieve your full potential in the future.

One of the advantages I appreciated when I was a young graduate was that, if an emergency came in such as a road accident or a caesarian on a Sunday evening, it was likely to be the only case at that particular time of day and so I could give it my full attention without any other distractions. I saw some really interesting and challenging cases and the management of them was completely down to me unless I felt that I really could not handle it on my own. Calling a colleague who was meant to be off-duty really was a last resort and our colleagues' time off was respected and protected unless absolutely unavoidable. This meant that I did perform caesarians and emergency soft tissue surgery such as splenectomies and GDVs relatively early in my career.

It was a steep learning curve but very interesting work and the more experienced I became, the more competent I was and the greater my belief in my own abilities. Each time I did a completely new procedure, my increasing confidence reduced the stress I experienced and on the next occasion when I would hear a client say on the phone, 'his belly is all swollen and he's trying to be sick but he can't', or I was faced with a collapsed dog, I felt more capable of dealing with the challenge.

Your first years in practice should be filled with firsts; the first caesarian, the first foreign body and enterotomy, the first tomcat with a blocked bladder and the first diaphragmatic hernia. Working out of hours means that these interesting cases are not whisked away from you for someone else to do and you will surprise yourself at how well you can perform when you put all your veterinary training into action; it can give you the opportunity to become more proficient relatively early in your career.

I have met some vets who have been qualified for over ten years and have still never done a GDV or a splenectomy because they have worked daytime hours only and there has always been a more experienced colleague available to perform the exciting surgery. This may be the direction in which some general practices are going, where everything other than a routine or minor procedure is referred for treatment to a dedicated referral centre, but there are still opportunities to work in traditional practice where you can gain experience and learn a great deal.

I would suggest that if you want to become proficient in dealing with complex medical and surgical cases then you need to be in a position in practice where those opportunities are going to arise or you could find yourself five years qualified and more without having gained these skills. If you feel you would be happier working without the challenge of performing emergency surgery, then that may be the choice that you make but, if it is just because of the circumstances in the practice you are in, then it could mean a restriction of the spectrum of your competencies which could last further on into your career. It might take you many years to achieve the same breadth of experience as a vet in another type of practice and is another reason to carefully consider your choice of the first job you take as a new graduate.

If you work daytime hours only, then you can be assured of a reasonable amount of sleep and for many vets who now no longer expect their work to rule their lives, the attractions of only working daytime shifts are obvious. It is argued that vets who are not tired from working during the night perform better and that tired vets make more mistakes, but I think this depends on many variables, such as the expected daytime workload. If I were to consult all day without a break, then I suspect I would be much more tired by the end of the day than I would be if I had attended a night call but worked less intensively during the day. There are many occasions throughout life when we are sleep-deprived for one reason or another, often self-inflicted due to social activities, and although sustained sleep deprivation is definitely not ideal, it is possible to function after a night on call and still do a good job. There needs to be a pragmatic approach to working in practice and if you personally feel that there is an occasion when you are not safe to work due to lack of sleep, then you should speak to your employer or supervisor.

I am certainly not underestimating how hard it is to work a full day followed by a night on call during which you had little sleep, and in every practice there will arrive the night from hell where the phone rings non-stop and you are up all night. The frequency of calls out of hours is partly a matter of chance, but also a numbers game, because in a practice where 15 vets are employed and there is a 1 in 15 rota, you are obviously responsible for the likely out of hours workload for 15 vets. In a rota covering so many vets' work, you are more likely to be called out in the night or at the weekend than if you work in a smaller practice where four vets work.

I lost many more hours of sleep with my children when they were small than I ever did by being on call. I am not saying that I always liked being on call, but I perfected the art of answering the phone, going out on a visit, coming home, getting back into bed and immediately falling back to sleep – a skill that has stood me in good stead over the years. Some individuals are not so lucky and struggle with broken sleep patterns and insomnia, so personal factors will have an influence on the working patterns you choose.

The one thing I am sure of is that it is much harder to start working in an out of hours rota if you have previously enjoyed every night and weekend off and I still appreciate that feeling when I wake up on a Saturday morning and don't have to go off to work.

One night when I had been out on call once and had left my clothes in a pile on the floor by the bed, I was called out again and as I hunted about could not find my knickers anywhere. I shrugged and put on another pair and drove to the surgery where I saw a very charming and rather good-looking police dog handler with his German shepherd. He heaved the dog onto the table and held it while I bandaged its cut foot and we chatted away about one thing and another. I thought he seemed to be finding something very amusing for one in the morning and it was only after he left that I realised that a pair of my knickers

*had been lying on the floor next to him on his side of the consulting room
table throughout the consultation. They had been lurking up my trouser leg
and worked their way out as I walked past him into the surgery and round to
the other side of the table. He was very tactful and when he came back to the
surgery two days later for the dog's leg to be redressed, nothing was said
by either of us, but I could never see his dog again without remembering the
embarrassing sight of those knickers lying on the surgery floor.*

Personal safety

If you have taken a job where you are working out of hours, then do keep your personal
safety in mind and follow the practice protocols which are there to keep risk to a minimum.
You may be working in a sleepy village where the risks are relatively low or in a difficult
inner-city area, and you need to be aware of the practice provisions such as alarms and
internal locking doors and use them. It is easy to become lax about security after weeks and
months when nothing happens and eventually you stop locking the internal doors or making sure someone knows where you are at night. Because we are working with the general
public from all walks of life, you will inevitably come across the criminal elements of society from time to time. We are working with drugs and it is common knowledge now that
vets have ketamine and other substances in the surgery, so we do need to be vigilant and
take care.

Your practice should have a protocol for lone working and for being in difficult situations
with a challenging client and it is very wise to find out about it before you need it. Some
practices never allow lone working at all, but this will depend on many variables such as
location and logistics and there may be times when it is inevitable that you will be working
on your own. It is worth finding out exactly what this entails and what security measures
such as panic alarms are in place. The advent of larger practices and of many practices having
a vet and a nurse working at night has reduced the number of times vets have had to work
alone, but there are still small practices, especially in rural areas, where you may be working
on your own and you need to be aware and look after yourself.

Many people assume that it is women who are especially vulnerable, but men can also
have bad experiences going into difficult situations on their own and the risk is not confined
to female vets. Male vets may, in fact, be more likely to be physically assaulted by an angry
client than a female vet.

You are categorically not obliged by the RCVS Code of Conduct to endanger yourself in
order to attend a sick or injured animal, so never put yourself into a dangerous situation
thinking that you had to for fear of being disciplined for failing to attend to an animal. Your
safety transcends all other considerations and is the main priority and if you genuinely feel
unsafe, then take yourself out of that situation. There may very rarely be situations where
you cannot help an animal because it is not safe for you to do so.

The Suzy Lamplugh Trust at www.suzylamplugh.org provides practical support and guidance about fear of crime and strategies and skills to help you keep safe.

General advice when working on call

One of the most helpful things you can do before you spend a night on call is to prepare yourself well so that you are ready for that emergency phone call.

If you are expected to respond to emergencies from your own home, then find out exactly what the procedure is for taking the calls and try to make sure someone knows that you are going to the surgery or out on a house call. It is important that someone knows where you are.

Make sure your phone is fully charged and that the settings are loud enough to wake you up from a deep sleep.

Many vets will have experienced answering the phone and then just closing their eyes for a few seconds only to fall back to sleep again, so I used to have my phone far enough from the bed that I had to sit up and move in order to answer it. This also means that your brain is in gear and you are not so sleep-befuddled that you cannot think straight.

Have a pen and paper next to the phone to note down salient points of the rather garbled history that the owner is likely to be giving to you. Some practices have an answering service to screen the calls before disturbing the vet, but it may be that you are speaking directly to a member of the public and it helps to be able to make a decision about what needs to be done having noted down all the important points.

Clients with an emergency in the middle of the night are often distressed and worried and you need to calm them down in order to obtain the information you need to help them. They expect you to leap into the car and charge to the rescue without further discussion and can appear irritated or even angry that you do not immediately come to their aid, but are talking about costs and asking for more details.

You will need to ascertain what the presenting signs are and any relevant history, and very importantly, who they are, where they are and their contact details including a phone number.

Some practices have an answering machine that informs a client of the costs of an emergency call-out but others do not, and the client needs to be informed how much it is going to cost them before you go out and that this will be for the initial treatment only. Some clients will exaggerate the severity of the symptoms because they want their pet seen, and some will think carefully about it once they realise that they are going to have to transport them to the surgery and also pay a substantial fee. Sometimes an enquiry and an initial request to be seen does not result in a call-out and, although the owners of genuine emergency cases will still need to be seen, the clients who want to bring a dog which has been limping for two days may decide that it is not an emergency after all and can wait until the morning.

It is always difficult discussing money in the case of an emergency and there is no easy way to do this without occasionally being accused of caring more about the money than the patient but it is important that you do. If you do not advise them of the fees then the client has not had the chance to make an informed decision and may subsequently refuse to pay because 'no one said how much it would cost'. This applies more commonly to companion animal emergency calls and rarely to farm call-outs where the farmer usually knows the fees incurred.

If an owner is uncertain whether to opt for a call-out or if you feel that the case does not sound urgent enough to need seeing out of hours, then I would advise you to always make sure that the owner is made aware that they can call back and ask to be seen if they think it is necessary. They are the ones sitting next to their animal and the decision as to whether or not they need to be seen should usually be theirs. Do not leave yourself vulnerable to receiving an accusation at a later date that 'the vet said it did not need seeing, and would not come out' but always leave the ball in their court with the chance to call back if they are not happy to wait until the morning. If you do decline to see them, make brief, contemporaneous notes about what has been said and transfer them to the client records in the morning.

In my experience, if a client is worried enough to call you out of hours and really wants you to see them and is willing to pay, then I would usually agree and go. It may be that the case could wait until the morning, but the distress of the owner needs to be taken into account too, and there must have been a reason for them to go to the effort of contacting the surgery. There is always the chance that if you refuse and the animal deteriorates, you will worry about it and later regret not attending. I also used to find it difficult to go back to sleep if a case sounded borderline in urgency and I preferred to go willingly rather than worry about it during the small hours, or have the client phone back for a call an hour later, having lost even more sleep.

A client's perception of the severity of the presenting signs of their animal can vary hugely. One person's description of 'blood gushing out of its paw' can be a tiny nick in the pad while another person's may be accurately describing the complete severing of all the flexor tendons and various blood vessels. Ask for specifics, such as whether it would soak a bath towel or just a flannel, and asking for a photo on a mobile phone can give you a more accurate assessment of the severity than a description. It can be helpful if the client videos an apparent fit while it is happening and can show you when they get to the surgery.

Clients often neglect to apply first-aid measures so advise them what to do before you see the patient. If a dog has a badly cut paw and you ask if they have put a bandage on, you will be surprised by how many will say no and are just watching the wound gushing blood.

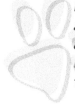

It can be quite surprising and worrying how little people know about basic first aid for themselves or their animals. I had one client put an Old English sheepdog with a badly cut leg into a bath of warm water 'because it was getting blood all over itself and the house'. It nearly bled out and the owners genuinely thought they were doing the sensible thing.

Some cat owners with an emergency may have no cat basket, so you may need to advise them on the best compromise to transport the patient in the middle of the night. A strong cardboard box with air holes punched in and strapped up with gaffer tape, a fishing basket or even a strong pillow case may be preferable to bringing them loose and completely free, bouncing about the car on the dual carriageway on the way to the surgery. Make sure they know they need to allow air for the cat to breathe and if possible, to bring someone else with them to attend to the patient while they are driving the car.

If an animal has swallowed any medication or a toxic substance, ask them to bring the bottle or container. The Veterinary Poisons Information Service is invaluable and your practice should have access to it, so make sure you have the contact details at hand.

It is a good idea to have pre-prepared directions to the surgery easily accessible if you need to give directions to clients. Have the postcode for the surgery to hand as clients may not be familiar with your location.

If an animal is on medication already, ask them to bring everything with them as you may not have easy access to medical records if they are registered with another practice or are on holiday.

When you are on call in both large and small animal practice, you will be asked to attend cases that should have been seen during the working day and which have been ignored or delayed for no apparent reason. Even though it is very annoying to be dragged out of bed after a long day at work, put a smile on your face and do not point this out to the owner. You are going to have to see it anyway, so smile and do not let the irritation fester because you will be the one who remains in a bad mood, so smile and be gracious.

You will also be woken up by clients who assume that you are sitting by the phone wide awake and that it is acceptable to call at 3 a.m. to make an appointment for the next day or for trivial advice that could have waited for the morning. As you try to go back to sleep, you will be thinking of all the brilliant one-liners you could have used to vent your irritation.

Illegal drugs

If a client has a dog that has eaten illegal drugs then they will probably be reticent about telling you the truth because they are worried that they will get into trouble and possibly face legal action, or just because you will think them careless. It is surprising how many dogs have 'eaten a plastic bag with some powder in it while out on a walk' or are presenting with symptoms which the owner cannot explain despite you having a strong suspicion of the dog being off its face on something and seeing pink elephants. Your patient is your priority, so you need to impress upon the client that you are not a police officer but need to know what the animal may have ingested in order to come to an accurate diagnosis and administer the correct treatment.

Naively, when I was first in practice an owner told me he was worried because his dog had eaten some grass. I blithely told him that dogs often ate grass when out on a walk and not to worry.

'Not grass, grass', he said.

'Yes, grass is fine for dogs to eat although they sometimes vomit it back', says I confidently.

'No love, I'm talking about grass, you know, weed. I'm not a bloody gardener.'

'Ah, I see', says I, as the light dawned.

Small animal house calls

Clients often expect us to go to their house to attend to an emergency with their animals out of hours and this rarely provides the optimum means of treatment for the patient but is very convenient for the owner who doesn't even have to get dressed. You know that you can treat them far more effectively at the surgery with everything you might need at hand and it is rarely satisfactory to try to deduce or guess what you might need and take it to the house of the client in the correct quantities.

Many clients will initially ask for a house call but can usually be convinced that a more practical, effective and economical option is to bring their pet to the surgery.

You may need to explain that you need access to the surgery facilities and it may be that you cannot leave a case you are currently treating. You may come up against considerable resistance from the client as we are very fortunate in this country to have the ambulance and paramedic services for humans and some clients expect the same level of service for their pets. You will need to stay sympathetic and polite and clearly explain why it is best for their pet to come to the practice. Repetition can help in the face of accusations of not being caring, so repeat that you can understand how worried they are, but that you will be able to help Fluffy much more quickly and effectively at the surgery.

It is not uncommon to be asked for house calls for all sorts of emergencies where it is clear that you cannot help at all by attending their home address. Clients will ask you to attend a road accident or a whelping bitch and you need to be able to quickly and succinctly explain why they need to come to you in order to save time and possibly the life of their pet.

Emergency euthanasia house calls

Requests for emergency euthanasia house calls happen quite frequently and it is worth discussing what to do in the event of this situation with your employer. They may have guidelines or protocols for this and you will need to take responsibility to do what you believe to be right for the relief of pain and suffering of the animal. I suggest you read the supporting guidance for the Code of Conduct for veterinary surgeons on the RCVS website. This is never an easy situation and each case will need to be assessed and decided on depending on the circumstances. It is still true that it is generally easier to perform euthanasia at the surgery where you have access to sedatives should they prove necessary. It is easier to arrange disposal of the body and this is a consideration for an owner with a very heavy dog. There is no onus on you to risk injury in carrying a heavy body to your car and though you may wish to help the client in what is obviously a very difficult time, your relief of the suffering of the animal is the pressing matter out of hours, not the disposal of the body.

Clients with no transport

Clients with an emergency and no transport can present a problem for vets on call because the client assumes that you will come out to their home, but many areas will have access to a local taxi or a pet taxi and it is always useful to have the number of such a service close to the phone when you are on call. If it isn't critically urgent then clients can organise transport themselves, but this can take longer than you think if they are asking a relative or a friend for a lift. Ask them to ring you back when they have made the arrangements so that you don't sit for an hour twiddling your thumbs in the surgery at three in the morning.

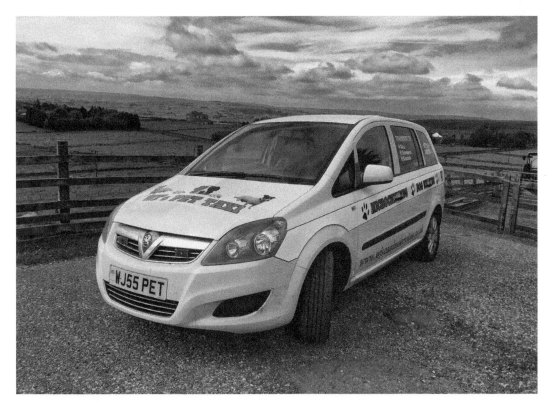

Pet taxis provide a great service not only because they can transport animals to and from the surgery, but also because they are usually run by people who know how to handle animals. Always keep the contact details of the local pet taxi easily accessible as this can help the animals owned by clients with no transport reach you promptly.

Seeing an emergency at the surgery

If you have an emergency coming down to the practice, you can spend the time waiting for them to arrive in preparing for what you might be likely to need. When you are on call you may need to lay your hands on a vital piece of equipment that you rarely use, so make sure you know where the stomach tubes are stored and how to access the controlled drugs. You might be lucky enough to have an experienced nurse on call with you, but because of shift patterns and staffing changes you cannot always rely on them knowing where everything is. If you know where important items are kept in advance, then it will help you to stay calm and focused rather than ransacking the surgery for the equipment while working out how to turn the burglar alarm off after the client has arrived. It is often not any lack of skill as a veterinary surgeon that can make you look incompetent, but the other, unforeseen eventualities such as not knowing in which cupboard the obstetric lubricant is stored, resulting in the frantic opening and closing of 20 cupboards searching for it.

Remember to get consent forms signed with the figures for the estimates filled in before embarking on a procedure and if a client is leaving an animal with you then ensure you have all the correct contact details. Let them know that there is no point in them phoning you in ten minutes' time because you will be too busy looking after their animal and that you will phone them as soon as you have some news. Follow up on your promise of phoning them back as it is a very worrying time for an owner and they need to be kept informed once the immediate pressing emergency is attended to.

You may have to convince the client to leave their animal with you and leave the room or even the premises because you need to be able to concentrate and you cannot attend to the patient and a frantic owner. Your support staff will probably attend to the clients but there may be occasions where you have to do it yourself.

In a large hospital practice with several members of staff on duty out of hours, all these considerations may be attended to without your involvement, but there are still practices where a nurse is not on call to help but who is only available when a surgical procedure such as a caesarian is performed and you might be seeing an elderly, collapsed dog on your own without anyone to help apart from the owner.

Prioritising

When you have an emergency before you, the main priority is to stabilise the patient and provide pain relief. If you feel you cannot perform a procedure then you may need to call a colleague for help; this is not an admission of weakness for a recent graduate but the right and sensible thing to do.

A good practice will provide support for a new graduate and will expect to help you with the more challenging cases, so ask for help when you need it. On the other hand, do not ask for help if you can reasonably deal with it yourself by using the skills you have acquired and your training. Stay calm, fully assess what needs to be done and make a decision as to whether it is within your capabilities.

Decision making is one of the hardest things to do when you are starting out as a vet and it is easy to think that there is one right decision and a host of wrong decisions which you might make. It is very easy to dither and not make a decision at all which helps no one, causing delays in treating the patient and leaving you still in the same situation.

Look at the evidence, make a plan of action and work through it systematically without panicking or rushing. It might be that you make a decision to do nothing and to observe the patient or perform further investigations and that may be the sensible thing to do. Do not rush into something without thinking and planning; working as a vet is all about making decisions and observing outcomes and changing course where warranted. Vets are continuously learning from their own and other vets' experiences with cases and there is not always a right way and a wrong way of doing things.

When you have worked on a case and perhaps operated on it, or admitted it, treated it and sent it home, then do write it up at the time even if it is three o'clock in the morning because otherwise you will forget something. By the following morning, you may well have forgotten what disposables you used or which leg it was that was bleeding and your recording will be more efficient if you do it at the time. It will not take that long and you will keep a far more accurate record and avoid subsequent errors on the clinical records.

If you see an emergency case out of hours and it is admitted for further investigation and treatment by another vet, then take the time to find out what happened and how it turned out. This is the way to learn from the experience and also will give you job satisfaction. Clients really appreciate you showing an interest in their pet and calling an owner to find out how the patient is progressing a day or so later goes down really well. There may only be one occasion in that pet's life when they needed a vet in an emergency and that client will remember you and will appreciate what you did for their pet. It is one of the best parts of being a vet, that feeling that your work has made such a significant difference.

Reward

It can be hard work and stressful being on call in a first opinion practice as a new graduate but it is also incredibly interesting and rewarding. You will see a diverse array of interesting cases and will have the opportunity to put your training into practice. You will experience some lows when animals die despite your best efforts after accidents or due to disease processes, but you will also know just how great it is to help an injured or sick animal and to have the opportunity to save a life and make a difference.

> My partner and I used to go to our local cinema and we would leave the number of the cinema with the nurse who was taking the phones. If there was an emergency, they would call the cinema and the cinema usher would stop the film and make an announcement asking for us. My first viewing of Star Wars was curtailed in this way thanks to Dennis the boxer dog charging through a plate glass window and lacerating his jowls.

Dennis was the most accident-prone dog I have ever met who, in addition to the plate glass window incident, also managed to get a four-inch twig up one nostril, two cut paws and a peach stone foreign body all within the first couple of years of his life. Mrs Hyde would phone and I would recognise her voice immediately as she said:
'It's Dennis again!'

Keep well

It is even more important when you are working nights and weekends to look after your health, to eat properly and to get decent amounts of sleep when you are not on call. You will experience sleep deprivation and erratic meal times and when you are working and driving around you need to do everything you can to keep yourself mentally alert. Most practices will be reasonable about rest time after on call, especially if you have had a particularly exhausting shift and will make sure that you use that rest time to recuperate. It is tempting to think that we are invincible when we are young, but vets have crashed their cars due to exhaustion and it may make more sense to get some sleep than to go clubbing if you have had a hectic night on call.

Working out of hours does not suit everyone and although some vets find it exhilarating and exciting, you may loathe every minute of it. There is now much more opportunity to choose the type of work and the work patterns you prefer if you are willing to look for the right position and go for it. It is much more important to find the job in which you are happy working than to continue to work where you find the work too stressful and the work patterns detrimental to your mental and physical well-being.

I remember to this day when, within six weeks of qualifying, on my first weekend on call I was called out to a cow calving, my first caesarian and a suspected foreign body all on the same evening. I was in the on call rota straightaway and I lived on adrenaline and just worked, slept and ate. It was expected of new graduates then, and it was treated as a rite of passage which in these more enlightened times has fortunately been discontinued. At the time, and with the relatively small number of women vets in practice, I wanted to prove that I could do the job as well as a man and I did what I was expected to do.

I carried on working in practice and although I still had days when I felt under intense pressure, I learned techniques and coping strategies and work became easier as I gained experience.

There is an element of seasonality to emergency work and you will find that when Easter comes, so do cases of chocolate poisoning; around Bonfire Night and New Year's Eve we see firework phobia and Christmas is a time when the home contains more food hanging around to be stolen by hungry Labradors. Christmas decorations and presents under the tree are also a temptation for the dogs of the household and clients seem to think that their gun dog's nose will not detect that a wrapped present under the tree contains a box of chocolates for Auntie Flo.

There was a case of repeated, unexplained urticaria in a dog in our practice which turned out to be caused by the dog eating the lurid-coloured candles on the Christmas tree; one Dobermann ate most of the tree decorations and a pair of Christmas socks plus some underwear in one sitting. I have spent an entire Boxing Day with an Irish wolfhound called Norah who had eaten the goose carcase and on another occasion a dachshund broke into the fridge and ate a huge chunk of Stilton cheese and a joint of ham. He lay on his side wheezing gently, looking like a small inflatable with all four legs off the ground until nature took its course and he scatter-gunned the kennel with varying colours and consistencies of diarrhoea.

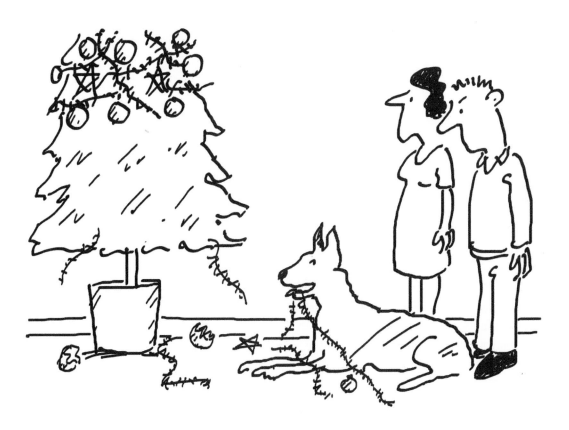

CHAPTER 9

Clients: the good, the bad and the ugly

It is likely that you chose to be a vet because you like the idea of working with animals but, as every vet very soon comes to realise, every animal you meet has a human attached to it. The human may be at the end of a lead or in the stable holding the headcollar or carrying a bucket in the farmyard, but you will always have to communicate with a homo sapiens somewhere along the way.

I have often been asked why I became a vet rather than a doctor and sometimes people ask if it is because I prefer animals to humans. I think there is an element of truth in that because although I cannot think of an animal which I have ever taken a real dislike to, I can think of quite a few obnoxious examples of our own species. I have had to learn to like humans too over the years of being a vet and become more tolerant of people and their individuality, and I enjoy the varied and sometimes frankly odd behaviours of people which somehow seem to be enhanced around animals.

Your patients may not be able to speak to you themselves, but you are going to have to communicate with those pesky humans every single day of your working life, be they owners or the vets, nurses and other support staff in the veterinary team. If you don't find it easy to communicate with people you need to learn how to very quickly if you want to be a successful vet in practice.

Most of our clients are lovely people who immediately have something in common with you because they are the ones who care enough about their animals to have made an appointment to come and ask your opinion. You will rarely see the truly hideous animal owners who don't care about their animals because they don't consult a vet at all if they can avoid it. It helps if you start with a willingness to like the people you meet and to approach each interaction with a positive attitude.

You will often inevitably meet owners at a very stressful time in their lives when their pet may be ill or injured, but many people also feel anxious just attending for a routine consultation or for an elective procedure such as a vaccination or a spay and it helps to have some understanding of how they might be feeling.

Understanding your patients and their owners

There have been many words written about the human–animal bond by people far more qualified than I am and these are my own, very personal, views from my observations as a practising vet. During my 40 years as a vet, I have seen a huge number of animal owners and been privileged to be in a position to see the relationships which exist between all kinds of animals and their owners. I believe we see human beings at their best and also their worst in their interactions with animals and it can indeed be an indicator of the way in which they behave with other humans. It was no surprise to me to hear that animal abuse is so closely allied to domestic violence and cruelty to children.

It may be that you grew up with a family pet who is or was very important to you and a significant stimulus to your own ambition to be a vet. You may have owned a dog, cat or horse yourself or lived on a farm with cattle and sheep and seen the local vet with your own animals; many vets in the past were children of farming families. It is possible and not that uncommon nowadays, however, to qualify as a vet having had quite limited personal experience of the bond that can exist between animals and humans.

As veterinary surgeons, we need to understand just how important our patient is to the human who is presenting them to us. I believe it is by understanding and recognising the importance of this bond that we can look after our patients' best interests by working towards positive outcomes in collaboration with the carer or owner of that animal.

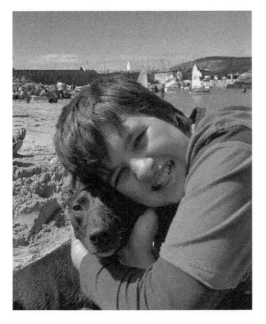

My son Jamie with our dog Gnasher enjoying a seaside holiday. Jamie was born with autistic spectrum disorder and language delay and so found it difficult to communicate with other people and play with his peers when he was a child. Our dogs provided unquestioning companionship for him when he was lonely, and they looked to him for commands which stimulated communication and made him feel more confident. Dogs give unconditional love and acceptance and their benefit to people who have problems in their lives has been well documented. Working in partnership with animal owners in all aspects of pet ownership, but especially in keeping assistance and support dogs healthy, is one of the many ways vets can benefit society.

Bagheera, known as Baggy, much-loved companion to my two autistic sons and a very special member of our family.

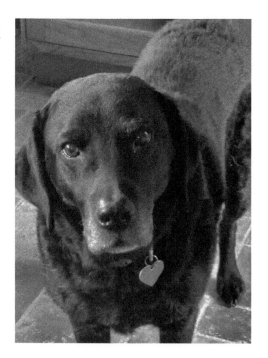

I am writing these words knowing that my elderly Labrador is in the last few days and possibly the last hours of her life. I am in that grey area of indecision with a much-loved dog with a chronic disease who is unlikely to die peacefully but will need putting to sleep in order to avoid suffering in her final hours. I am deliberately writing this now because at this moment my understanding of the importance of that relationship between an animal owner and a veterinary surgeon is uniquely enhanced and for once it is I who am the owner and relying on a vet when the time comes to say goodbye.

I want the vet who helps me at this time to be sensitive to my feelings but most importantly, I want them to make my dog's comfort and best interests their first priority. I want them to be professional and objective and help me make the right decision for the good of my dog who is their patient. I also want them to empathise with how I feel and to help me at this incredibly difficult time because it is a very complex and painful place to be in emotionally and, even though I am a vet myself, it is incredibly difficult to be objective and make that decision. I am very lucky because the vet is my personal friend Helen, but this experience is giving me a true sense of how it feels to be a client and dependent on the skill of a veterinary professional. I feel really vulnerable and quite embarrassingly needy and, however well qualified I am, just now I want someone to help me to do the right thing with this very precious member of my family who has been with me through some very significant life events and who I am going to miss very much.

When you interact with your clients, try to be empathetic towards all the emotions they may be feeling about their animals and understand that you may need to be tolerant of their actions and reactions when under stress. While it is true that we must remain objective and professional and make logical and dispassionate decisions, I believe that the best vets retain that awareness of the significance of the human–animal bond throughout their careers and never lose sight of the effect our actions and attitudes may have on our patients and their owners.

In my first job, a client who was a six-foot coal miner used to come in with a fluffy, black toy poodle called Princess dancing along at the end of a pink lead. This minuscule dog was about the same size as one of his massive, gnarled, coal-engrained hands which were each the size of shovels. He used to lift Princess up onto the table in one of his great, meaty paws and nudge her towards me in an offhand manner, mumbling something about her being his wife's dog, before giving me a detailed history and all the while gently caressing little Princess' ear. Princess used to repay him for this attention by trying to bite him all the time and he had no control over her whatsoever. We had to resort to taking her into the back room to give her any treatment, whereupon she would behave like an angel. When a minor ailment was diagnosed you could clearly see the relief on his face but to maintain the illusion that he did not adore this little dog, he used to say something like, 'Oh, nothing terminal then, eh? Better luck next time,' before leaving the consulting room and having a really good moan to the nurse about vet bills on the way out. As a parting shot he would be saying, 'I'll have her put down next time, she's costing me a fortune.'

This was all for the benefit of any of his coal mining mates who might be in the waiting room and we all knew he loved that poodle with a passion, but this was in the days when men hid their feelings much more for fear of being branded a softy. It would have been easy to assume on first meeting that he was an uncaring, hard-hearted brute, but Princess was indeed treated like royalty and there was no doubting who wore the trousers in that relationship.

Clients' behaviour in the waiting room

Many of our clients only come to see us when they are worried about their pet and the way in which they behave when they come in to the practice can be quite challenging on occasion. Stress and uncertainty can have varying effects on different people and some individuals can be awkward and even belligerent when they are worried and frightened of what could happen to their animal.

Try to imagine the visit from their perspective; this may be their first pet and they may have never had to deal with a sick or injured animal. They may never have been to the actual practice before and may have found it hard to locate under pressure to make the appointment time. It may have been a challenge even getting their pet into the car. They may be feeling nervous because, although they are familiar with their local doctors' surgery, they are uncertain of what the procedure is and what they should be doing in a vet's waiting room. They do not know how to check in to let you know that they have arrived or where they should be sitting while they wait for their appointment. Worried humans out of their comfort zone can present as prickly individuals, illogical and sometimes erratic and abrupt without meaning to be.

Hopefully, you will have the services of an excellent receptionist to rely on, who will help them to follow the procedures and who will also assess if a situation requires immediate attention, such as an animal bleeding or having difficulty breathing. Receptionists do a wonderful job and their expertise is often underappreciated. It is helpful to be aware of what could be happening in the waiting room and to realise that the client experience there can have a bearing on the demeanour of the client when they enter the consulting room. There are some practices where they ask their new vets to spend an hour or two on the receptionist desk so that they appreciate the skill involved and the effect the receptionist can have on a busy waiting room.

It is not unusual to have a frantic client burst into the waiting room with a dog in their arms expecting to be seen immediately, and on these occasions clients sometimes behave in what appears to us to be a really foolish manner. They may bring the dog in without it attached to a lead, or with a cat squirming and struggling in their arms and not in a cat basket. Their animal may be bleeding profusely but they have not thought to stop and put on a bandage and it is easy for us to be quite judgemental in circumstances like this.

In a situation such as this you need to be able to take charge and assume control for the sake of your patient. Stay calm, give clear direction authoritatively and reassure them and guide them through the whole experience with tact and consideration.

What clients really want

A veterinary practice cannot survive without a continuous supply of predominantly contented clients. There will be a core number of loyal clients who have been coming to a practice for years with a variety of animals and who would never go anywhere else unless something really bad happened or they moved out of the area. There is also a pool of potential new clients who may choose to give their custom to your practice or may choose to go elsewhere. They may be new to the area, have newly acquired an animal or be wavering in support of their current practice for one reason or another. Keeping existing bonded clients happy and acquiring those new clients and making them want to continue to bring their animals to you is what makes a practice thrive.

When I first qualified, clients tended to be much more in awe of the doctor or the vet than they are now and were far less informed about their own and their animals' health. We were given no formal training in communication skills and we learned by watching other vets during our time seeing practice and from working with other vets. I could see that the approach of some vets in practice was different to others and that different clients wanted and expected different things from their vet.

Our clients have complete freedom of choice and they can go to whichever practice they like as long as they are willing to pay the bills. There has been much research on the reasons why a client chooses a practice and these include conducting Internet searches for good reviews, how convenient it is to get to the surgery, word of mouth recommendation from family and friends and factors which may seem quite trivial such as ease of parking or even just the fact that they have driven past a practice on the way home from work and know where it is.

The veterinary profession has an excellent reputation in the eyes of the general public and historically has enjoyed very high levels of trust, so the general assumption is that most vets are fundamentally good people, capable, professional and well regulated. This is a really valuable reputation to have and our profession should safeguard this as much as it can as once a good reputation is lost it is rarely, if ever, fully recovered.

Once a client has chosen a practice they will be highly likely to remain a client both for the reasons they chose it in the first place but also because it takes some effort on their part to change to another practice. Unless the client experience falls short without reasonable resolution by the practice, or the costs of treatment are considerably higher than those of a neighbouring practice, then they are likely to continue to remain as a client.

Cost is often cited as a reason for changing vets when in reality it is some other factor which has disenchanted a good client and prompted them to move on. They are more likely to look elsewhere for veterinary services for reasons which have nothing at all to do with money but because of a negative experience such as a curt response and refusal when phoning for an appointment, offhand treatment of them or their animal by a vet or nurse or some other breakdown in communication.

It is rarely the premises or the equipment which make a client change practices but usually an occasion when they did not like the way in which they were spoken to or the way their animal was handled, which affects how much trust they have in the vets and nurses. It is a sad fact that one bad experience for a client can override a previous succession of positive experiences and years of good service can be ruined by one episode of thoughtlessness.

Client loyalty

I always approached my consultations with the desire to give the clients the best of my abilities and I trusted my vets who I employed to give the same high level of service to the clients too. The majority of the vets I have worked with have been dedicated professionals who go above and beyond client expectations and I am proud to be part of a profession that cares so much about the job that they do.

Now I am retired from practice, I have become a client myself and I realise that I never fully appreciated just what it was like to take your dog or cat to the surgery or call a vet to see your horse. Some animals are owned by people who are not emotionally attached to them, but the majority of our small animal clients now consider the animals in their homes as part of their family, and horses and other pet farm animals can be of significant emotional value to their owners.

The trust and confidence between a client and the vets and nurses in a practice is an immensely valuable thing. It means repeat custom and revenue for the practice but also that the client puts their trust in you when you advise a certain course of treatment. That trust and the partnership between a vet and a client to ensure the health and well-being of their animal makes your interaction with the client easier and more enjoyable. If a client trusts you, then you will be the one insisting on giving a cost estimate for treatment while the client is saying that they are very happy for you to do whatever you think is right because they have complete faith in you.

As an employed veterinary surgeon, you play a huge part in bonding your clients to the practice, not only benefiting the practice and you as the employee, but also all the animals that are the patients of that practice. If the entire client experience is successful, then everyone benefits including the animals, because the bonded client will trust the vets in that practice and be willing to comply with suggested treatment. They will enjoy excellent veterinary attention for their animals in a well-equipped practice which employs highly trained staff. They will feel that the practice cares about them and their animal and that they are getting the best attention and value for money. They will tell all their family and friends how wonderful you are and go on social media praising you and have complete faith in you. This trust and confidence makes every subsequent interaction you have with that client so much easier. They are a pleasure to have as a client because they trust you and your recommendations and will show their appreciation with their continued custom and by being a pleasure to work with.

Clients, cash and value for money

As an owner of a practice, I was understandably keen on seeing the client numbers go up and the money come in because I knew that increased profit meant that we could continue to maintain good levels of pay for ourselves and for our staff and to continue to reinvest in the practice.

We cannot ignore the massive factor that finances play in veterinary practice and the fact that some clients simply do not have the money to pay for all the treatments that might be of value to their animals. Some clients have the necessary finance but choose not to spend it, and this is much more likely to happen if we have not delivered our advice in an effective and convincing manner. The size of the pet food market and the pet paraphernalia that is on sale, such as novelty dog outfits, toys and special organic diets, illustrate that many people are willing to spend a considerable amount of money on their animals but may not choose to spend their disposable income on veterinary services. The choice of where they spend is theirs, but we should make sure that they value veterinary services for maintaining the well-being of their animals and are willing and happy to pay for it.

Vets will say that they are professionals and not salespeople and that they find selling to people demeaning, but caring about animals and having a veterinary degree is not enough to make you a successful vet in general practice. Clients need to feel reassured that they have spent their money wisely, have received value for money and that their custom has been appreciated. The way we conduct our consultations with our clients is hugely important, and no clients = no practice income = no job. It doesn't matter how brilliant you are as a vet, you need happy clients who trust you and who seek you out and are willing to follow your advice.

Trust and honesty

Trust is the most important factor in the relationship between a vet and their client. They want you to care for the health of their precious animal and there is no way on first meeting you that they can know if you are a good vet or a mediocre vet. They can like you as a person and other clients can recommend you to them, but ultimately they are putting their animal in your care in the belief that you know what you are doing and will be honest with them.

When you examine and assess their pet and recommend a course of treatment or an investigation, a client trusts you to recommend the necessary treatment, and you are also trusting them to fulfil their side of the bargain by giving you complete and truthful information and then to follow your advice and pay you for your expertise. If that mutual trust breaks down between a vet and a client, the relationship becomes dysfunctional and in many cases can never be repaired.

Being on their side

Clients need to know that you are working with and for them and for the good of their pet and are 'on their side'. Sometimes a client may feel that a vet is not really engaged with helping them and is not listening to what they are saying, or may believe they are judging them negatively and looking down on them.

Perhaps they have let their dog become badly overweight and not kept them on the lead after surgery or stopped a course of antibiotics halfway through and it can be maddening when this happens, but clients need to feel able to come back and see you without losing face and have the reasons for compliance explained again. The worst thing you can do for an animal owned by a gormless or inadequate owner is to make them feel so bad that they stay away from veterinary surgeons altogether to the detriment of the animal.

Friction or disconnect of any kind between the vet and client does not make for a good working relationship and makes the clients much less willing to come back for follow-up treatment or a new condition which may arise; they certainly do not want to pay to be told that they are falling short. If you persevere with communicating with a client and gain their cooperation, then the satisfaction of relieving the pain of an obese, arthritic old dog or easing the itchiness of a chronic case of atopy is extremely rewarding.

Client complaints

This is why client complaints can be so traumatic for both parties involved and this is sometimes not fully comprehended by a client. It is soul-destroying to know you have done your best for a client, and even more so when you have gone beyond the call of duty for them, to be faced with a complaint. In the present climate of enhanced awareness of consumer rights, it seems that complaints are increasingly common in all areas of service provision and it appears we vets are just going to have to get used to it too. Customers are far more likely to complain about what they perceive as poor service such as a bad meal or a delayed flight, and inevitably some will take advantage of this and will also use the complaint system as a means to avoid paying for a satisfactory service. A proportion of client complaints are not genuinely about the standard of care but are triggered by a reluctance to pay the bill, and it is hard not to take this personally when it occurs.

Clients are not aware just how devastating it can be for a vet to receive a written or formal complaint and how the confidence of a vet can be damaged even when a complaint is found to be unfounded or based on a misunderstanding. A complaint from a client, if handled sensitively, may not result in the loss of a client but is usually extremely time-consuming and emotionally draining for everyone involved. A bad experience shakes the confidence of that client and if it is not resolved successfully then every subsequent interaction after that is an uphill struggle based on mistrust.

Some clients may not fully understand why they should have to pay for investigation and treatment if their pet did not survive, and they may be encouraged by friends or relatives who do not know the full story to avoid paying or to seek compensation. Despite a complaint appearing to be a personal attack on the vet, it often arises because of other drivers that are in play and we need to develop a thicker skin and learn not to take it personally because there is nothing we can do about the culture that exists.

Everyone has a justifiable right to complain and it is right that we as professionals are held to account, but a bedrock of trust and good customer service significantly reduces the likelihood of complaints and we can do something about that.

Your clients

Clients come in every guise, shape and form, the old and the young, the intelligent and the ignorant, some resentful or angry, some smiley but deaf, others sad and scared and you can see all these variations and more in the course of just one consulting session. Vets have to be able to glean information from each and every one and impart information back to them because those animals in our care need us to use our skills to get the message across and help them.

As a vet, you will constantly be surprised by people and have your perceptions challenged regularly. Some owners are in awe of you as a vet and will be worried about being judged by you and some are like Jekyll and Hyde, giving the receptionist or nursing staff a really hard time then coming into the consulting room all sweetness and light.

Some clients are worried that you will use really big words and that they will feel foolish and uneducated. It can be difficult at times to pitch the discussion at the right level and to make sure that you are explaining yourself well without being patronising, but you will soon learn how to change your delivery as the consultation progresses if you are careful to assess how well the client understands what you are saying. If there is a misunderstanding between the vet and the client, then the mistake is likely to be ours in not making sure that we have delivered comprehensible questions or instructions, so be aware of how much your client understands you.

> *A client came in to see a colleague of mine with a dog which had injured its tail which was hanging limply down. The vet asked the owner, 'Can he wag his tail?' and the owner solemnly took the dog's tail in his hand and wagged it from side to side himself.*

A three-hour consulting session is the veterinary equivalent of going on stage for a dramatic performance and you will develop a routine in the way in which you conduct your consultations, which will become second nature. You will also need to subtly change and adapt to the challenges of each consultation, making nuanced changes for each client who comes in.

Some clients want you to be hyper-scientific and analytical and others will be more responsive to giving you the information you require if you are more informal and gently ascertain the relevant information without sounding like the Spanish Inquisition. This is the art of consulting in general practice and it takes practice, good communication skills and empathy.

You will have clients who are scared and present as irritable and angry, and clients who are intent on telling you what they think you want to hear rather than the true facts. Some anxious clients exaggerate every symptom because in a weird way they think that by doing so you will take them more seriously and they will receive better treatment such as 'stronger antibiotics'.

If you ask a leading question such as, 'Is Gnasher drinking a lot?' they will say, 'Yes, loads', even if she isn't, because obtusely they think that that is what you want to hear. Always ask open questions such as, 'What is Gnasher's water intake like?' which often elicits the client worrying that they do not seem to drink much. The current obsession with humans constantly drinking litres of water whether they are thirsty or not can create concern when an animal is just listening to its own body and thirst mechanisms. I often had to reassure a client that low water intake is not an adverse symptom.

Others will hear you say a phrase with their ears but completely misunderstand what you actually said with your mouth, which is why in some cases you have to repeat the important information several times. If you ask some clients to starve their dog for 12 hours, they will not think you really mean that nil by mouth includes the treats they give while they are watching TV, so be clear and check that the client has understood.

It is a great gift for a vet if they actually enjoy meeting people with all their quirks and differences, because you will spend a lot of your life interacting with people you do not know and may never see again for just ten minutes at a time. Add a bouncy dog and a couple of hyperactive children into the mix and you will need to be able to think on your feet and take charge of that consultation with a total stranger.

I believe one of the most important factors when consulting is that you show that you appreciate their animal. The worst way to get off to a bad start with a client is if they think you do not like their cat or dog and, although the snarling Chihuahua with the halitosis is not a thing of beauty to your eyes, you must find something positive to say about him even if it is to compliment his impressive snarling technique, and say how clever he is because smart dogs recognise a vet when they see one.

Every client is different but there are certain personality types who you will see time and again in practice. This is by no means an official analysis and I know some of these are rather unkind stereotypes but most vets in practice will recognise them and I include them here as a little light relief. You will note that discussions about money and the ability to pay is a recurring theme, but this is the blunt reality of first opinion veterinary practice in many areas. Our clients would probably love us much more and be incredibly nice to know if veterinary treatment was free for everyone.

We frequently see the lovely Motherly Melanie who is the mum of a family and the caregiver and who looks on the pet as a member of her family, not quite equal to another child but not very far off. She spends the most time with the pet, feeds them and is really good at providing accurate history, noticing a loss of appetite or a limp immediately. Although she is very busy with her life, she makes time to come to the surgery; we see a lot of Melanies in the course of our work and they are a real pleasure to have as a client and should be cherished. Melanie is frequently empathetic and understanding towards you as a young person starting out on a career as a vet and she generally wants what is best for the patient; she lifts your spirits when you see her name on the appointment list. She may have children approaching the same age as you and will be wanting you to succeed and is the bedrock of general practice.

Working Will is married to Melanie and unless he works from home he doesn't see the animal during the working day but he might have been asked to bring it to the surgery because Melanie is busy with the children or working herself. He has been told to bring the dog, but he has no idea if it has been eating or not, what its motions are like and whether it has been depressed or not. Phone calls to Melanie from the consult room may be necessary. Will really likes the patient too, but he is perhaps a little more worried that veterinary treatment is going to be very expensive and is likely to want an in-depth analysis of potential costs. If push came to shove, however, he and Melanie will most likely agree to the treatment of the family pet and Melanie and the children will give him hell if he doesn't.

In some cases, it is Melanie who works and Will who is the caregiver and stays at home with the children of course, and you can transpose the behaviours as appropriate! I would remind you I am illustrating deliberate stereotypes based on my own experience!

Tracy Teenager may well accompany her parents and be very attached to the pet though she may not be as keen on it if it is vomiting everywhere or smells really bad. She will probably be involved in the decision-making process to a variable extent and should be included in the consultation and in the explanation of what is wrong with the family pet. Most teenagers are calm and sensible and will be the good clients of the future, but others are not so predictable and may be an unwelcome source of complication and drama. Tracy may shriek and recoil when she sees blood or any other bodily fluid and although she insisted on coming to the surgery, she may be prone to bursting into hysterical tears at times of crisis and flounce in and out of the consulting room like a drama queen until she receives a message on her phone, whereupon she may be completely focused on texting her friends.

Designer Dionne regards her pet as both a fashion accessory and a substitute baby who she dresses in pink romper suits and bootees and takes everywhere with her and never allows the paws to touch the ground. She will coo over the ferocious, snarling, drooling Chihuahua as it sits in its designer handbag wishing it could live the life of a proper dog. She may even present her 'fur baby' to you nestled well down into the deep valley of her substantial orange cleavage. For purposes of health, safety and decorum, do ask her to extract her pet from between the twin peaks before attempting examination without being savaged or accused of anything inappropriate. She will often be a reasonably compliant owner and vet bills may

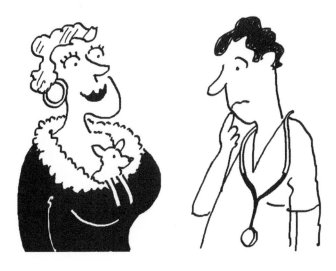

seem quite moderate to her compared to the thousands she has spent on accessories such as diamanté-encrusted collars and fancy dress for her pampered pooch. She might not be so keen when anointed with bodily fluids such as the contents of anal glands or vomit on her white leather jacket or if she is told that dogs should actually walk around from time to time rather than being carried.

Angry Anthony may present quite a challenge to you in the consulting room and you can usually tell that he is tetchy as soon as he comes in. He may have had a bad experience with a vet elsewhere and is determined to make you suffer for it, but there is also the possibility that he may just appear angry because he is worried about his pet and is feeling vulnerable.

Nervous Neville can masquerade as Angry Anthony and his emotions make him come out fighting like a cornered porcupine. He may resent waiting for his appointment even for two minutes and does not seem to be listening to a word you say and is unwilling to follow your advice. He wants the problem with his dog or cat sorting there and then and he thinks he can get his own way by being belligerent. You must not react to his confrontational manner but remain professional and polite and even try to charm him out of his anger. Do not be goaded into retaliating with outraged indignation because you will achieve nothing but an escalation of the situation. The best outcome is when you convince this client that you are actually on his side, you are listening and that you will be doing the best for his animal. You will need to explain everything pleasantly but make it clear that you may be unable to sort out the problem in one single visit to the vet. He will resent it if he feels you are being patronising or trying to make him look small.

There are times when it is appropriate to stop an abusive or foul-mouthed Angry Anthony in his tracks by saying very firmly that you are not prepared to be spoken to like that and to refuse to continue the consultation. If it becomes a trade-off of insults and invective then you have not achieved anything and it is a waste of time in continuing the exchange.

Single Sarah and Bachelor Brendan are young professionals who are building their careers and live alone or with a partner but without children. They have a pet who they think the world of and who they envisage being the perfect family dog in the not too distant future. They may employ a dog walker and go for 12-mile walks every weekend with their partner and they are usually really good owners and a pleasure to see. They often arrive at the end of evening surgery because they work such long hours and you will probably identify with them because you know what it is like to be working all week and finding it difficult to get to appointments. Cherish these clients because they are often long-term bonded clients who are willing to follow your suggestions and will often ask to see you again because you are on the same wavelength. They are often fellow professionals and can be relied on to agree to necessary investigative work, follow instructions with medication correctly and come back for follow-up treatment when asked.

Internet Ian may fancy himself as being a bit of a scientist and demand an in-depth explanation and even a full lecture and explanation on every disease process. He has been doing research at home and comes in with a wad of printed information, most of which has been written by some nutter in a bunker in Oregon. He has already decided on the diagnosis of some outlandish disease only known in the Galapagos Islands and the required treatment, and expects you to be impressed by his knowledge and his diagnosis. He thinks any fool with access to the Internet could be a vet and although he hasn't gone as far as buying the drugs illegally, he has been tempted. You will need to make a thorough examination as always and explain your findings without being drawn in to imparting an entire veterinary degree in the course of a consultation. You may need to use tact and diplomacy to convince him that he may be basing his diagnosis on false information and perhaps does not have as much knowledge as he thinks he does.

Alternative Therapy Agatha will bring her animal in because she has tried various herbal remedies and they have had no effect. She may have her friend Homeopathic Harriet with her who is insisting that antibiotics are the scourge of the universe and tell you that she had a dog with pus dripping out of one ear which was successfully treated by her friend up the road with a few drops of diluted water and a couple of crystals. If an animal is really ill this can be a tricky situation and you will need to assess whether you need to act immediately on welfare grounds to convince her to have the case worked up properly to achieve a diagnosis and start conventional treatment. If the situation is not too serious, it might be reasonable to make a diagnosis and ask her to seriously consider your advice because you all want the same outcome which is for her animal to get better. If she does not feel that you are pressurising her into using conventional treatment or ridiculing her then she may listen and eventually reluctantly acquiesce and allow you to treat the animal.

It is usually no use getting into a heated discussion about the merits of alternative therapies because it pushes clients like Agatha into further entrenched positions. Some followers of alternative therapies are akin to religious devotees and you will never change their minds with scientific logic about the efficacy of water diluted a million times. Leave the door open for the client to think about your advice and hopefully come back and agree to appropriate treatment if their pet does not get better. If you browbeat Agatha about her beliefs then you back her into a corner and she cannot return to you with her dignity intact for that course of antibiotics if they become essential. Most alternative therapies do no harm per se and so can be given in addition to conventional medicine where the owner allows.

Agatha will, of course, always believe that it was the homeopathy that cured Trixie and not the treatment you prescribed for demodex. Some cases which are just about to recover anyway due to a prolonged course of conventional treatment annoyingly make a full recovery just after the client consults a homeopath or tries Great Auntie Marigold's patent remedy. You treat a cat for flea allergic dermatitis conventionally and the day before it stops scratching the owner has given a one in a squillion dilution of stinky, scabby, bonkers weed and once again the efficacy of homeopathy is confirmed!

A considerable percentage of clinical cases can and do recover from disease without any treatment whatsoever and this will continue to confirm the value of those alternative therapies to some clients. I think that you might just as well run around a toadstool 16 times as use homeopathy, but despite the cost being so much more expensive than conventional medicine, clients still go back for that water diluted a thousand times. Instead of being infuriated by their beliefs, we should ask ourselves why they continue to do so and alter our approach to consultations for some clients and try to work with them. Many consultations with homeopathic vets are considerably longer than conventional vet practice consultations and the clients are listened to at length and given respect and attention. Homeopathic vets always warn that things often get worse before they get better, so they manage the client's expectations. They prepare them for a case to take a relatively long time to resolve and they ask the owner to come back and be listened to at length again. This is clearly what these clients want from their medical practitioner and we should learn from this and not be annoyed with Agatha and Harriet, but look out for their pets' interests as best we can by engaging with them.

Elderly Edward or Senior Sue will often present with their beloved companion who is their pride and joy and their only company on a cold and lonely evening in December. They may have lost their spouse in recent years and this elderly pet is their main reason for keeping their house warm and for getting up in the morning. Often their pet is an extremely important part of their lives and for many pensioners, it is the cat that keeps them company when they can't sleep and the dog that makes them go for a walk and keep mobile.

Most importantly, please never assume that just because someone looks old, or is hard of hearing, or takes a while to process what you are saying to them, that they are also stupid and talk to them as if they were an idiot. Speak to them with respect and tactfully ascertain if they are hearing you and understanding you because you might be speaking to a retired doctor with all their faculties intact. The ageing process sometimes means that while everything in the brain works, it can take longer to process and digest the salient points and compose a reply. It can become difficult to make decisions as we become older and to an older person the pace of life can feel very rushed and this makes them feel insecure. When we are pressed for time, it is all too easy to gallop through a consultation at speed and this can be very hard for older people who leave the consulting room feeling bewildered and short-changed.

I love talking to elderly clients because if you like people and social history as I do, they often have fascinating tales to tell and have led such interesting lives. Older people are all too often ignored in our society and lead very lonely lives and they love to have a reason to leave home and come to the surgery and have a chat to you during a consultation, so if you do have a little spare time for them then make their day with a little conversation.

I remember one lady with a budgie coming to me and I noted her name was Mrs Partridge. I remarked on the fact that she had the name of a bird and had also brought me a bird and she said with a twinkle in her eye, 'Eh love, I'm a Partridge now but I was a Throstle before I got married, you know,' and we had a bit of a giggle about Miss Throstle and Mr Partridge getting together on the dance floor all those years ago. It was lovely to see her smile and was one of those little moments that brighten up the day and make you appreciate your fellow human.

Elderly clients may not look very affluent but do not jump to the conclusion that because they are pensioners they will therefore not be able to afford the optimum treatment. They may appear shocked by the cost but that is probably because they have no terms of reference for the cost of veterinary treatment. I have often been in the middle of feeling terrible about the cost of a necessary investigation being £500 only to have an 80-year-old client in a worn old coat tell me they thought it was going to be twice as much or bring out a massive roll of notes that they have been keeping under the mattress for a rainy day.

Some older clients may be relatively unaware of the advancements in veterinary treatments and may be surprised by how much is available now to improve the quality of life of their pet. They should be given a choice of the recommended treatments just as all our clients should be and then they can decide which level of treatment to opt for, so make no assumptions.

Older people and those who have a disability may find it difficult to administer treatments and you may be able to help by offering the services of a nurse to put drops down ears or to give tablets. Choosing a long-acting injection might be a better alternative for an animal with a frail or disabled owner who might struggle to medicate a cat on their own. These clients might struggle to bath a dog with a skin condition and appreciate this being offered as a service by the practice, because holding a soapy, wriggling dog in the bath for the required length of time for a medicated shampoo to work is taxing for the young and fit, let alone a frail old lady living on her own.

Some clients may have poor memories, so write instructions and a request for re-examination appointments down on paper where appropriate. Booking repeat appointments for the daytime when the surgery is not as busy and you have the opportunity to take a little more time with them can be much appreciated. You have an opportunity to make a real difference to the lives of elderly pet owners and this can give you such a reward in job satisfaction.

Goggle-box Gemma arrives and has been watching *Supervet* so she now wants major surgical intervention for Barney the Bulldog with the bandy legs, who she has rescued from 'a friend'. She says she is crazy about animals and likes everyone to know just how amazing she is for adopting Barney from Romania and now expects you to come up with a treatment just like the supervet, but which does not involve a large bill because 'it is not really her dog'. She has four other animals which she has rescued and already has an outstanding bill which she cannot pay. Good luck with that one!

Skint Sid and Entitled Angie want everything doing for their pedigree dog but have no means of paying for it whatsoever. They bought the dog as a puppy from a man in a car park at a motorway service station for £500 but present it to you two weeks later saying they cannot afford a puppy vaccination. They want to know why they have to pay anyway, because they had their babies' shots done for free at the doctors' and all their prescriptions at the chemist are free, so it's not fair that they should have to pay and why do you vets say you love animals when you expect people to have to pay all the time? They have another two dogs at home and think you should treat all animals for free and it's just not fair and you are condemning their puppy to be unvaccinated and it is all your fault if it dies of some disease they saw on the telly. If their dog suffers an injury on a weekend, then they insist you must come to the house and fix it right away and they have had too many shots of vodka to drive and they cannot leave the kids and they do not care what it costs and if you don't come it is terrible because what kind of a vet are you? They do not care what it costs because they do not intend to pay and they are intent on making their choice to have a pet that they cannot afford into your problem and to make you feel bad.

I have deliberately included this rather cruel stereotype because it is very difficult to feel sympathetic towards clients who behave like this and vets naturally have strong beliefs about the responsibility of animal ownership and welfare. You will find this situation very difficult and if you are not careful then this will be a source of stress and distress to you. It is hard for vets to see an animal that does not appear to be cared for well or receive the treatment it needs and be told that this is your fault and your responsibility because you are a vet. You must hold on to the fact that you cannot be responsible for all the animals that you see during the course of your work and you cannot take it upon yourself to fix other peoples' problems and if you try to do so, then you will damage your own well-being.

Take care also that you do not leap to any prejudiced opinions about a client who may appear to fit this stereotype and automatically leap to assumptions based on appearances. You might be completely wrong and they may confound your negative perceptions so treat them just as you would any other client. Try not to alter your manner or talk down to them and be dismissive and confrontational with this client because they will know that this is what you are doing and they will have experienced professionals sneering at them before. If you treat them with courtesy and kindness they may surprise you, because they often go through life without anyone in any position of authority being civil to them.

Explain the fact that private veterinary practice charges fees at the point of delivery and tell them what you propose for their animal and the likely costs, just as you would to any other client. They may have access to the necessary funding in some other way and be able to contact a friend or relative who can pay or they may qualify for treatment at an animal charity such as the PDSA or RSPCA.

If you are finding the consultation difficult, then do go and ask for help from a more senior member of staff who will have previous experience and will know the options that may be available. We cannot assume responsibility for social ills but must focus on doing what we reasonably can for the animals presented to us and build resilience to protect ourselves when faced with situations which we cannot make right.

I know it can be very difficult and very frustrating to be in this situation and I have always felt more conflicting emotions when faced with ignorance rather than with deliberate animal neglect. We should resist the temptation to judge someone who has not had the same benefits of education and opportunity as we have and concentrate on doing what we can for our patient. I used that consultation as a chance to help improve the lot of that animal in whatever way I could at the time and hope that at least they might continue to go and seek help from a vet if they needed to.

Histrionic Hilda can be very wearing in the course of a busy consultation session. Lots of tears and wailing and tales of past disasters when vets did not understand the needs of her very special pets. If her dog has diarrhoea, she voices suspicions of poisoning by the long-suffering, aggrieved neighbours and it cannot possibly be a result of the pound of greasy sausages she gave to Sidney the Schnauzer last night. She shrieks and flails around when Voldemort her feral cat doesn't want to come out of the wicker contraption she has fashioned from a fishing basket and two pieces of string. Every consultation with Hilda takes twice as long as it should as you navigate through her dramas and her tendency to go off at a tangent on another weird symptom she has just remembered.

Hoarding Hermione seems to acquire a new addition to her rapidly expanding cat colony every month. She has a limited budget and often works for an animal charity too in her spare time, where she adopts all the hopeless cases with chronic disease which she then introduces to her existing colony to perpetuate the problems. She struggles to pay the bills and you find it difficult because although she is very well meaning she really cannot afford all these needy animals which are suffering from all the infectious diseases that unvaccinated cats in a colony are bound to have. You can only do your best in this situation and treat as well as you can within her budgetary constraints; you may be able to direct her to charities to help with spaying and treatment. It will be a benefit to the cats she already has if you try to gently discourage her from acquiring any more before the time comes when she reaches the point where she really cannot cope any more and loses them all. Hoarding of animals can be a mental health-based problem and a more complex issue than it appears and such clients can need medical and social help.

Friendly Fiona and Happy Harry are the best of clients to have; they are responsible animal owners and make up the greatest proportion of your clients. They take care of their animals supremely well, train them appropriately, are well informed and expect to provide for their animals' health and work with you in maintaining their well-being. They will also defend you to other clients who might criticise you in the waiting room or in the pub and they recommend you to their friends and relatives. They try not to use or abuse you by phoning you out of hours for a mild lameness, always keep their appointments and try their best to do what you ask of them. If you see them in a social setting, you are genuinely pleased to see them and if they see you in a restaurant they do not insist on interrupting your meal to tell you about their dog's bout of diarrhoea that morning. They ask your advice about what sort of a dog would best suit them when they are looking for a puppy and they even buy you a bottle of wine at Christmas just because they appreciate you.

Do not lose sight of Fiona and Harry when you look back over a difficult day's work, because they are the clients who make it all worthwhile. At 3 a.m. you will worry about the one Angry Anthony who upset you when you will have seen 30 clients like Fiona and Harry, so remember that most clients are reasonable, courteous and friendly, follow your advice and are a pleasure to see. Try not to dwell on the one or two who are difficult and keep your sense of humour when the more challenging ones come in because one of the joys of life as a vet is the people and the surprises – life is never boring where people and animals are involved.

We should never make a client feel foolish because of a lack of knowledge because we need them to keep coming and seeing us for the sake of their animals and there will be times when people will astound you by how little they know about animals and what is normal and abnormal.

> *I was contacted by our local vicar who rang me one night and after the preliminary greeting posed the question:*
>
> *'Clare, do guinea pigs hibernate?'*
>
> *'No', I replied.*
>
> *'Oh dear,' came the reply, 'he has been lying motionless for two days and we thought he must be asleep or hibernating.'*
>
> *I would have thought that recognition of death would have been part of his day job but it seems that recognising a deceased guinea pig was out of his area of expertise.*

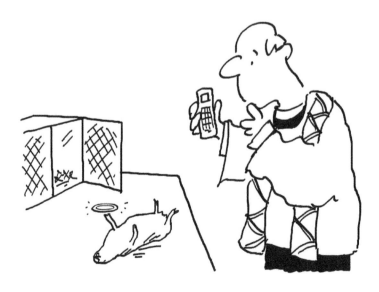

Children

Children in the consulting room can be a real challenge for a busy veterinary surgeon but I advise you to get used to them because they will always be a part of your life as a vet. Try to include them where appropriate because, even though it may require some extra effort from you on a busy day, being nice to children is part of your job whether you like it or not. It is perfectly reasonable to bring a well-behaved child to the vet with the family pet and it can be a positive experience for all concerned. The children are the clients of the future and if they are involved in the discussions then the enjoyment of an interesting visit to the vet may remain in their memory. They may even decide to become a vet themselves as a result of seeing you in action. If you are kind and chatty to their children, clients really appreciate it so it also helps to bond the client and increase their goodwill towards you. One day you may also have children and be glad of the understanding and kindness of a sympathetic professional, so look on it as another form of training for the future and smile at those little darlings when they come in.

There will undoubtedly be times when children in the consulting room make it far more difficult for you to concentrate and perform your work effectively. Parents can have their attention distracted because they are managing their own pet who is most likely on a lead or in a cat basket. Meanwhile their children are completely free-range and may be more or less out of control, and although it might be tempting to lock them all in the walk-in kennel out of harm's way, this does not go down well with the parents.

You may wonder when you are childless why parents bring them to the surgery in the first place, but you have to understand that clients often treat a visit to the vets as an enjoyable family outing. They may also have no alternative but to bring them because they have no childcare available but often it is because they have a bizarre view of it being an animal-themed family activity.

Small children often assume that every animal is like their own and they may never have come across a dog which might bite them if they throw their arms round them and poke them in the ear or eye. The dogs in the waiting room are often nervous because they are in the vets and in close quarters with other dogs and may be even more defensive and less tolerant than usual to a small child in their personal space. A hyperactive, inquisitive, overconfident child with a distracted parent in a confined space with a nervous animal is likely to be a dangerous combination and you cannot always rely on the parent to know this. Hopefully, you will have someone observant and efficient on reception who will maintain safety, peace and harmony in the waiting room but once the client enters the consulting room they will most likely bring their children in too and they are then on your territory and your responsibility.

Some small children will make a beeline for your side of the consulting room table which looks extremely interesting with all the shiny instruments, syringes and stethoscopes and they want to pick up all your instruments and try to put their hands in the sharps bin or pick disgusting things up off the floor. One of the benefits of keeping the consulting room tidy and disposing of any syringes or bloody pieces of cotton wool is that not only does it look much better to the client when they enter, but there are also fewer things for a small child to find and stab themselves with or put in their mouths.

Try to maintain control of the situation and tactfully suggest and then insist that the children stay next to their parent and warn the parent if appropriate that there are things in the consulting room which should not be touched. Some parents resent their child from being discouraged from doing whatever they like and seem to think that the vet's consulting room is an animal theme park or a potential hands-on learning experience.

If necessary, tell children clearly and firmly where to stand and not to touch anything and tell them why. Some children respond much better to the authority of a stranger than they do for their parent who may be very glad that you have taken charge. The parent who objects to having their little monster told not to touch is usually keener to comply if you point out how many filthy ears the auroscope has been down in the past hour and that things 'might be contaminated'. No one wants to see a child injured or put something unspeakable into their mouth and if they do, then suddenly it will be all your fault. A favourite for toddlers seems to be chewing the edge of the consulting table, the surface of which will have been cleaned but may still have the odd crusty bit of unidentifiable debris underneath the rim. Mmmmmm, tasty!

Children who are included in the consultation are often less likely to look for their own entertainment and can sometimes be more reliable at giving history than their parents when you ask what the dog may have eaten to cause the projectile vomiting. They will spill the beans and tell you that the dog stole some chocolate or fell in the canal the day before.

It is important to be aware of the presence of children in the room when discussing the prospect of death and dying and you may be aware that you need to deliver bad news while the owner is oblivious to the potential distress for a child who is listening. Check with the parent that they are happy to continue with the child in the consulting room before making any major pronouncements about potential surgery or worse. Teenagers will sometimes have picked up on the direction in which the discussion is going before their parent has, so you may need to think ahead and employ great sensitivity. Illness and death of a pet may be the first experience children have of a life not lasting forever and we need to keep this in mind and be as kind and understanding as we can, especially when imparting bad news.

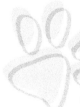

Having said all this, it is not uncommon for a parent to tenderly tell their child all about how Smoky has gone to sleep and will be with Grandpa in heaven and for the child to say, 'OK, how sad, can we have another kitten?' Small children often may not understand the concept of death and be less affected than the parent, but my advice would be to let the parent handle the explanations.

Communication difficulties

There may be times when, for various reasons, you find communicating with a client quite difficult. If a client has a hearing aid or appears to have compromised hearing, make sure you offer the use of hearing loops and speak clearly facing them so that they can see your lips moving but do not shout at them. Shouting at someone with a sensitive hearing aid can be extremely painful for the hearer and make things even harder to distinguish and so clear enunciation rather than volume is often what is needed.

Some clients will arrive at the surgery under the influence of either drugs or alcohol, especially out of hours, because an emergency with an animal can happen at all hours of the day or night. It may be that the accompanying inebriated human is not very easy to talk to and may find it difficult to understand the procedures which their animal may need. Your personal safety takes priority over all other considerations but there are also steps which you can take to help in situations such as this to make sure that the consultation proceeds. It may help to ask another member of staff to come into the consulting room with you so that you have a witness to what has been discussed and you might feel it appropriate to ask the client if you can call anyone to be with them and support them.

Bear in mind that a client who is ataxic and may appear to be drunk may in fact be suffering from an illness or condition such as multiple sclerosis or a disability, so take care not to jump to conclusions but concentrate on facilitating the transfer of information between you and the owner for the benefit of your patient.

If it is obvious that someone is having considerable difficulty in understanding you, do not overload them with information and unnecessary wordiness but concentrate on the essential facts they need to know; write things down for them and offer a means of communicating with them at a later date. Try to obtain informed consent with a witness present if possible, especially when the situation is life-threatening, and attend to the immediate needs of the patient with emergency treatment such as pain relief and support as appropriate, though you may need to defer non-urgent treatment until you are sure you have been given informed consent.

Careless talk

When in the public areas such as the waiting room or behind the reception desk in a busy surgery, members of staff sometimes forget to be mindful of clients who may be hearing their conversation. You must of course be very careful about maintaining client confidentiality and it has been known for a client to overhear derogatory remarks about themselves or a relative or friend while waiting at the reception desk. Case discussions should always be confidential and private and if you start chatting to the receptionist or veterinary nurse in or near the public areas, then the subject under discussion may concern a patient or an owner who is known to someone in the waiting room. Try to keep in mind who is within earshot when you discuss the deterioration in the condition of an inpatient or an impending euthanasia. You may need to take an urgent call in the prep room and your conversation may be audible at reception if doors are left open, so be careful and transfer it to a more discreet area of the practice if necessary.

The waiting room will often have a steady stream of clients who are waiting in silence and can hear the conversations you and other members of the vet team are having behind the scenes which can sound flippant and unprofessional. When you are in the middle of the job you can become so habituated to the comings and goings in the surgery that you forget how it may appear and sound to a member of the public. If a client hears you laughing and joking in the background when they telephone to talk about their severely injured dog or ask when they can collect their pet's ashes, it can inadvertently create an uncaring impression and any vet who has been on the phone discussing euthanasia with a client while a loud party appears to be going on round the corner will recognise this scenario.

If you are in the middle of having a conversation with the receptionist at the desk and a client walks in, greet them and smile and acknowledge their presence rather than blank them and carry on your own conversation. You may recognise this scenario when you have been in a shop and two shop assistants behind the counter carry on discussing the details of their night out as though you were invisible.

You will be faced with situations where something hilarious happens and you may have to keep your face straight in the face of considerable difficulty. Working with the general public can have its downsides but more than makes up for it in entertainment value.

> *A receptionist of ours called Liz was an expert in keeping her cool even when faced with a client whose name reduced the other members of staff to mass hysteria. Mr Proudcock rang every month to discuss ordering and collection of prescriptions for his dog and to arrange various appointments and the phone was always passed over to Liz while everyone else dissolved into sniggering and giggles. He was on first-name terms with the vets and was a very good client who came in often with his dog which was epileptic. After a few years, the lovely Mr Proudcock rang to say he was moving to another part of the country and would be transferring to another vet practice. As usual Liz took the call and she was sorry as she heard the news because she had come to enjoy her conversations with the client who was always very charming.*
>
> *'I am so sorry to hear that you are leaving us, Mr Proudcock,' said Liz.*
>
> *'So am I, Liz, but I think it is now the moment,' he replied, 'to tell you that my name is Mr ProudLock, with an L and not ProudCock with a C.'*
>
> *He had clearly been aware all the time and enjoying the joke.*

Continuity of care

It is a great feeling when a client asks for you by name because it means that they have appreciated your treatment of their pet and you have done a really good job. You will build up a strong rapport with certain appreciative clients and they will be bonded to you and to the practice and you get pleasure from knowing them and their animal. Clients really appreciate continuity, especially with the treatment of a continuing case and if they have a good experience with a vet then they will prefer to see that vet again and will ask for them.

One of the most common complaints clients have about a practice is that they see a different vet every time they come, however while this is inevitable to some extent, there are ways in which you can help to give them continuity of care. Be aware of when your next consulting session is and if it is at a reasonable interval then encourage them to come back and see you, or actually make the appointment for them at the time. It is much easier to re-examine a dog and get an accurate picture of progress if you are the vet who saw it the last time and it is also really rewarding for you to see an improvement as a result of your diagnosis and treatment plan. Continuity of care and positive feedback are factors which make the work of a vet a pleasure and I would encourage you to foster those bonds with the clients and their animals. It is so much easier to work with a client who you are familiar with and who has trust and confidence in you and it makes the experience better for all concerned.

It can backfire if a client becomes so attached to one vet that they refuse to see other vets in the practice, so also convey to the client that all the vets in the practice are good vets and never imply that seeing another vet is a second-best option compared to you. If you have to book them in to see a vet who is new to them then say something positive about the vet such as, 'Will is an excellent vet, he will look after Fang really well', a recommendation which gives the client confidence even though it is not you who they will be seeing next time.

> *The relationship between you and your clients can become very close, especially if there has been life-threatening illness or injury and you have seen them through very traumatic times in their lives. Occasionally, clients feel that because you are a medical person they can share their own most intimate, personal, medical details.*
>
> *I have unfortunately been forced to hear far too much detail about a client's prostate problems before I managed to stop him in full flow and on one occasion was asked if I would check a client's nipples because she feared her nipple piercings had become infected. I managed to hastily prevent her from this inappropriate and alarming act of oversharing but it never ceases to amaze me how much personal detail clients are willing to divulge.*

The overall message I would like you to receive about clients is to encourage you to embrace the diversity of the people who you meet in consultations and recommend that you resist the mindset which considers that being a vet would be great if it were not for all those horrible clients cluttering up the place. Some vets will say that they feel worn down over the years by the behaviour of some members of the public and there is no doubt that you will see some really bad examples of the human race on the other side of the consulting room table, but the majority of clients are really agreeable people just like you or your family and friends.

Keeping a sense of proportion, remembering that the unpleasant clients are in a minority and deliberately looking for the good in people does help make you feel positive about your job. Building resilience is a very popular concept and we each need to adopt ways in which to protect ourselves from becoming disillusioned with working in general practice, but we also need to remember that it can be very entertaining and rewarding too.

CHAPTER 10

How to get on with the rest of the veterinary team

Some of my best and most enduring friendships have been with the nurses and support staff with whom I have worked over the years. They have been there for me at 3 a.m. with a caesarian and helped me with euthanasia of aggressive dogs who wanted to bite my head off. They have clung on to ferocious cats to stop them savaging me despite being clawed to shreds themselves, and laughed despite being sprayed with various bodily fluids during enemas and operations. They have comforted and supported me when a case went badly and with the ones with which I had become too emotionally involved who eventually died in my arms. They have been there silently encouraging and calming me when I couldn't find the vein in a difficult euthanasia consult or when I was searching for that elusive uterine horn in a cat spay. They have also been there celebrating the good times, became friends with me, enjoying social events, attended my wedding and supported me working during two pregnancies. I have become really close friends with some of the people I have worked with and remain so to this day.

The team you work with will see you at your very best and at your worst, day in and day out, and the experience of working a really busy exhausting day in practice can be made so much better and enjoyable by the people you work with. Working in a practice where you trust the people you work with to look after you and work with you as a team, passing you instruments before you realise that you need them, making coffee when you are flagging or lightening the mood with a smile or a joke, makes all the challenges you face as a vet worth it. I really hope you experience that camaraderie because it is like no other and enjoying your working day with like-minded colleagues is priceless.

When you start your first job in a practice it is important that, even though you may have qualified with honours and you have a brain the size of Stephen Hawking, you accept that at this particular moment you know less about everything related to this practice than just about everyone else, including some of the clients. You may have been top of your year at vet school but now you are going to really need the goodwill, help and support of all the people you work with and nobody really wants to help an arrogant smart-arse who thinks they are a gift to the profession.

The cooperation and guidance of the nursing and support staff is invaluable and if you are wise you will be approachable, open to advice and will take guidance from those who may be lesser qualified than you, but who are very experienced in veterinary practice and especially in this particular practice and its clients.

The nurses and receptionists know where everything is, who everyone is, which clients are really difficult, which vets should not be spoken to until after eleven o'clock, where the chocolate biscuits are and which are the best pubs. Your vet colleagues are very important and may be your clinical mentors but in practice you often spend much more time with the veterinary nurses and support staff and they can make your life so much easier if they feel warmly disposed towards you. You might have the veterinary degree but they know far more than you about being in practice and they can ease your path and prevent you making mistakes, helping you when you are struggling and shielding you from potential danger. A new member of staff who is unappreciative or rude or offhand to the nursing staff will live to rue the day, so make a special effort to connect with them and be part of the team.

Despite the fact that the nurses may initially know more than you do about their practice and have seen a cat spay so many times that they could probably perform one more easily than you can, it is still you, the veterinary surgeon, who holds the position of authority when it comes to the animals in your care and the buck always stops with you. The clinical decisions and the responsibility for those decisions is yours and so you will find yourself having to give instructions and directions to the nursing staff. The way in which you do this will set the tone of your relationship with them for the foreseeable future and it is entirely possible to assume authority and be assertive but remain respectful and friendly. You don't need to bark orders and stomp about without listening to the nurses to let them know that you are making the decisions and to gain their respect. A nurse who is on your side and feels appreciated will go out of their way to help you but a resentful nurse who has been snapped at when they tried to help you and treated as a lesser being can make your life a living hell.

There will probably be times when a well-intentioned nurse may question your decisions and hopefully they will do this in a tactful and helpful way. It may well be that they are in fact right and are trying to prevent you from making a mistake, so make sure you are listening to what they are saying, consider the facts and make your decision explaining why, if appropriate. You are going to be spending many hours with one another over the coming months and a little tact and diplomacy goes a long way to producing a happy working environment.

Listen to feedback from them and ask for their opinions because they are watching vets work all day, every day and they see how different vets do different things so they will have useful advice to give you if you are willing to listen. Be considerate in your demands on them and think about how you impact on their workload, and do not expect the impossible from them but be prepared to change your plans or wait when necessary.

Some members of the nursing and support staff will have been in the practice for years and will be considerably older than you and may be of your mother's or grandmother's generation. They may challenge your decisions and may be resistant to new ideas, especially if you want to change things to do it your way. When you are a new or inexperienced graduate this can be very difficult and undermines your confidence, but there will always be a way to exert your authority in a pleasant, friendly way and you should always preserve their dignity even when you decide not to do things their way. Many practices have a matriarch who has been there for years and she is often the one who drives you mad half of the time while offering immense support and kindness the other half. Just watch them swing into action when a client steps out of line and criticises you unfairly, when you will see them bring their significant arsenal of dignity, life experience and assertiveness into action to defend you, and observe the shock and awe.

Minimise distraction

It is essential that you are able to concentrate on what you are doing and although many vets and nurses do chat about anything and everything over the operating table, it can be very distracting if there is a lot of background noise so do ask for silence when you need to focus. Just politely request that everyone stops talking so that you can concentrate and explain why you need peace and quiet for a while. If they do carry on chattering about their exploits that weekend, do not give way on this but insist on silence. Some people enjoy background music as they operate whereas I do not and it is not unreasonable to make sure the environment is conducive to your ability as the surgeon to concentrate on the job in hand.

Vets and support staff work very closely together and share experiences which draw them together over long hours at work, making sharing of confidences, opinions and information very easy. This camaraderie and sharing can be a good thing and a great source of support for members of the team, but equally can be a terrible breeding ground for gossip and bullying. Don't get drawn in to any backbiting of any kind and if you see someone being bullied or picked on then you should challenge the perpetrator. Silence from you when someone else is being picked on or bullied can be taken for acquiescence and you may find yourself drawn in to an 'us or them' situation. This is particularly true when you first start work and you don't know everyone very well as you will not be aware of the practice dynamics and you need the support of everyone. It is so easy to fall into the trap set for you by a manipulative member of staff following their own agenda at this stage, so without wishing to be melodramatic, beware the cliques and the playground bullies!

It may seem obvious that you need to get on with your work colleagues but it is surprising how frequently vets seem to go out of their way to upset the support staff. Here are a few examples of how to get right up their noses:

❖ Talk incessantly from the moment you arrive about yourself and how great you are without bothering to ask about them and their lives.

❖ Make sure they know they are really lucky to have you there and that you really wanted to work somewhere else that was much better and that this practice was not your first choice.

❖ Ask everyone's name but don't bother to make any effort to remember it.

❖ Remind everyone that you are the vet and and refuse to listen to any suggestions or advice.

❖ Never clean up after yourself or anyone else including the patients.

❖ Don't ever do what you consider to be a nurse's task even when you can see they are really busy and you have nothing to do at the time.

❖ Never dispense your own medicines even though the other vets do.

❖ Tell the nurses what they are doing wrong in their work but be incredibly offended if they suggest a different way of you doing something.

❖ Speak to the staff in an offhand manner in front of the clients and put them down to make yourself look really important.

❖ Be friendly one day and then really grumpy and moody the next without any apparent reason.

❖ Moan all the time.

❖ Moan about your financial position even though you are making more money than they are.

❖ Moan about the other vets.

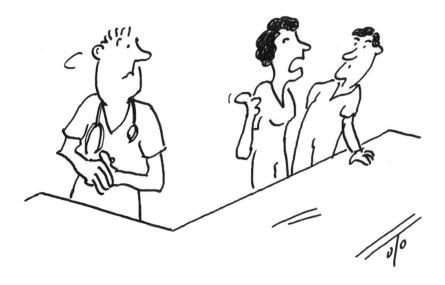

- Moan about your rota.
- Moan about the boss.
- Moan about the clients.
- Moan because the milk in the kitchen has run out even though you never go and buy any.
- Ditto the chocolate biscuits.
- Tolerate something one day and then moan about it the next day depending on your mood.
- If something goes well and it was a team effort, make sure you claim all the credit for it.
- If something goes badly, blame everyone but yourself.
- Have special favourite individuals amongst the nursing staff and make it really obvious that you prefer to work with them and are disappointed if you have to work with someone else.
- Criticise one nurse to another nurse and join in when someone is on the receiving end of snide remarks.
- Repeat negative comments that someone may have said in passing to those concerned.

Personality clashes

Some of the worst behaviours in the workplace are very subtle and they can taint the team spirit in a practice to the extent that people really do not want to go to work any more and may even be driven to leave. There are many different personalities in any workplace and it is inevitable that you will like some people more than others and prefer to spend time with them. Working with someone you do not have a rapport with can be really difficult and you will find some individuals really hard to work with, but this is part of life.

At vet school and in your private life you had the freedom to choose who you spent time with and, although you will have had to work in rotations with students whose company you did not particularly enjoy, the chances are that you could avoid them most of the time and keep the contact with them to a minimum. This is not the case when you are working in a small practice and the staff rota will throw people who do not particularly like each other together for many hours and in stressful situations.

You need to accept this and make the best of it, and avoid making it obvious that you prefer working with someone else as this can damage confidence and be very hurtful, just making matters worse. It is important that you go out of your way to develop and maintain a good working relationship with everyone in the team and, because you are the veterinary surgeon and the professional in a position of authority, even more is expected from you in setting an example to the support staff.

Some nurses and receptionists will be more experienced and better at their job than others and working with them makes your life much easier. You might grab every opportunity to work with that experienced brilliant nurse rather than another more recently qualified but it is very undermining for the confidence of a nurse who is not preferred and who is made to feel second best. That is often a student nurse or an inexperienced member of staff who is already lacking in confidence, so imagine how they feel when a vet makes it clear that they are trying to avoid working with them.

Having favourites can be really divisive and hurtful, causing unhappiness and division, so try to avoid it and treat everyone the same as much as you can. It is not unusual to see one member of the team who is popular with the senior vets and management being allowed certain liberties or having certain behaviours tolerated, simply because of who they are and this can cause resentment and discord within the team.

Never allow yourself to criticise one member of staff to another because that puts the listener in an impossible position. They may feel compelled to listen because you are a vet in a position of authority and it is inappropriate and unprofessional to put them in that predicament.

There will be sometimes members of staff who are just plain mean and nasty individuals but if you are courteous, fair and reasonable in your dealings with them then they cannot bring you down to their level no matter how hard they try. Even if they don't change their ways, you will have the reassurance of knowing that your own behaviour has been above reproach.

Your attitude to and handling of the animals

I am sure I do not have to tell you that you should never treat any animal you meet with anything other than kindness and respect. You have chosen a career in which to do anything else would be abhorrent but there have been cases where a vet has disrespected or ill-treated their patient, perhaps because they mistakenly thought it was funny or because other members of staff have created an atmosphere where offhand attitudes and ignorant behaviour has been tolerated. Most nurses have chosen their career because they want to look after animals and animal welfare is extremely important to them, so they will be justifiably horrified if they see anything but a caring approach to the patients.

One of the greatest compliments you can ever receive in practice is when another member of the practice asks you to treat their own animal because they have seen the way you work and they have faith in you and the way in which you relate to animals.

Talking about your salary to other members of staff

The support staff in a practice usually earn less money than the vets and it is very insensitive to complain about how hard up you are when your take-home pay is likely to be significantly greater than the people you work with. You are a highly qualified individual and have been to university for five years and quite rightly earn more money, but you do not need to rub their noses in it. They work extremely hard too and put in long hours, often cleaning up after you, so talking about your financial woes is just tactless.

If you are given gestures of appreciation from clients such as chocolates, then do not take them home to guzzle alone but share them with the staff. Good support staff make you look good, so share the appreciation that comes from the clients who often overlook them when the presents are being handed out. Once in a while, buy some cakes and don't be stingy about chipping in to the collections for people who have had a baby or are getting married.

Pitching in to help

Some days in practice, the support staff can be really busy and under pressure from a heavy workload while the vets might have much less to do for an hour or so. It may be that you have phone calls to make or urgent paperwork to attend to, but if you are sitting around with nothing to do and able to help, then do what you can to help out. Answer the phone or mop up after that dog and make a round of tea and coffee and do not sit around playing with your phone while the nurses run around working really hard. It might not be your job, but you are part of the team and no individual is too important to get the mop and attend to the puddle in the waiting room. You need leadership skills as a vet in practice and it is never too soon to learn to lead by example and earn the respect of your team.

When things go wrong and mistakes are made, it should always be looked on as an opportunity to prevent it happening in the future and not a time to apportion blame. If there

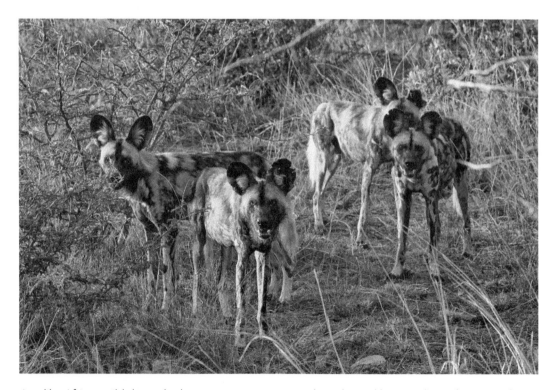

Just like African wild dogs who hunt as a team, more can be achieved by people working together in harmony, cooperating with one another. Make sure you are a valued and respected member of the pack by maintaining good working relationships with your colleagues.

is openness, honesty and understanding of the occurrence of human error then everyone feels empowered to speak up to avoid mistakes and the whole team takes responsibility for improvement of procedures rather than blaming individuals. Sometimes it is best to simply apologise to a client, even if it was at least partly someone else's responsibility and if you stick up for and protect other members of your team rather than dropping them in it simply to shift the blame, this will not go unnoticed and will be much appreciated.

Teaching

Most nurses learn through work placements and so it is likely that you will have student nurses working with you, also vet students and perhaps school children seeing practice. Be generous with your time and attention, as it was not so long ago that you were training. Teaching is an integral part of being a vet, whether it is educating the clients or mentoring and teaching those in the team less experienced than yourself. We should never stop learning from others and passing on our knowledge to each other in practice.

Socialising and more!

It is highly likely that you will become good friends and socialise with the support staff in your practice and while it is great to go and have fun together, it can bring its own potential problems. You will spend many hours with the people you work with and when working emergency out of hours shifts you often become very close to one another. It is inevitably an intimate environment and the circumstances and nature of the work we do brings us closer still.

Vets and nurses have often formed relationships at work with one another and, as in every workplace, this can present its own problems, especially if things turn sour. It is very awkward for everyone else if friends fall out and especially so if it is a couple who have fallen out and then have to work together. You are old enough and mature enough to know that you should not bring personal grievances into the place in which you work and if you do form a relationship with a colleague, be careful to have clear boundaries in place and keep your private life as private as you can without oversharing the ups and downs.

I have seen nurses become completely besotted with vets who do not recipro-cate their feelings and vets fancy nurses who do not feel the same way and vets fall in love with other vets and nurses likewise. It can be like a really bad soap opera with all the jealousies and recriminations played out in the practice when a fling turns sour and someone is nursing a damaged ego.

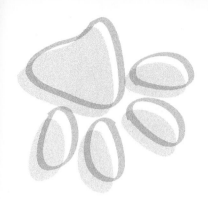

CHAPTER 11

How to get on with other vets

You have just spent five or six years with your fellow vet students, enjoying close friendships during your time at university and cementing those relationships over practical rotations and maybe some pretty wild parties. The important friendships which you make as a student will often continue after graduation, although you may need to make quite some effort to keep in touch. If you value those friends, you will continue to provide support and companionship for each other even though you go your separate ways. The relatively small size of the profession makes it likely that you will continue to maintain contact on social media and meet up with your peers from time to time at congresses and CPD meetings, but some friendships will inevitably fall by the wayside and new ones will be made.

There is as wide a spectrum of personality in vets as in any other group of people and there will be those individuals who you like and wish to spend time with and inevitably others who you do not. When you are a student, there are individuals who you warm to and others who you actively avoid and it is relatively easy to do this in the vet school.

Once you start work in general practice, you will be working very closely with other vets and you may find yourself working day after day with some people whose company you would not normally seek out. You just cannot avoid the vets who are working in a team with you and you will need to communicate with them effectively and build a relationship of trust. Even if you do not like a colleague, your working relationship with them needs to be nurtured and looked after and may require some effort from both parties.

There are countless ways in which we human beings contrive to irritate and annoy each other and in a busy practice there are all too many opportunities during a busy day under pressure. It is easy to fall out with a colleague when you are working in such close proximity and are passing cases on to each other. Friction between you and a colleague you work with will cause both of you pain and also impacts on everyone else in the veterinary team.

You might find you intensely dislike a colleague but it is important that you maintain a professional working relationship with them and do not indulge those feelings in the hothouse environment of the veterinary practice. When vets are sniping at one another all the time it creates a toxic environment to work in and can ruin the camaraderie in a practice. Most people have some good aspects to their personalities if you look hard enough, and there can be all sorts of reasons for someone's bad behaviour, such as anxiety or a lack of confidence, which, while not being an excuse, is at least an explanation for it. Always try to give a difficult or bad-tempered colleague the benefit of the doubt and make sure the way you behave is above reproach even if they are giving you a hard time. You might even be able to help them to improve the situation and everyone around you can breathe a sigh of relief.

You may have received the impression while at university or seeing practice in a state-of-the-art referral hospital that first opinion practice is full of ageing vets who are out of touch. The realities of life mean that there are compromises which have to made between the 'gold standard' which you may have seen as a student and what is feasible in first opinion practice in a poor area with a case with multiple pathologies owned by a client on a limited income.

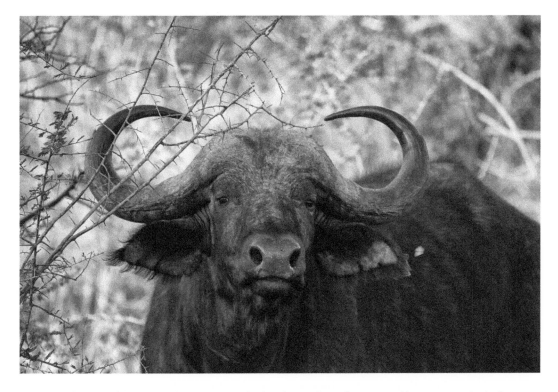

There is often an older vet in the practice who has been there forever and has a great deal of experience, and who may appear formidable. Such vets are walking repositories of knowledge, advice and tricks of the trade, and there will be few challenging situations that they have not previously encountered. Do not hesitate to ask them for help and for a second opinion on a baffling case. Despite their leathery exterior, they are usually more than happy to help.

Learn from and respect your experienced colleagues, because they possess multiple and varying skills which they have acquired from working in practice over the years. They may seem old to you and seem like wrinkly, battle-scarred dinosaurs, but they have survived the years and are still doing the job, and have a bottomless fund of knowledge and experience for you to tap into if you keep your ears, eyes and mind open. They should also appreciate your having up-to-date opinions and the knowledge you have recently acquired at university, especially if you present it in the right way with tact and diplomacy.

Golden rules for working with other vets

- Never, ever, ever, *ever* criticise another vet's work to an owner by a word or a look.
- Never, ever criticise a fellow vet's work to another veterinary colleague unless it is required of you by your employer for the benefit of the vet concerned and his patients, or is unavoidable on grounds of animal welfare. The only reason would be because you are actually trying to be constructive and never intentionally to undermine another vet's reputation within the practice. If you strongly disagree with the treatment a vet has performed or proposed, first of all approach the vet concerned in private as soon as you can and be willing to follow it up face to face and explain your reasoning.
- Never criticise a member of the support staff to another vet or to another member of support staff or to a client.
- Never book a heart-sink client or a really difficult case back for another vet without doing your best to personally warn them so that they are prepared for it and can read through the notes and think about it in advance. This includes your superior or mentor because even though they may be very experienced, it still helps to be forewarned when that stinker of a case is heading over the horizon.
- If you can make the life of a colleague better by a small or large act of kindness, then do so and be generous with your time and attention. It will be repaid many times over.
- Never score points or make yourself look better at the expense of a colleague.
- Do not gossip about the people you work with. If someone tells you a tasty titbit of information keep it to yourself and do not feed the gossip dragon. It is probably a half-truth anyway.
- Do not gossip about or bad-mouth the boss. They will know!
- Do not listen to or believe any tittle-tattle and reports of what anyone might have said about you. There are mischief-makers in practices who love to sow the seeds of distrust.
- Always give your fellow vets the benefit of the doubt if you are surprised at an action they have taken. You were not there at the time and might have done exactly the same in the circumstances.
- Say thank you when another vet helps you out or gives you some advice.
- Compliment your colleagues on a job well done because we all like positive feedback however senior we are.

Having told you how to get on with your fellow vets, here are some examples of how to really upset the people you work with and get right up their noses:

- ❖ If you see a case seen previously by a colleague, change the treatment and say you would not have given the original treatment as you always find X works much better.
- ❖ Increase your personal turnover figures by doing all the high-value work and leaving the low-priced hard slog to others.
- ❖ Even worse, write up the work that someone else has done to increase your turnover and your bonus.
- ❖ Avoid all the difficult cases or the ones which are lots of work for little recognition.
- ❖ Take no responsibility for a case which is not going well because 'it's not my case'.
- ❖ Refer a difficult case to the vet on duty at 5 p.m. on a Friday for X-rays and exploratory surgery, having dithered about with it all day or even all week.
- ❖ Leave on the dot at the end of your shift, every time leaving work undone for someone else to clear up because your social life is more important than anyone else's.
- ❖ Refuse to swap shifts but always expect others to swap with you.
- ❖ Moan all the time about how tired you are and how you have too much work to do.
- ❖ Moan about how you don't like the clients, the nurses, the other vets, the boss, the hours, blah blah blah. No one wants to listen to Moaning Minnie or Complaining Colin.

If you make a negative comment about another vet to an owner then sooner or later there is a very good chance that the vet will get to hear about it. You do not have to say very much, just a vague, off-hand remark that you would not have chosen that ear drop or antibiotic because you think another one is better, or an expression of surprise that a blood sample has not been run the last time the cat was seen. You may think that you have made an insignificant comment but that will not be what the client hears, and they will feel no loyalty towards you that would make them keep this to themselves. In their minds, they will hear you say that the first vet got it wrong and made a mistake or an omission, and they will make sure they relay this fact to the next person they see, especially if it is the original vet or the boss!

If the vets in a practice all trust one another completely and never denigrate or criticise the work of one another, then everyone is in a much better position when a malicious client tries to stir up trouble because you know for a fact that your colleague would never criticise you to a client. A collective confidence in one another exists so that you know that a client must be bending the truth; this gives power and resilience to all the vets in the practice.

It promotes more confidence in the practice for the clients too, because they do not have their confidence undermined by any hints of disagreement or infighting within the practice team. They become less dependent on seeking out their favourite vet and experiencing disappointment if they cannot see them if they are not at work for some reason, such as when they are on holiday.

If a client speaks negatively to you about a fellow vet, including one from a different practice, then do try to defend them as far as is appropriate or at least refuse to enter into a discussion about what they did. Never use the client's opinion as a means of inflating your ego and making you feel a better vet than a colleague who might have had a very good reason for doing whatever he or she did at the time. The client who flatters you now while having a go at another vet, will be the same one who metaphorically stabs you in the back next time your treatment is not immediately effective.

If you backbite about another vet to a veterinary colleague, then be under no illusion that this will stay confidential. Sooner or later that vet will hear a version of what you have said via the practice grapevine and it will probably be related to them completely out of context and will be very inflammatory. The person listening to you mouthing off will also think poorly of you and will be thinking that you are just as likely to denigrate them one day. It is so easy with the benefit of hindsight to perceive a colleague to have made what you might consider to be a blindingly obvious mistake or a misdiagnosis; the retrospectoscope would be a very useful tool but has yet to be invented.

Learning from mistakes

Vets are humans and vets do make mistakes; if something does go wrong, then you should support your colleague as much as you can, always giving them the benefit of the doubt and backing them up. I do not mean that you should conceal the facts or lie about anything and if you genuinely feel that there is a serious issue which needs addressing, then of course you need to act, but do this through the correct channels and discreetly. If you do think that a colleague has made a significant mistake, speak to them first in private and, if at all possible, in as friendly and supportive a way as you can.

The correct handling of an error should result in a learning experience for the whole team and an atmosphere should exist where mistakes can be admitted, corrected where possible and, most importantly, learned from and shared. The health and welfare of the patient is the primary concern and this should never be a time for petty differences and point scoring which prevents people from having the confidence to report near misses.

If you do have a serious concern about the performance of a working colleague, then you should speak about it to your employer, because there is a risk of compromising animal welfare. Anything you say to your employer should be regarded as confidential and there are times when we need to speak out to protect the well-being of our patients and the rest of the veterinary team. You should never go public as a whistle-blower unless all other avenues have been explored.

Working together

There are so many positive actions that we can take to help our colleagues and this usually makes for a happy practice. Look out for your fellow vets and take the strain when someone is having a bit of a bad day or struggling with a challenging situation. At the end of a busy day, helping a colleague with a case when you are not officially still working gives you the opportunity to learn and will be really appreciated.

There is a great Yorkshire saying, 'what goes around, comes around', which is so very true in veterinary practice. It is so much appreciated if you are willing to swap a shift to allow someone to attend a social event even if it inconveniences you and you would rather not do two Saturdays in a row. One day you will have a wedding to go to or there will be some event that you do not want to miss. If you swap with someone now so that they can go to a party, or if you put yourself out a little to help with a caesarian or a foreign body or step in when someone is running late, then it is far more likely that when you need a favour in return, that someone will step up and help you as you helped them.

Spare a thought for those vets with children or with other caring obligations such as elderly relatives to look after. They might always seem to be in a rush to leave at the end of their shift because of child minders, and afterschool clubs and carers are waiting. You are probably free of such obligations at the moment, but one day you will most likely be in the same position and will really appreciate a young graduate saying they can cope with the last-minute vomiting dog which has just arrived at the end of surgery.

Some readers may be thinking that I am stating the obvious and advising everyone to play happy families, and that they already have the social skills and common sense to know how to behave. The fact is that not everyone is blessed with this instinctive emotional intelligence and may not realise that flexibility and compassion oils the wheels of goodwill in the practice team. They may struggle to maintain good relationships with the people they work with and be bewildered by the fact that they are unpopular and that they might have upset people by their actions. They do not understand why no one wants to change a shift for them to book their holiday and they forget that they have never themselves said yes to any similar request in the past.

One of the saddest things I have experienced is to see more than one good vet leave a practice because they have experienced personality clashes and problems with the people they work with and they feel their only choice is to leave and start again. This can cause a great deal of heart ache for everyone concerned and any friction at work when you are already coping with the stresses and strains of your first years in practice is an extra complication that you can well do without. Follow a few ground rules right from the start, and this can really help you to work in a happy and collaborative atmosphere.

There are vets who definitely do not want to be everyone's friend and who prefer to come to work and do their job without engaging with other members of the veterinary team on anything but a professional level. The longer we are in practice then the more choice we have about where and with whom we want to work and we can choose the right work setting for us, but as a new graduate still learning our craft, we may have to compromise a little more and learn to fit in.

I know of excellent and highly successful vets who are aware that they do not work well with other vets and have chosen to work alone as much as they can. They may have made this career choice after experiencing working in a multi-vet team and finding that it is not for them. Some thrive much better in a one- or two-vet practice than in a big practice, even setting up their own practice after some time because they have very strong views and beliefs about how they wish to work and are often dynamic individuals whose clients appreciate their single-mindedness. Vets come in many different personality types and clients will gravitate towards vets who they respect and there is a place for everyone.

Being a square peg in a round hole

There are some personalities who are simply not suited for work in small animal first opinion practice and it is not the right working environment for every vet.

I once worked with a vet who seemed very relaxed at interview and who was well qualified and extremely keen. On starting work, however, it transpired that he was an adrenaline-fuelled, coiled spring and rigid about his expectations of both humans and animals alike, finding it very difficult when things did not always go according to his plan.

If he entered the feline inpatient ward, every cat in there, however sick, took one look at him and assumed fight or flight mode. A large proportion of the dogs he came into contact with also seemed to have an uncharacteristic desire to attack him and I have never known anyone get bitten and scratched and have so many near misses with animals that were usually docile and cooperative. He used to get really impatient with the animals and although he tried to suppress it, they reacted negatively, presumably because they sensed his inner tension and assumed attack was the best form of defence.

He was very keen and enthusiastic about his work and wanted to cure everything yesterday, and so was infuriated with any hesitation on the part of the owner to comply with his suggestions for investigation or treatment. He ricocheted around the practice like a commando on speed, amazed that no one took his advice or seemed to be moving as fast as he thought they should.

He had received all the training and passed the exams but possessed none of the finesse and innate empathy with the animals that the clients and the rest of the practice staff were comfortable with and were used to. Many clients saw him just once, then refused to see him again and the rest of the vets and nurses hated working with him, which was devastating both for him and for the practice. He referred to the inpatients as 'the pyo' or 'the bitch spay', as if they were inanimate objects and had no concept of them as being anything other than a challenge to diagnose then make compliant with his treatment plans. He was not a bad person but certainly not cut out to be a vet in a first opinion small animal practice at that time, and he left after a short time much to our relief.

There is far more to being a good vet than being a brilliant diagnostician or surgeon. Eventually, this vet did find his niche in a large animal practice doing a lot of testing and enjoyed the physical challenges of the work. Gradually, he must have altered his behaviour and acquired the skills he needed to work with his colleagues and clients. It is always possible to learn better techniques and interpersonal skills even if they do not come as naturally to you as to others.

Getting along with your mentor

Your practice may have, and indeed should have, provided you with an official mentor from whom you can ask advice and who will look after you at work and guide you in your first months. Some larger organisations have formal, organised support in place for new graduates which may include the allocation of a dedicated mentor, but this may not always be the case in the smaller practices where there are fewer vets and support is on a more ad hoc basis. If the practice has not officially designated a mentor for you, then it is worth asking as it may just not have occurred to them.

A really good mentor or a work buddy can make such a difference to you in your first job and beyond and some vets really enjoy mentoring new graduates and teaching them. The demands you make on your mentor must be reasonable too, as this individual is most probably supporting you in addition to managing their own substantial caseload. They are not there to do your job for you but to enable you to do it yourself, so do not make their job unnecessarily arduous by not putting the required effort in yourself. Thank them for their time and trouble and be considerate and they will be happy to help you.

Making decisions is part of the job

Every day in practice, vets have to decide what treatment to advise for their patients and the making of these decisions is a fundamental part of the job and carries a great deal of responsibility. Vets make treatment plans all the time and have to live with the outcome of these decisions, even when things do not go according to plan.

The weight of this responsibility is hard to appreciate when you are a student but once you start work you realise the significance of the job that you are doing. When you advise a surgical procedure or you reach for a sedative to give to an animal, your decision really does matter and if you miss something or make a mistake with the dose of a drug, it can have serious consequences. It is not surprising that newly qualified vets who may be lacking in confidence in their ability are reluctant to make decisions and are tempted to continue to defer to a more experienced colleague, just as they did when they were an undergraduate.

There are many occasions when it is absolutely the right thing to ask the opinion of a more experienced colleague and they will be glad that you asked for advice rather than making a mistake. There is also, however, a temptation to continue to ask even when you really know the answer and to continue to reassure yourself by just checking. This comes from a natural, subconscious desire to avoid ever running the risk of making an error, but do try to resist the temptation to ask your mentor time and time again to double check absolutely every single decision you make, however trivial.

Look things up yourself and make a plan and if you need to ask a question, make sure it is at a convenient time and not in the corridor in the middle of a busy surgery unless absolutely unavoidable. If you go and look something up yourself, such as the dose rate of a sedative, you are far more likely to remember where that dose chart is located the next time rather than asking your mentor every day for a month. Every vet was a new graduate once and understands how much there is to learn and wants you to know you can ask questions, but do not abuse their goodwill just to lighten your load.

You may become a mentor to a new graduate yourself within a few years of being qualified because in some big practices a new member of staff is joining the team on a regular basis. You will be on the receiving end of the questions from the new graduate wet behind the ears and you will understand just how they are feeling. Give your time and kindness freely when it is your turn to be the mentor and remember what it is like to be the new kid on the block with so much to learn.

Team work

Never underestimate the value of team work in a veterinary practice and the benefits it brings to everyone associated with it, including the staff, the clients and the patients. Some of the most soul-destroying, stress-inducing, destructive words in practice are 'it's not my case', 'it wasn't me', and 'it's not my job'.

The best days in practice are often those when the workload is high, but everyone is working together like a well-oiled machine; those are the days when you arrive home with your legs aching but with the euphoria of having made a real difference and having achieved so much. If you have a good relationship with your veterinary colleagues, you will constantly learn from one another and the team as a whole becomes much more efficient. You can feel the buzz as you work in a successful team and it is like no other experience. A successful practice is only as good as the collective effectiveness of the veterinary team, otherwise it is just another variation on herding cats.

CHAPTER 12

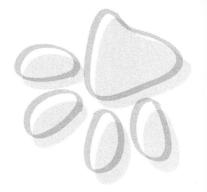

How to get on with your boss

When I speak to my fellow vets, most of them remember their first employer and continue to remember them all their lives, usually with affection and gratitude but occasionally, unfortunately, for all the wrong reasons.

A bad experience in your first job can cause catastrophic damage to your confidence and self-esteem, which cannot be overstated. Some graduates have even left the profession within a year or two of qualifying, with all their aspirations to work in practice destroyed after a bad start in a poor and unsupportive practice with an uncaring employer.

Hopefully, you will have chosen a practice with a really good boss who is willing to support you in your first job, will make sure that you have an excellent mentor and recognises that you need nurturing. The BVA supports an initiative to inform and remind employers about the importance of mentoring new graduates and many larger practices have put substantial systems in place for induction, mentoring and support for their new graduate employees.

For the purposes of this book, 'your boss' is the person who is in charge of you in the practice in which you are working. This may be the owner but could equally be the clinical director of the practice if owned by a company rather than individuals. These large groups of practices, often referred to as corporates, are increasingly more common as practices are bought out and come under the ownership of companies. The clinical director will still rely on the loyalty and performance of the employees in the practice for its success and hence their own personal success, and so to all intents and purposes has similar interests to an owner in your progress and performance.

You and your boss should have the same aspiration for you, which is to be happy, healthy and enjoy your work. Contented vets are far more likely to come to work with a smile on their face and perform their jobs well and be a pleasure to work with, whereas miserable vets are more likely to moan all the time and are less likely to make the clients happy. Unhappy, disillusioned vets may do just enough work to fulfil their obligations but may not go out of their way for the benefit of their patients, their clients or their practice. They are more likely to ring in sick, cannot wait to leave the building at the end of their shift and, while they may not neglect their job, they never do more than they need to do, rarely smile and can be soul-destroying to work with. I have no doubt that many vets work very hard at pleasing the clients and perform well, even though they are hating their job for various reasons.

If your expectations match those of your boss and you are enjoying your job, then it can only be good for the practice; a contented employee is unlikely to bring many problems to their employer. It does help, however, if there is give and take on both sides and so you too have a role in ensuring that you try to get on with your employer and you should play your part in maintaining a good relationship.

From day one in practice, you have a major influence on the financial performance of the practice in which you are working. You will make a difference to the productivity of the practice and because you are an employed veterinary surgeon and drawing a salary, you now have financial responsibilities to your employer as well as to your patients and their owners. Reinvestment in equipment and premises is generally dependent on the financial success of the practice, whoever happens to own it, so if you want to work in a well-equipped and well-maintained practice, then you should work hard to increase its chances of success. Salary levels for the employees of a practice are dependent on the profitability of that practice, so if you want to be well paid, then you need the practice to make a reasonable profit.

From an employer's point of view, most new graduates rarely earn enough money to cover more than the cost of their salary and other associated expenses for at least the first six months of employment, if not longer, and so it is a significant financial investment from your employer when he or she employs you as a new graduate.

It is also quite a big investment from the boss personally, because employing a new graduate is a bit like adopting a puppy. You want the new addition to be housetrained quickly but you expect the odd mess to clear up, and you are prepared to invest quite a lot of time and effort in training so that you can enjoy the pleasure of a well-trained companion. You enjoy observing the youthful enthusiasm and learn quite a lot yourself from the experience but there are days when you shake your head and wonder why on earth you took on the responsibility.

When I meet my first boss, he never fails to remind me that in the first six months of employing me I managed to completely write off the brand new practice car. It was a dark-blue Chrysler with vinyl seats that were the colour of calf diarrhoea, but that is still not a good enough reason for the treatment I meted out to it. In my feeble defence, I had only passed my test a few months before graduation and so had very little driving experience before he just handed me the keys, and I started work in a mixed practice in South Yorkshire with a brand new car and very few miles of driving experience.

In those days, I had to drive between three small branch practices which were 'lock-ups', surgeries in converted shops with no nurse to help and with open surgeries with no appointments. We just arrived and unlocked the door in front of a queue of clients, consulted, dispensed the drugs from a visit bag, took all the money and dished out the receipts ourselves. Between surgeries, we did a round of house calls and so I was driving over a hundred miles a day around Sheffield and Rotherham either side of the M1, and frequently going under or over it and around various roundabouts.

This large amount of mileage combined with my lack of driving experience and the pressures of being a new graduate was a recipe for disaster and I drove up the back of a lorry at a roundabout while thinking about a challenging case. I repeated this again on at least one more occasion before finally rolling the car over onto its roof in a snowstorm on the top of the moors and condemning it to the scrapyard. Thankfully, I survived and my old boss can laugh about it now, although he was not laughing at the time and nor was I!

Appreciate your boss, warts and all

It can very tempting to consider the boss to be a heartless person who may be a vet like you but who has gone over to the dark side and doesn't have any understanding of your lot!

It is the evil boss who put your name on the rota to work late on Christmas Eve and who is in final control of the holiday allocations. They are the one who says no to your request for a day off and the one you have to see when things have gone wrong and a client complains. They want to know who dropped the endoscope and why the place looks like a bomb site, and who asks you to attend that meeting next Tuesday for your review.

It can be hard to feel much sympathy for the boss but consider just for a moment what they may be dealing with in the average practice. Veterinary practices are very complex organisations and at any one time depending on the size of the practice, your boss is likely to be dealing with a number of challenges of varying degrees. They may be worrying about the latest new practice opening up down the road, a recent drop in turnover and the two staff pregnancies they have just been told about; there may be a vet off sick, the mysterious discovery of the expensive, broken endoscope and a practice standards inspection looming, and they may have just been informed that three grumbling clients each want a phone call.

It may seem to you that the boss is an aloof and soulless individual who employs the seagull form of management, that is, they fly in, make a lot of noise, dump on someone from a great height and then leave. We can all agree this is not good, but before you hasten to judge them remember that even the boss is a human being and can have bad days.

Many practice owners or clinical directors are under a great deal of pressure to deliver and cannot just arrive for work, do what they have to do that day and then go home and mentally close the door on their work without a care in the world. They will have a continuous stream of concerns and their life can be a little like managing constantly spinning plates with them moving round the practice making sure everything is running smoothly.

It can be quite lonely being the boss and as the practice leader, they need to maintain a certain authority and be the one who sometimes has to deliver unwelcome direction and information. Even the boss answers to somebody, even if it is the bank manager or a regional director and it is not all sitting in the office with a cup of coffee and your feet up looking at spreadsheets and gloating over your bank balance.

You do not have to become their friend, but it does help if you get on reasonably well with them and there are many ways in which you can have an excellent working relationship with your boss.

What you should expect from a decent boss?

- Respect
- Honesty
- Fulfilment of the terms and conditions stated in your job offer and contract
- Support while you are becoming proficient in your first year at least
- An allocated mentor
- Concern for your well-being
- Protection of your rights as an employee
- Protection from abuse by colleagues or clients
- Support in fulfilling the obligations of the RCVS Code of Conduct
- Opportunities to learn and advance your knowledge and skills.

But, remember that the boss is human too.

What can they expect from you?

- Respect
- Honesty
- Fulfilment of the terms and conditions in your job offer and contract
- Good attendance and enthusiasm
- Respect for other members of the practice
- Respect for the clients and a desire to provide excellent service for them and their animals
- Respect for the equipment and property of the practice
- Respect for the fee-charging structure
- A positive attitude.

What they want most from you is an employee who has the interests of the practice at heart, who expects to work hard during the hours agreed in the contract and who will be honest and a pleasure to be around. They want to feel that you will behave like a responsible professional and respect them, their other employees and the clients and not abuse their trust.

Bosses will love you if you are willing to be flexible

If you and your employer have been completely honest when negotiating your job then there will be few surprises once you start work. There will be times, however, when the unpredictable nature of veterinary practice means that everything works better when people are prepared to be flexible. If it is exceptionally busy, then a willingness to work until the work is done, and an acceptance of reasonable requests to go beyond the exact minute that your shift is meant to finish, will be much appreciated. I do not mean night after night of late finishes without any change to the staffing levels but under special circumstances when that day from hell arrives, as it always does, and everyone needs to work a little longer to get the work done.

Your support and help will be appreciated so much on those occasions where they are experiencing staffing difficulties, such as during a flu epidemic or when an emergency comes in just as you are about to leave at the end of your shift. Some people are never willing to work more than they have been contracted to and will always say no to any request to help. When faced by multiple problems in a crisis, it can make such a difference to a boss if you hear your vets say, 'I can do that if you like', and offer to help you by covering a shift or swapping to help out.

When, one day in the future, the time comes that you yourself need a helping hand or a bit of a favour, they will definitely remember the times when you were willing to step up and help out when they were struggling. A good employer who sees that you have been willing to step up when needed is likely to ensure that when things are quieter you can leave early and will see that your willingness to go the extra mile is rewarded. If there is a promotion in the offing in the future, then someone who volunteers to take extra responsibility and contribute time and effort towards the good of the practice will naturally be taken into account.

How to be fair to your boss

If you said at your interview that you were content to work weekends and nights then it is unreasonable to complain about it once the job starts. Make sure that you check your job offer and check your contract for exactly how many shifts you are contracted to do before insisting that you are working too many shifts and complaining about it.

If there is a genuine problem with your shift patterns or your on call rota, then do not moan about it to all and sundry, and put up with it while seething with resentment, but go and talk to the boss about it. If you feel sure that what was promised to you when you took the job has changed, then it is only fair to give them the opportunity to address the problem and they might have made a genuine mistake. If you are being asked to do more than is in your contract by a third party, then make sure the boss is not oblivious to this and the last to know, only finding out when you leave. Complaining about a grievance to everyone but the person in charge is not helpful and is not going to change your lot.

It might be that circumstances beyond their control have resulted in your work pattern changing temporarily and you might be asked to do something extra as a short-term solution to keep the practice running. It is completely reasonable to expect to be paid adequate recompense if this is in addition to your contracted work and not covered by your job description and salary as stated in your contract. Your help and cooperation will most likely be appreciated very much by your harassed boss but make sure you have some idea of how long these extra duties are likely to be expected of you so that it does not become a permanent fixture. There should be open communication between an employee and employer or manager and these discussions should be civil and polite.

Tell your boss straight away if you make a mistake

There will inevitably be times when you make mistakes and the first thing to do is to tell your boss without any delay. Never be tempted to conceal or lie about anything that has gone wrong as there will be very few disasters that the boss has not seen before and they will know what to do to minimise the damage and deal with the aftermath. The sooner they are notified, the better, and your boss will not be surprised because every new graduate makes mistakes, as indeed does every vet, so give them the facts as soon as you can. To err is human, but to lie about it is foolish, unprofessional, counterproductive and a far greater threat to you and your future as a vet than any mistake. It is at times like these that you will really appreciate your boss and you will always remember that time when something went wrong and you needed a helping hand and someone to back you up, and it was there for you.

Speaking up when things are not right

Most good employers much prefer it if you talk to them about anything you are worried about either in your work or in the practice as a whole. It is far easier to help you to prevent something going further wrong than to be asked to sort it out a long time after the event. There is so much to learn in practice at first that it is bewildering, and you may not know what to expect or how to extricate yourself from difficulty, but if you are experiencing a problem then you will be surprised at what your employer can help with if it is brought to their attention.

Every practice has its own way of doing things too, so you cannot always assume that what happens in this practice is the same as in the practice in which you saw EMS. You will most likely have been assigned a mentor or buddy in the practice and the nursing staff will help you too, but if you need help, do not hesitate to speak to your boss direct.

You definitely need to involve your boss when you have a serious problem with a client or another member of staff. Your employer has a responsibility to all employees as regards bullying and discrimination, so if something significant happens to you in the workplace, go and speak to them privately and immediately. Don't tell them about it days later when there is no evidence and nothing they can do about it.

If a client is rude or offensive to you then you need to speak up as soon as possible and you should not be expected to tolerate it, particularly if they are verbally or physically abusive. Inform the client that you are not going to listen to any further abuse and remove yourself from the situation and tell your boss immediately, giving them all the facts. I used to descend on any client who was abusive like a Valkyrie; I would not tolerate such behaviour to my employees and had no hesitation in telling those clients to seek their veterinary services elsewhere. It is a bad habit of some clients to be much ruder and more offensive to support staff and younger vets than they are to older vets like myself, and it used to make my blood boil if the same client came in to my consulting room all sweetness and light after I had heard them rudely blasting the receptionist for something trivial. They were made aware in no uncertain terms that such behaviour would not be tolerated and that unless they changed their ways, they were not welcome.

There will be occasions in every workplace where friction arises between work colleagues, especially when people are under pressure and the work is relentless and stressful. You will need to make your own judgement as to when you can deal with a situation such as this yourself and when you need to ask for help from a senior member of the team. No one can give you a formula for this and there has to be give and take and tolerance when working with other members of staff, but you should not have to put up with unreasonable behaviour just because you are new to the practice and younger. Vets can be bullied by support staff just as easily as nurses by vets, and if you allow certain unreasonable behaviours towards you to escalate without dealing with it, then it can be very difficult to regain a good working atmosphere. If bullying is not brought to the attention of the management promptly and nipped in the bud, the situation can deteriorate so badly that it can be hard to remedy and all parties suffer.

If you are unable to work

If you are too ill to work then, unless you are unconscious, phone in yourself and give as much notice as you can because someone else is going to have to cover your shift and it takes time to organise another vet. You either are too ill to work, or you are not, and you do not need to feel any guilt or worry about who is going to cover your shift if you are genuinely ill.

The following may sound harsh, but please don't put on a pathetic, childlike, whimpering voice demanding sympathy when you ring in sick because you are an adult and it is not necessary and is also very annoying. Your boss may sound distracted when you tell them about your terrible cough and this is not because they are unsympathetic or do not believe you, but because they are already thinking desperately about how they are going to cope with being a vet down. They are just not going to be as sympathetic to your woes as your mother would be, so do not think they are being uncaring, just tell them what the problem is. Your boss will completely understand that you are unfit for work and will not want you to give a virus to everyone else, so if you are too ill to work then just say so and try to give as much notice of how long you are likely to be off, if possible.

If you have a serious medical problem, then do not try to bravely carry on working when you are unwell as this will be bad for you and potentially harmful for your patients. Vets are notorious for not seeking medical help when they are unwell and for feeling they are indispensable and have to soldier on for the good of the patients, but your health both mentally and physically is more important than anything else at all. Your employer wants to help you to keep well, both for your own sake and because when you are feeling good and enjoying the challenges of your work, you will also be performing at your best.

Throwing a sickie

Please don't lie about being ill either and skive off for the day, because this is not worthy of an intelligent professional person. In these days of ubiquitous social media and the close relationships between members of staff, it is highly likely that your boss will find out. However good an actor you are, your boss is likely to be very astute when it comes to identifying insincerity even in a phone call. Be honest and do not let your boss down by having a duvet day because you think they can easily manage without you. You may think you are the only person off that day and be completely unaware that two other really sick people have rung in that you didn't know about and appointments are being cancelled. I could always tell when someone was genuinely ill and when they were borderline, and I could definitely tell when they were lying. The usual culprits tend to be repeat offenders and though they think they are very clever, the chances are their boss will know.

It is often the case that colleagues will be affected if you are off sick and they will offer their help in covering shifts at short notice. If they find out that their goodwill is repeatedly being taken advantage of by a fellow worker pretending to be ill, then they will be extremely annoyed and will often be the ones who will bring this to the notice of the employer.

One of my employees popped round with a bunch of flowers to the home address of a fellow sick employee who was a suspected repeat offender who had phoned in with gastroenteritis. She suspected she was being economical with the truth and sure enough, when she arrived at the house she found her just about to get into the car in her running gear.

Another nurse who rang in sick after a heavy night out announced to her friends on Facebook that she was 'dobbing off work with a bit of a hangover and going shopping' which was rather foolish as she was 'friends' with the head nurse who was incensed at having to work the late shift for her.

Be fair to your employer and do not deliberately and cynically book six weeks off for elective surgery just at the time when it is your turn to work the week of Christmas, so that some other poor vet in the practice has to cover for you. Some people can behave in this way and justify it to themselves as being someone else's problem, but it is surprising how selfish behaviour can rebound on the perpetrator somewhere down the line. Employers and colleagues soon notice a pattern of being ill on a Monday or a Friday and this will be taken note of with many practices requesting attendance reviews for repeat offenders.

Talking about problems with your job!

If you decide you need an important conversation about your work, then do ask to meet with your employer but arrange a suitable time to talk in private and without any time pressures. If you are having a problem with your job itself, then it is much better to talk to your boss and not bottle it up until you reach crisis point. There may not be anything they can do about the situation, but most employers will seriously consider reasonable requests, especially if you have thought of a solution. Do not accost them in the corridor between operations on a hectic, busy day to tell them you are thinking of leaving because you are unhappy or to announce that you are pregnant. If it is a job-related issue or a complicated request, it may be helpful to email your boss setting out a brief résumé of what it is you want to discuss so that they have some thinking time and don't have to make a knee-jerk reaction to a request.

Employers have already invested money and time in advertising, interviewing applicants, recruiting you and inducting you into the practice and if you are a good vet, they will want to keep you if they can. If you feel something is not working for you then if it is feasible have a reasonable solution in mind, but be aware that you may be one of several vets in a team and that agreeing to one request can set a precedent for your employer. This can mean that they may have to refuse what may seem to you to be a very small concession. In some cases, however, it may be that adaptations are possible and if they can keep you happy by being flexible then they are likely to try to do so.

I had a situation where a new graduate I had employed full-time felt she could not cope with the pressures of a full-time job after all, and we came to an agreement to reduce the number of her days at work until she felt better able to cope. Within a year, she felt able to increase her hours when the opportunity arose and she went on to become a very successful and valued member of staff. There was, of course, a reduction in her salary when she was working reduced hours but it was much better for her than leaving altogether and looking for work at another practice with the stress of having to settle in all over again when she was feeling vulnerable. Requests for flexible working patterns when it is possible to accommodate them are good for everyone, as long as the business and other members of staff do not suffer any ill effects and I believe it is the way forward for veterinary practice.

Money

Money is definitely a very important matter for employers, not because they are all money-grabbing, cut-throat swines as often portrayed, but because they have to balance the books at the end of the month or perhaps achieve the targets set of them by the management team.

You may be the owner or the manager of a practice one day yourself, but even if you are never responsible for controlling the costs of running a practice, having an interest in practice finances will enlighten you and will earn your employer's respect. There are often threads at CPD events about practice management and finance which you may find very interesting.

Am I being underpaid?

If you have been in your job for a while and you feel that you are now worth more in salary, then it is not unreasonable to ask to talk to your boss about your work and payment prospects. I have known a vet leave a job because they saw another one advertised elsewhere for more money, even though they have not actually asked for a pay rise at their existing job. It is always worth asking and if you are a valuable employee, your boss will be keen to keep you and if they cannot or will not pay you more, they can always say so. Some companies have set salary levels with no leeway but there are still some where the rate is negotiable and so it is always worth asking the question. If they say an increase is not possible, you will at least know where you stand and can make an informed decision as to your future plans and at least you will have given them the opportunity. I think that in the past, women have perhaps been less likely to ask for a pay rise for one reason or another, and we should be just as willing to enter into this discussion and close those pay gaps between men and women doing the same job.

How to make your boss sad

Bad-mouthing the boss is a very popular pastime for employees in veterinary practice generally and to a certain extent is inevitable. Your boss, however you may feel about them personally, deserves your respect and cooperation and the relationship you have with them should be one of mutual confidentiality and loyalty. Just as you have the right to be treated with consideration, and it would be completely inappropriate for your boss or manager to discuss your personal matters with other members of the team behind your back, so you should also confer the same degree of consideration upon them. Try not to join in with any backbiting, gossiping and personal criticism about your employer as it is unprofessional and bad for everyone's morale. Avoid commenting about any work issues on social media in the heat of the moment as it is disloyal to the practice and you may later regret it.

> *The fact is that the boss always hears about such things from one source or another, and for years I knew of a nickname that I was given by my employees of which they thought I was unaware. In our practice, my veterinary partner and I were nicknamed the Duke and the Duchess so, if I had called in at a branch as I sometimes did with a box of cakes to sweeten some feedback on the figures, then they would say to their colleagues that the Duchess had popped in. It could have been worse and there are far more unpleasant names to be called, but I suspect that they had no idea that I knew. We were also aware of a good*

proportion of the low-level flak directed at us of the type that I expect exists in every practice. I meet practice owners who think that this does not happen in their happy band and that they are all close friends with their employees, but I suspect that once a practice reaches a certain size, it is inevitable that some form of hierarchy exists. This can take some vets by surprise when they become branch managers or clinical directors and are in charge of other people. It is very true that you should treat people you work with well right from the beginning, because if they like and respect you when you are a new member of the team then it is much easier to have a good team working for you some years down the line.

How to make your boss really hopping mad

A few things are quite unpleasant but tolerable about being the boss, but there is nothing worse than feeling confident that you have complete trust in your employees only to find that they have been dishonest.

Giving stuff away free doesn't sound nearly as bad as stealing, but in actual fact that is exactly what it is when you take something off the shelf to give to your own animals or those of your friends and family without writing it up and being willing to pay for it. It is theft and is dishonest, and is no different to shoplifting a packet of dog food in a supermarket because it is practice property and not yours to take. It is also theoretically theft if any employee fails to charge for goods or services deliberately or takes time off without permission. It is not a question of the amount of financial loss that has occurred, but the loss of trust and it happens quite often, so just make sure you don't do it 'because everyone else in the practice does'.

I recently spoke to a practice owner who only discovered after her practice manager had left that there was a secret system in place where each member of staff was given a day off to go Christmas shopping on full pay and which she as the practice owner knew nothing about. The members of staff tried to justify it by saying they all covered for each other and so they thought it was all right because everyone was doing it and it had been going on for years, but this must have constituted a considerable expense for the small business and was completely dishonest. The owner was more upset by what she quite rightly regarded as a betrayal of her trust than the loss of the money.

The drugs in the dispensary are the property of the practice and they are worth a lot of money. You might think this is obvious and that you would never do such a thing as to steal, but unfortunately stock 'shrinkage' is widespread in practice. Make sure you are never tempted.

A vet who worked for me agreed to vaccinate a litter of puppies belonging to the practice nurse for free using practice vaccine. The facts only came to light because a third member of staff felt they owed their loyalty to the practice rather than to their dishonest colleagues.

Investing your time and ideas

An enlightened employer will be delighted to hear if you have constructive suggestions which can make the practice better and it is equally rewarding for you to make a difference to the practice in which you work. If you have a really good innovative idea or a suggestion as to how something could be improved, whether it be a new protocol or a way of reducing waste, then do suggest it to your boss.

It is often the case that we older vets work away in a practice doing the routine things the same way we always have and until you arrive with your new perspective, we have never thought to change our ways. People do tend to be resistant to change and so it may take a little tact and take a little while until the boss and the other members of staff see the logic of your suggestions, or there may be a good reason why your proposal would not work, but a good boss will really appreciate your taking an interest. A willingness not just to criticise the way things are done but to come forward with a plan for improvement is the best way to approach change, and learning from new graduates happens all the time in forward-thinking practices.

Organise your thoughts and make a good case and then present it to your boss at a suit-able time. Try not to jabber on to the other members of staff about how terrible the present system is and how you have a much better idea for how things can be managed without actually coming up with a plan to make things better. People can be quite defensive about their practices and will leap to defend the status quo before you have had a chance to make a reasonable suggestion.

If you are thinking of leaving

If you have a problem and are thinking of handing in your notice, then please do not let your employer be the last one to know. The chances are they will have heard a few rumours that all is not well, and it is courteous to let them know what is happening in their practice and also to give them the opportunity to put things right if that is an option.

If you have agreed to work a specified notice period then it is professional to honour that commitment if requested and to work your notice diligently and hand over cases to another vet so that no patients are left in the lurch by your departure. It will be much appreciated and remembered, and the way in which you left will be remembered when you ask that employer for references when you apply for another job at a later date. You never know what the future holds, so even if you feel very aggrieved and angry or hard done by, I would recommend that you remain courteous and professional to your employer and colleagues and try your best to leave on good terms.

Confidentiality and speaking up

Do not discuss your salary with anyone else at work as this can cause division and ill feeling. Someone usually gets the wrong end of the stick and makes comparisons without consider-ing all the factors involved and so ends up feeling aggrieved.

If there is something going on in the practice which is illegal or worse still, against animal welfare, speak to your employer about it in confidence. No other member of staff should expect you to keep quiet about the mistreatment of an animal or another member of staff and while it can take a great deal of courage to speak up, we have a duty as professionals to speak out. The practice owner should not be the last one to know and maintaining silence of that wrongdoing is condoning what is happening.

If you are being bullied or treated unfairly by another member of staff, then do not hand in your notice and move on without speaking to your employer as they need to know what is happening within their practice and take steps to protect their employees. They may be very glad to have concrete evidence that bullying has occurred as there may have been previous unconfirmed episodes and the employer can only take action against a bully with firm evidence. Your employer should respect your confidence and make the resolution of any problems in practice their responsibility. If your concerns are not addressed or confidentiality is broken, then this is not the sort of practice you want to work in. Make sure your facts are accurate and do not just sound off at the end of a difficult day about trivial incidents. You know what is fundamentally right and what is wrong so do speak up for yourself and for any other member of staff who is being unfairly treated.

In our practice, we had a horrible experience where a young graduate was led into a situation which was very painful for her. Older members of staff in one of the branch surgeries had a culture of what they referred to as banter but which was in fact a practice of insulting one another using very inappropriate and offensive language. Because the new graduate wanted to be part of the team she joined in and was also on the receiving end herself of what were purported to be 'jokes' at her and everyone else's expense, and to which she responded in kind. The problem arose when there was a falling out over another matter and an accusation was raised against the new graduate of her having used sexist and racist remarks. This was reported to the practice management and of course an investigation had to be undertaken.

Once the magnitude of the situation was realised by those concerned, they wished to withdraw the complaint as they said it had just been expressed in the heat of the moment when they had had an argument over something else, but because an official complaint had been made it was necessary to ascertain the facts. I am giving this illustration of a very painful past experience for my previous practice because it shows how easy it is when working in a very small team with big personalities to fail to observe the rules of respect towards fellow workers. Do not be drawn into a culture of being party to actions or behaviour which you know in your heart to be wrong.

When you become 'the boss'

I became a vet because I wanted to work as a practitioner, but during the years after becoming a partner our practice expanded rapidly and I found myself having to manage a significant number of people, in addition to working as a small animal practitioner. I did not have any training in management for this formidable task and I am sure I made many mistakes on the way and I learned from some bitter experiences.

It is very likely that there will be times in the future when you are in charge and you will need leadership skills, so take every opportunity from the start to learn how to manage people. This can be as simple as the first time you are asked to supervise a school student on work experience or a student nurse; the leadership and team-building skills you gain early in your career may ultimately be used if you have your own practice or are clinical director for your own branch.

The ability to manage people may help in the future if you choose a different career path, for example in industry or in mentoring new graduates, so do watch and learn all the time. If you attend congresses it can be very interesting to listen to some of the speakers discussing

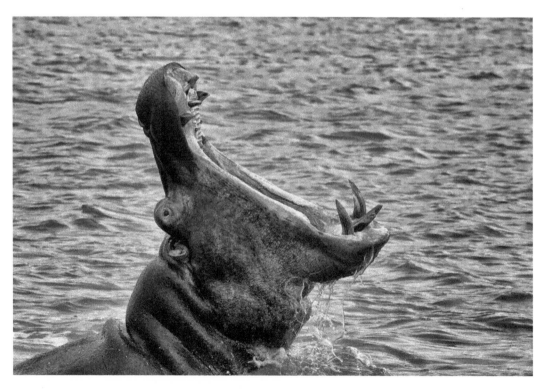

In every practice, there has to be someone who is in charge and though they may not win a popularity contest, they may not be as formidable as they appear. It is far better to enjoy a good working relationship with your boss than to be a thorn in his side. Even a hippo needs small fish to clean his teeth and prevent toothache, so cooperation is the name of the game.

the psychology of different personality types and how to communicate with them, and this can also help with your consulting skills. Business management and human resources management or at least an awareness of it is now included in the veterinary course, but the subject is as vast as the veterinary degree and infinitely interesting with new theories coming along all the time.

Finally, I hope you now have some understanding of what it is like to be the boss and to appreciate the responsibility that comes with that role, and the way in which you as an employee can affect the experience of the boss in a positive way. Often, the same individual is working as a practising vet doing clinical work at the same time as managing everyone in the practice, and is continuing to work at home when the working day is over. You do not need to be a sycophant but just remember that your boss is human too, and if they are as irritable as a hungry hippo on occasions, cut him or her a bit of slack because it is not always as much fun being the biggest person in the pool as you might think.

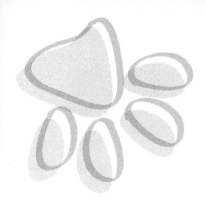

CHAPTER 13

How to get on with yourself

You will probably always be your own fiercest and most unforgiving critic throughout your veterinary career and many vets are very hard on themselves. No matter what you may think, every vet has moments of self-doubt and everyone makes mistakes, even those who are very experienced and those who may appear the most confident. It is the way in which you deal with those mistakes and learn from them and move on which makes you a good vet and enables you to continue to work in such a challenging job and remain well balanced.

Many veterinary surgeons choose our profession not only because they are interested in science and medicine, but also because they want to heal and improve the lives of the animals in their care. Ours is a job in which you can really make a difference to the quality of life of animals and their owners and what a privilege that is. You will see and experience at first hand the unique bond between humans and animals and you will have the reward of practising the art of veterinary medicine and changing lives.

You will see tough, gritty men crying with relief at not losing their cat after a road accident and you will help to save the life of a dog who is the only companion in life of a disabled person living alone. You will meet horse owners who rely on their horse riding for their mental health and children whose lives are so dysfunctional that the only constant in their lives is the love and attention of their dog. You will be in the unique position of possessing the skills to make a significant difference to many peoples' lives through keeping their animals alive and healthy. This may sound overly dramatic to you now, but during my career as a vet in practice I have witnessed so many special situations where animals and humans touch each other's lives and I will always remember them and feel so fortunate to have been able to make a difference.

It is a great profession to be a part of, but it also brings a huge amount of pressure on us as individuals and in order to be able to continue to pursue your vocation and enjoy life, you need to stay healthy and look after yourself.

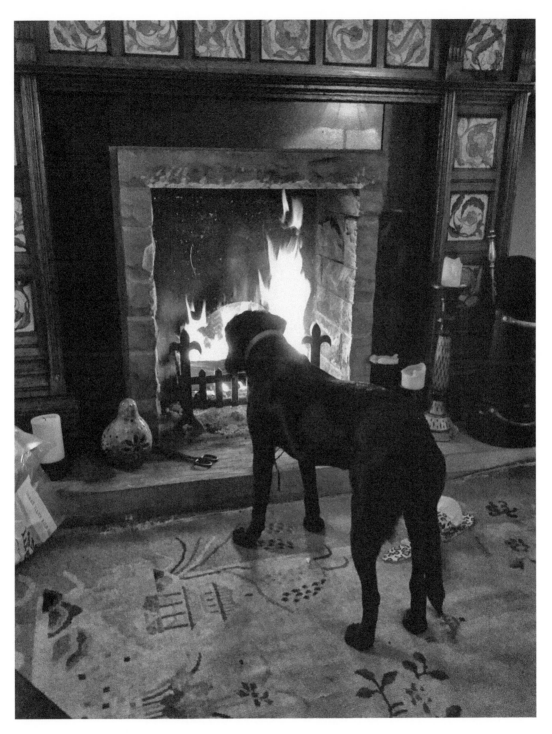

When you spend hectic days caring for your patients and their families, always remember to make time for yourself. Think about what makes you happy and prioritise some time for you to care for your own well-being.

If you experience burn out and leave the profession early, then not only will you bear the disappointment and the emotional scars of having lost the career you dreamed of, but the veterinary world will have lost a highly trained and motivated individual who could have been a great asset to the profession. It is crucial that right from the start you take care to look after yourself and avail yourself of all the help and support that is there to ensure that you stay well and motivated and happy in your life. Some of our colleagues will say that it is just a job to them and that they can separate it from the other parts of their lives, but for me, being a vet has been an intrinsic part of my life and has had enormous influence on the person I am now.

I have never regretted being a vet, despite the fact that my work used to build me up and then smack me down on a regular basis. Just when I felt I was getting to grips with what I was doing and feeling as if I might be a half-decent vet after all, along would come a case or a challenge which would knock me down to size. I think this happens to every vet in practice and it is the resilience and the ability to bounce back which protects you from permanent damage. Some people are naturally resilient and have the ability to shrug off adversity and forget those things which did not go according to plan, while others will be distressed when things go wrong and may dwell on difficult experiences, going over them again and again, which is not good for their mental health.

Ours is a profession which can present you with situations and problems which can trip you up and make you question your ability on a daily or even hourly basis. We are dealing with living creatures and they do not always respond as they should, or present as a classic case in the textbooks and this can be very challenging but it is part and parcel of the job. There are also financial constraints and time constraints which may prevent you from doing what you know you are capable of doing for a patient and vets often have to compromise and make the best of the time and resources available. Many vets are perfectionists and find compromise hard, especially when they know that they could achieve higher standards and do a better job with the right resources.

Seeking perfection is admirable, but I think the key to resilience is that sometimes we have to settle for a compromise which, while it is not perfection, is good enough for the job in hand and attainable within the circumstances in which we find ourselves. This can be hard to accept when you have very high standards and when you feel passionately about the animals in your care, but we cannot always achieve perfection in our imperfect world.

I am a bit of a worrier by nature, but I had to accept that sometimes things went wrong, and I had to learn from it and move on, leaving it in the past and using the experience to help me to do better in the future. It did not come easily to me to accept that there were occasions when I didn't do a perfect job or made a mistake and I had to learn to become resilient and forgive myself. I knew that if I wanted to continue to be a vet in practice, then sometimes I must put that poor performance down to experience and learn from it and do better in the future without beating myself up about it. If I had not learned to draw a line under a negative experience or a mistake and move on, then I don't think I would have been able to continue to work for over 30 years in practice and still be glad that I made that choice of career.

You will be aware that there is a great deal of understanding nowadays about the effects of stress experienced by vets in practice and much more is known about ways to protect yourself. We all cope with stress in different ways as individuals, and it is widely accepted that a certain amount of stress is an unavoidable factor in many jobs and it can indeed be beneficial to experience some pressure in our lives. While I would never seek to minimise the problems some vets face, I think it is important to recognise that the career we have chosen is by its very nature not predictable and it is not possible to cushion ourselves completely from the effects of being in this type of environment.

We have to build the capacity to do the best we can, and to work in less than ideal conditions and cope with difficult situations and events without becoming so traumatised that we cannot perform our role and live with the aftermath. We have to learn to develop a positive attitude to life and to recognise opportunities and reasonable compromises and adaptations to the circumstances in which we find ourselves.

We should also not accept unreasonable demands and conditions of work from either our employers or our clients without speaking up and trying to change things and if you are in a bad situation for whatever reason, there are many more avenues for you to seek help.

That six-monthly kick in the teeth

During my first six months in practice, I grew in confidence each day and every week I felt I was a slightly better vet than the week before. I passed a lot of milestones such as the first house call, the first euthanasia, the first caesarian, the first prolapsed calf bed and the first splenectomy, and after six months I felt I was really getting there as a vet. I felt rather pleased with my progress and I was full of confidence and enthusiasm, only for the biggest nightmare of a euthanasia consult to bring me right back down to earth with a crash.

Nothing went right with this case from start to finish. It was the middle of the night and I was on my own on a house call with the client who was in hysterics and with an uncooperative patient who was an old, semi-collapsed but aggressive Border collie. The owner kept letting go, I was scratched and bitten and there was not a vein to be found, and because the client was becoming more and more hysterical and was demanding that I call my boss, in the end I felt it best to capitulate. He came out immediately and of course he found the vein first time and the owner said he was wonderful and I crawled away to lick my wounds or at least to bandage my bleeding hand. My ego was the major casualty and my confidence had taken a real battering as the doubts rolled in as to whether I could cope and do a decent job or was a useless failure. I went back to work the next day and it was such a busy day that there was no time for navel gazing; the memory eventually faded over the following days but I have never forgotten that night and was a humbler person as a result.

A pattern seemed to follow and every six months or so, something would happen that I had not anticipated which would remind me that veterinary practice will regularly deliver a metaphorical slap in the face. I grew to realise that this was in fact normality and that it was something I was going to have to live with if I wanted to continue to be a vet. Over the months, it did become easier and I learned that I could bounce back and live with myself and that cases would go wrong, injustices would happen and people would behave badly, but I would survive.

The demands of experience

The more skilled you become as a vet, the more difficult cases will come your way and the risk of something going wrong is still ever present and may even be greater, despite you increasing in experience. If you look at the workload of your more experienced colleagues, you will probably find that they see a greater proportion of the longstanding and complicated cases and they often have to see the more difficult and demanding clients too. This is the inevitable result of being around for longer and the reward for being a better vet can be being asked for by name by a demanding owner because Tricky Woo just has to see you, and only you, every time. Every vet has one or two heart-sink patients whose names you dread appearing on your client list because they are so demanding. You have become a victim of your own success and though it is a compliment when a demanding client asks for you by name, it does not always seem that way at the time if the client is high maintenance.

I used to see a client with several animals who always kept a notebook and jotted down everything I said like a matronly Sherlock Holmes on a difficult case. She insisted on seeing me every time and flicked back through the pages during the consultation, appearing to be on the verge of saying that I was contradicting a pronouncement I had made previously which had been recorded by her three months earlier. As time progressed, I grew to like her and her dogs and cats who were a delight and very well cared for and I used to enjoy her visits because she always wanted the best for her animals. The notebook eventually disappeared, and I never really knew what it was that had triggered her suspicions and made her feel the need to record evidence but was very happy to have earned her trust.

The cycle of everything going smoothly followed by a bit of a bumpy ride is normal for the life of a vet in practice. Experienced vets may become better at coping when things do not go according to plan, but this is a job where the unexpected happens frequently and we have to deal with the variety and the uncertainty.

Perfection and compromise

Accepting that you are not going to perform every single consultation and procedure perfectly is going to make all the difference to you as a vet. I don't mean that we should become complacent with doing things badly but there are times when we have to do the best we can in the circumstances in which we find ourselves and not beat ourselves up about it when things do not go according to plan. Vets frequently have to settle for things being good enough but not perfect, and thankfully the innate ability of the body to heal helps us immeasurably by working with us to produce a better outcome than we may feel we deserve. The natural healing processes of the body are a wondrous thing and they are the vet's friend in a world where people cannot always afford state-of-the-art investigation and treatment. Our patients may not treat their surgical repairs with respect but chew their bandages off, rub their eyes on the furniture, take their own stitches out and scratch themselves until they bleed.

I am not advocating that you drop your standards or become careless, but you do need to be able to live with yourself when circumstances prevent you from delivering perfection. Most of all, you must be as understanding and kind to yourself when things go wrong as you would be to a friend or a colleague if things went wrong for them. Beating yourself up about it and putting pressure on yourself to deliver only the best every time, will make you unhappy and sometimes actually ill.

Do not become obsessive

There is a great temptation, especially for all those of you who are perfectionists, to become obsessive and to double check everything constantly and not to trust yourself to have done the right thing. By all means, take great care and check where necessary, especially in an unfamiliar situation but do not get into the habit of checking things multiple times or asking your colleagues to check up on everything you do. Find your own systems and routines, focus on what you are doing, avoid distractions, take ownership of the decisions you make and trust in yourself. You wouldn't have got this far if you were incompetent and not capable of doing the job.

Embrace feedback

Many practices have a system of regular appraisals to give you feedback on your performance, and it is equally important for you to give the practice feedback too on how you are finding the work and how things are going. Appraisals or reviews should be a mutual two-way exchange process between you and your boss and not a list of things which have gone wrong followed by admonishment. Prepare well for your reviews and appraisals and make the effort to fill in reports or feedback forms, which I know everyone hates doing, but they are a very useful tool for you to make sure your needs are being met and to make sure you do not go to the meeting without having given it some thought.

Sometimes, practices are not very good at scheduling regular appraisals for their vets and you may need to actively seek feedback about how you are doing and request a meeting. Ask the nursing staff and your colleagues how you are doing as well and if they offer suggestions for improvement, do not reward them for their honesty by being defensive. You will be reassured by the positive feedback and if you are given suggestions to improve then accept them with alacrity as a means of improvement and a learning opportunity.

Be brave

Organise yourself to make life easier and do not procrastinate but face challenges head on, taking all the help and support on offer for a new graduate. Do not avoid performing more complex surgery and the opportunity for more experience just because you are nervous or hesitant about your ability. You sometimes need to be a little bit out of your comfort zone and to push yourself to gain surgical experience, so be brave and step up when a chance is offered.

Shake it off

Do not compare yourself to others and do not be disheartened if one client complains and says they prefer another vet or a case baffles you. You will have clients who do not like you, and you will perform bitch spays which bleed, and there will be nurses who do not do as you ask, but these are not major disasters in life so shake them off. The real disasters in life are the death of a family member, or life-changing injuries from a car accident, not a minor mistake at work or a complaint from a client.

Try to remember that 99 percent of the things we worry about never happen and that in a year's time you will not be worrying about the issues you are dwelling on today, so learn from them and let them go.

Choose to be positive

There may be days when you are feeling really miserable and wondering why you ever decided to become a vet, but you still have to turn up and carry on working and seeing the clients. This is the time when you may need to make a conscious decision to change your attitude and actively decide that for the next few hours, you are going to forget about anything negative that has happened, slap a smile on your face, and start the next consulting session even though you may feel like running out of the building screaming. The clients neither know nor care that you have had a bad day and they are hoping and expecting to see a calm, confident professional who is going to deliver the best for their animal. You now have to act as if you are genuinely pleased to see them, be positive and cheerful, be really interested in their demonstration of their dog's cough and relish the delights of telling them all about the benefits of cat vaccination.

Often, you will find that by simply acting the part of a positive, happy vet, it lifts your mood and makes you feel happier in yourself. The clients respond to a happy, smiling vet by being pleasant themselves and they find it much more difficult to be grouchy or miserable in the face of positivity and friendliness. It makes for a more pleasant consultation all round and may remind you that being a vet is rewarding and can be fun and that most people are reasonable and good to know and so life is not so bad after all.

If you carry your bad mood and resentment into the consulting room with you, then you usually find that the clients react by being bad-tempered too and even the animals will sense your irritability and be harder to handle and less positive in their responses to you. The same applies in working behind the scenes and with your colleagues, so do not get sucked into the whirlpool of despair of miserable, grumbling moaners but seek out the company of the happy people as they will lift you too.

Coping with the day-to-day pressure and variety of practice life

I enjoyed clinical practice because I never knew what each day would bring and I enjoy new experiences, meeting people and the variety and novelty of a day in the veterinary surgery. Every day has some interesting aspects and what a pleasure that is in a world where in some other jobs people have to perform the same repetitive tasks day in, day out. There are routine tasks such as explaining for the millionth time about how to control fleas or the benefits of vaccination, but every animal is different and every client is unique and you never know what is going to happen next. It could be a cyanotic dog with a tennis ball lodged in the back of its throat or a patient in a critical condition after a road traffic accident or a whelping bitch. You might be examining a dog for a booster vaccination and detect the enlarged lymph nodes of lymphoma or spot a heart murmur and your knowledge and expertise might save a life. The unpredictability of never knowing what you are going to be faced with does bring its own problems and I am sure that the way I deal with the pressures of work will be different to the way you choose to deal with them. There will be things which you find easy which I found really hard and you will find certain tasks frustrating which I used to enjoy, but I do believe that our attitude and approach to our unpredictable life as a vet coupled with an acquired arsenal of coping mechanisms and techniques is what makes the difference in how we deal with the challenges and develop that elusive resilience.

A typical day in practice

Let us assume you are working in the right practice for you and have chosen the field of work which suits you best and that you are blessed with good health and are raring to go.

In vet practice, it is normal for a day which looks well organised and easily manageable on paper to have become complete mayhem by late morning. In this situation, some people react by staying calm, increasing their activity and becoming more productive, whereas others assume the headless chicken pattern of behaviour. They become agitated and make all the appearance of increasing their activity, but in fact become less productive because all their energy is in noise and bluster and ostentatious rushing around.

First of all, stay calm and assess what needs to be done most urgently and then concentrate on that task without being distracted by the huffing and puffing of the noisy members of the team who often do the least work and just wind up everyone else.

In an ideal world, every animal would be presented on time for their appointment with a clear and accurate history and with clearly identifiable symptoms, with an owner who has unlimited funds and an enthusiasm to allow all necessary investigations. Each patient would be amenable and cooperative, every owner would smile and appreciate you and everyone you work with would be happy, efficient and supportive.

Unfortunately, there will be times when your client will present without an appointment because their dog which is 'really ill and can't wait', comes in barking and snarling with its harassed owner and two small, free-range, wailing children. The dog will be so fat and noisy and aggressive that you cannot feel anything in the abdomen even if you could get near enough to touch it and everything you or the owner says is inaudible above the cacophony of dogs and crying children. You just manage to hear the client say that it has been ill for four days and that they have no money and that they usually prefer to see a different vet anyway.

It is very easy to feel resentful and downhearted in this situation and to feel that you have an uphill battle to do a decent job; there have been many occasions when this or a similar scenario has happened in my life as a vet. I am sure it will continue as long as humans and animals co-exist and veterinary practices continue to offer consulting services. This is the reality of what being a vet in first opinion practice can be like and our job is to diagnose disease and treat animals to the best of our ability and to manage it in the situation in which those animals are presented to us.

I am not saying that we should not try to change our working environment and encourage better behaviour from our clients and their pets, but if we accept that we will be faced with situations such as described above and manage not to allow ourselves to feel resentful, then we reduce our stress levels. Do the best you can at the time and follow the principles of good practice as far as is possible in an imperfect world.

Compromise is inevitable in general practice and we have to accept that on many occasions, the client's wishes and circumstances are not always the same as ours would be. There are some clients who may not agree to feed their animals a conventional diet, or prefer to try various useless alternative therapies before they come to you, or have insufficient money to pay for the level of treatment and investigation you wish to provide. They may simply not choose to spend any of their money at all on veterinary treatment, even though they have the funds. To some extent, you are not only a professional but also an advocate for your patient and you will need to use a certain amount of skill in communicating the value of what you can offer a client for their animal. Vets dislike feeling that we have to sell our services, but part of our job is in illustrating the value of what we can offer in the way of investigations and treatments to owners where these are in the best interests of the animal.

This is completely different to selling per se where the sole intention is to achieve targets and bonuses regardless of need, which is not professional for a veterinary surgeon. When you give a client a recommendation for a product or a procedure, it should never be for any financial reason and only that which is in the interests of your patients. It is up to the individual veterinary surgeon to decide what is the correct course of action for their patient and although a practice may encourage flea and worming product sales, and having regular dental preventative work is undoubtedly beneficial where appropriate, ultimately the clinical decisions and the responsibilities of giving a professional opinion are yours and yours alone.

Making mistakes

Vets are human and even the most well-intentioned and highly trained individual is not infallible and so there will be times in your career as a vet when you make a big and significant mistake. It is virtually inevitable, and it is the reason why every vet must make sure they have professional indemnity insurance from providers such as the Veterinary Defence Society. We pay for this insurance both to deal with the aftermath of our mistakes, when, if appropriate, they will compensate the owner or correct matters, and to defend us from unjustified accusations. When things do go wrong, contact them straight away, give them all the facts and let them deal with it and you will find they will be non-judgemental and extremely helpful as they deal with these situations all the time.

It is a truly awful moment when you realise that you have made a serious mistake and you will feel traumatised and terribly guilty, especially if an animal dies as a result. You did not become a vet to cause death or damage to animals but sometimes our actions or inactions have devastating results and we have to live with that knowledge. It is a horrible feeling and one that I and nearly every vet in practice or retired will have experienced in their time, and there is no reason why this should not happen to you.

The only comforting thing I can say, is that it is the way in which you acknowledge and deal with the aftermath of your mistake and the learning experience which you take away from it that is important in the end. Looking after the owner and the animal and providing any possible remedial action has to take priority over your emotions at the time, and the only comfort I can give is that you will not always feel as bad about the mistake as you do in the immediate moment. Time really does help to heal the wounds and the support of your colleagues and employer will make all the difference to you.

The most important thing of all after having made a mistake, is never ever to attempt to hide an error from a client or from your employer. Honesty really is the best policy, so notify your employer and the owner as soon as possible and acknowledge to the client that you are acting in their animal's best interests to find out what has gone wrong and why, and how you are going to correct it if at all possible. Do not rush in and immediately blame yourself without ascertaining the facts, but never be tempted to hide a mistake or delay in owning up. If you have injected the wrong drug, admit it immediately and find out what the consequences are, putting it right if at all possible; never lie about it or try to cover it up. It is not the making of a mistake that risks any disciplinary action by the regulatory body but the concealment of it afterwards that certainly does. It will most likely come to light sooner or later and you will lie awake at night in fear and dread waiting for someone to find out.

I am retired from clinical work now after 38 years in practice and I can tell you that during my years in practice I have made, and seen others make, some really big, serious mistakes and everyone survived to tell the tale and no one was struck off. If any group of vets gets together in a bar and they feel comfortable in one another's company, then the tales will be told of the errors these experienced and respected clinicians will all have made over the years.

Confession time

I have opened up a male cat for a cat spay at least once and I have injected antibiotic intravenously instead of anaesthetic when trying to anaesthetise a bitch for a caesarian and wondered why it was not losing consciousness but still looking me in the eye.

I once left a remaining twin calf inside a cow at a calving and had to go back with my boss and apologise for being careless.

I have put a cast on the 'wrong' leg on a young dog and not the one with the fracture.

Once, to my shame, as a new graduate I accidentally incised the top of a kitten's head through the wall of the uterus during a caesarian section and I had to suture the skin of the kitten's head after I closed the abdomen.

On each of these occasions, I have been completely mortified and felt like the worst vet in the world and wished the floor would swallow me up. I still cringe and find it hard to confess all these embarrassing mistakes all in one go here, but I admitted my errors at the time and dealt with the consequences and the world did not come to an end. It is never easy to confess to an owner, but I have usually, ultimately, been forgiven by them and although my employers have looked aghast at my confession at the time and were understandably unhappy, I was always supported and reassured by them. None of these cases, to my knowledge, went any further than the practice and the owner because in each case the aftermath was handled correctly and apologies were given where appropriate, and the owners of the animals were generous enough to forgive me and to understand that mistakes happen.

People do forgive mistakes more readily than we think, especially if we own up and are clearly sorry and do not try to squirm out of it. It is dishonesty and lying and the concealment of the truth that is hard to forgive and makes people seek retribution and compensation.

As an employer, I have known a vet who had vaccinated a puppy with cat vaccine, only realising at the end of the session and another who dispensed the wrong dose of medicines with catastrophic effects. I was not thrilled to hear their confessions, as you can imagine, but these vets had my complete support because they immediately told the truth.

Some mistakes are easy to remedy, such as the vaccination error, and the vet had the integrity not to keep quiet about it and risk the pup being unprotected, but to speak up so that we could put things right and make sure the puppy was called back to receive the vaccination that he needed. If that vet had not owned up, then no one would have been the wiser, but that pup would have remained vulnerable to disease despite the owner thinking he was vaccinated.

The worst case I know of was when a very able vet we employed amputated the undamaged leg of a cat instead of the badly broken leg. Even in this case, the owner forgave the vet because she went round to the house straight away and apologised for what had happened and was clearly devastated. The indemnity insurance cover paid several thousand pounds for the cat to have the badly damaged remaining leg repaired at an orthopaedic referral centre, which the owner had not been able to afford in the first instance. The cat healed well and lived a good three-legged life and the family remained clients of the practice and held no grudges against the vet concerned.

Always tell the truth when something goes wrong and sleep easy in your bed at night with a clear conscience. Do not let it prey on your mind if you can help it and, although the day it happens is painful and you feel things will never be normal again, you will come to terms with it. A mistake may rock your confidence in yourself but after a day or so, you will start to feel better and you will be a better vet who is highly unlikely ever to make the same mistake again. Not only will you avoid repeating the same mistake, but you will most likely be vigilant when others are in the same situation and be able prevent it happening again in the future to someone else.

The airline industry was one of the forerunners in deciding that, instead of having a blame culture for errors, which encouraged concealment and cover-ups and no learning, they would encourage pilots to speak up when things went wrong or when accidents were narrowly averted after pilot error. They could then improve the procedures and protocols and reduce the likelihood of mistakes in the future. Enlightened vets should do the same and in this way, fewer mistakes would be made and more vets would feel able to come forward and flag up potential hazards when they experienced a near miss.

The Royal College of Veterinary Surgeons

It is still widely and erroneously thought that a vet who makes a serious mistake risks being struck off by the RCVS, but making a genuine mistake is not the same as behaviour which brings the veterinary profession into disrepute.

If you lie about having made a mistake and conceal the facts, or alter or falsify the clinical records to deceive the client, then you do risk being disciplined because then your dishonest behaviour will definitely have fallen far short of that expected from a veterinary professional.

Many vets, especially new graduates, cite the fear of a complaint being made about them to the RCVS as a major cause of stress and concern in their professional lives, but if you follow the principles of the code and, even more importantly, you do not do anything which you know in your heart to be wrong or dishonest, then you have very little to fear. It is the right of the general public to have some recourse for complaint and the RCVS is the regulatory body for vets in the United Kingdom to which clients can address their concerns, whether these are ultimately proven to be justified or not. We would expect to be able to do the same if we felt our dentist had transgressed and drilled holes into a healthy tooth to make money out of us, or a doctor had knowingly used a cheap and faulty implant.

A number of vets will at some time in their career receive a letter from the RCVS saying that a complaint has been made against them, the majority of which come to nothing. The RCVS has to follow protocols and procedures and cannot discard a complaint without due consideration and this can take a relatively long time to resolve because both parties, the vet and the client, need to have their chance to submit their report of the events.

I have experienced receiving a letter from the RCVS telling me there has been a complaint against me and it is not a good moment when it drops through the letter box. Even though you know in your heart that you have done nothing wrong, it is disheartening to know that a client has gone to these lengths to complain about you. In the majority of cases, there is no case to answer and very few are taken forward to the disciplinary level but if you receive a letter, contact your indemnity insurer and your employer or supervisor and answer it promptly, giving the information requested. Do not panic and do not ignore it or fail to engage with the process as the matter will not go away and you will feel better once you have dealt with it.

The RCVS Code of Conduct is composed of guiding principles as to how a veterinary surgeon should behave and has a comprehensive amount of supporting guidance to help vets manage the myriads of situations they are faced with. It is constantly reviewed and updated and although there can never be an answer to everything, you will find it very helpful in many situations where you may be unsure of what to do. It is not in itself a set of rules and regulations, but if you follow the principles of the code and refer to the supporting guidance then you should prevent yourself from following a path which might lead to an accusation of unprofessional behaviour. Always ensure that you are not tempted or put under pressure by anyone to do what you know at heart to be wrong or dishonest, even if they are your employer.

Your own health

When it comes to looking after yourself, you are a healthcare professional and you know the score. Eat well, get some exercise and fresh air, and make sure you get enough sleep. It is the same advice we give for the animals in our care and if it keeps a Labrador happy and healthy, then it must make sense.

Try not to become reliant on alcohol to relax or sleep and of course no recreational drugs for the sake of both your health and your career.

Try to do some exercise in the fresh air because the effect of circulating adrenaline from being on high alert during the working day can be alleviated by exercise to some extent, and there is something inherently healthy about being in the countryside which makes us feel better about life.

Exercise can be difficult to fit into your busy days, I know, because working patterns may vary from week to week, but lack of motivation to exercise when you are tired is probably a greater barrier, if we are honest with ourselves. If you have been on call and feel tired when you get to the end of a busy day, you may think you are too exhausted to do anything other than collapse in a heap, but some exercise really will make you feel better. Small animal vets often spend all day, every day inside, in a warm and airless environment under artificial light. Go for a walk and get some fresh air and if you haven't got a dog then borrow one, because they are usually in plentiful supply around vets and nurses. You became a vet because you like animals, so make sure that you have some fun time with some healthy ones too.

Driving

I know this may seem to be stating the obvious, but do be really careful if you are driving when you are tired; as every recent graduate will know, you are going to feel more tired than you have ever been in your life during the first few months of working. Your mind will be bombarded by new information and challenges and if you are distracted while you are driving you are at a higher risk of being in an accident.

Adopting waifs and strays

I am going to give you some advice now which I know most of you will not follow. I know I would not have done so either, and I have been a serial offender in letting my heart rule my head when it comes to adopting animals through the course of my work.

If you are going to do as I did and adopt a waif or stray, then do at least get the right one for you and your circumstances. Resist adopting the dog no one else wants because there is probably a very good reason for that! I am currently looking at my rescue lurcher who had two broken legs as a pup and who is now just about housetrained at the age of 11. I think the world of her, but she has not been an easy dog and even now she prefers the comfort of urinating in the house if it is raining outside. How much more sensible would it have been had I adopted a more suitable candidate or even no dog at all?

> *The very first time I let my heart rule my head was in adopting a cat with a permanent head tilt, which was a case study at vet school. When we had all examined her, the lecturer said we could put her to sleep because her owner said she did not want a lopsided cat. Loppy Lugs came home with me to the student flat and accompanied me when I moved to my first job in practice.*
>
> *My second adopted waif was a whippet puppy who had been vomiting for a week and was so thin that it was possible to identify the foreign body in her small intestine as the teat from a baby's bottle. Emma lived with me for 16 years and accompanied me to work every day, travelling with me in the car out on call to the farms and coming out on calls at night as the most unsuitable, fragile bodyguard you could imagine.*
>
> *This was followed by a golden retriever called Sky which another vet in the practice left in a kennel for me with a luggage label on his collar saying, 'if you*

*don't want me, put me to sleep'. That vet was a master of manipulation as he
knew I would fall for this very obvious emotional blackmail.*

*I then adopted another supposedly untrainable, unwanted retriever and have
also adopted various cats of all shapes, colours and sizes and with variable
complements of legs, ears and eyes.*

If you do succumb and feel the need to have a companion, cats are much easier to own
because you can leave them to look after themselves but if you get a dog and you are working
all day, then that dog will need looking after and walking. If every single vet and nurse in a
large practice took their dogs with them to work, there would be no room for any inpatients
in the kennels so it can be a problem, and taking them with you may not be an option. Think
about how you are going to manage in a practical way with a dog before you fall for those
big brown eyes and be prepared to pay for dog walkers if you are determined to adopt that
three-legged, young Border collie.

Find an activity that you love

I expect you already know what makes you feel good about your life and what you enjoy
doing. Don't expend your energies doing something you think you ought to do but which you
find boring, like going to the gym perhaps, because the chances are you won't sustain it. Do
something you enjoy, and you will be motivated to find the time to go and make it happen.

Make a real effort to prioritise these out-of-work activities and put some effort into finding out how to fit them into your life. Join a book club or a cycling club or ride horses and
do everything you can to keep that activity going, despite being on call and late finishes.
Ask your boss and your colleagues for help to make sure you can get there, as a life outside
work makes all the difference to your life as a vet.

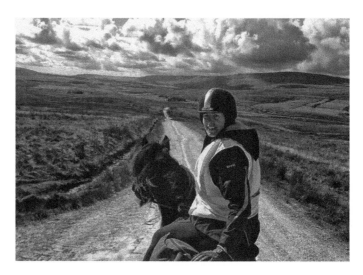

If you have an activity you enjoy,
then make a dedicated space
in your diary and tenaciously
defend that time as essential for
your health and happiness. It
could be cycling or running or
even just time with friends and
family, but it is just as important
as work commitments in your
busy life.

I have a friend who is a young vet and who found the first year or so in practice really difficult. She was working hard but also spending quite a lot of time alone and not really recuperating in her time off because even when she was off-duty, she was thinking and worrying about work. Fortunately, she is a really talented horse rider with a very understanding mother who realised that she was missing out on the activities she was previously reliant on throughout her time at school and university. She helped her daughter to organise access to riding when she was off-duty and she now has action-packed weekends riding in shows and schooling a horse, giving her a complete mental break from work plus getting exercise and making friends. We may not all be lucky enough to have this type of opportunity but think about what you really enjoy doing and make it a priority to balance your working life with your non-working life. It will take some effort and probably some sort of financial investment, but the benefit will be invaluable.

Most new jobs will mean moving away from your friends and family and it is particularly likely that you have left your vet school friends and your flatmates behind to some extent. You will be working hard and it will take a while to make new friends, but hopefully you will have been welcomed by those you work with and will develop a social life. Don't expect it just to fall into your lap though; you need to go and make an effort to find new friends so be proactive about it. It is very daunting when you start with a new practice and do not know anyone, but it will not take long to build up friendships if you make an effort and join in.

Keep in touch with your friends and family and do not become so immersed in work that you neglect your friendships and family relationships. Do phone your parents because they are your biggest fans and will be so happy to hear from you, whether it is a monologue of moaning or an excited blow by blow account of your latest success. They have probably gone through a lot to help you to become a vet and they will be so happy to hear from you. If you are having problems, then most parents will be only too happy to help you in any way they can, so even though it is great to have your independence, let them know how you are doing.

Contact the people you qualified with as they will be going through the same things as you and you can give and receive support from each other. They may have come across a solution to something that you are struggling with and that network of friends often has access to sources of information which you do not have, such as a colleague who has a certificate in some discipline or with experience in exotics. This can really help with a case that is baffling you and which the owner does not want to have referred.

Go to the new graduate congress if possible and if there is a local BVA young graduates support group near you, then join and attend whenever you can. There is nothing quite as encouraging as being with other vets from other practices where you can have a good discussion and come away feeling that you are not the only new vet in the village. Go to the VDS and SPVS supported new graduate weekend and exchange information with other young graduates.

The perils of being known to be a veterinary surgeon when you are off-duty

On a lighter note, the fact that you are a vet will be a great source of pride to your family and your friends. My proud father could bring the fact that his daughter was a vet into any conversation on any subject, especially if speaking to a medical professional or an animal owner. Lovely though this was, it also meant that in conversations with him I would receive second-hand enquiries about the health and ill-health of the animals of all his friends and acquaintances. It can seem that you are never off-duty when people know you are a vet and you may need to be assertive to protect your off-duty time.

In a social setting, be prepared for people to ask you all about their dog's ear problems or horse's bowel function over the table in a restaurant or at a wedding reception. When asked a question like this, it is tempting to try to help by offering an opinion but be careful about commenting or offering advice about an animal that you have never seen and are not likely ever to see. Imagine how you would feel as the person's own vet to hear that some cousin at a wedding diagnosed hyperadrenocorticism in your client's dog without ever having seen or touched the patient. It is unprofessional, and you may need to use all your tact and diplomacy skills to avoid passing comment in this situation, plus you are off-duty and meant to be relaxing so people should respect that. I usually smile and make noncommittal but sympathetic comments and say that it would not be fair to offer an opinion in the circumstances and then try to move away or change the subject.

I keep the fact that I am a vet to myself when off-duty or on holiday so as to avert a series of entertaining tales about Fido the dog or Diabolo the horse and his many ailments. My friends are very good at protecting me too if anyone tries to bend my ear at a party and one asked a local publican, who was asking me about his dog, if he would be as willing to pop round with a gin and tonic when his pub was closed. Living in a small community makes it much more likely that you will be recognised as the local vet, but most people will have enough consideration not to consult you in the street. Some vets I know hate being known

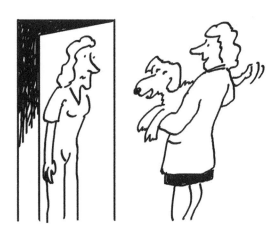

locally as the vet and like to keep their work completely separate from the place they live, but I enjoy being part of the community and it does bring positives as well as negatives.

Beware the neighbours calling round at your home with sick and injured animals too. You need to help them by informing them where they can access veterinary treatment but it is not incumbent on you to provide a mini vet service from your home. You would not refuse to bandage a gushing artery but you do not have to assume responsibility for a limping cat, or a dog with a lump on a Sunday morning off-duty.

My colleague and his wife used to crawl round on their hands and knees so that the clients did not know they were at home when they lived over the surgery premises.

The great general public, warts and all

There are occasions when the general public can behave really badly and seem to consider you fair game for very unpleasant and sometimes personal remarks, so be prepared for individuals telling you that all vets are money-grabbing swines who do not care about animals. Ignore the ones who say that all vaccines are a rip-off and be prepared for the ones who take great delight in telling you tales of woe about disastrous visits to the vet where everything went wrong and they paid thousands of pounds and the animal still died. It is painful to hear these remarks about your profession and these remarks are often made by someone driving an expensive car who earns three times what you are earning and who probably happily agreed to the treatment which was proposed at the time.

You do not need to feel you have to justify yourself to these people or apologise in any way for your choice of career. I usually defend the profession when I feel like it and when I reasonably can without getting into an argument, by responding that there is no NHS for animals and that vet fees have increased because there is so much more that we can do for them nowadays. There is no point getting angry about people who are being insensitive and rude, so instead of letting them ruin your evening, just walk away, brush it off and forget about them.

Your physical health

Make sure you look after your physical health as well as your mental health. You are not superhuman and there will be times when you are ill or injured but feel under pressure to carry on working when you should not. The nature of veterinary work and being part of a team means that conscientious individuals worry about how the practice and their colleagues will cope if they are off sick. If you are not fit to work, then the practice team will cope without you and it is far better to get well and return to work than to carry on when you are not fit. You are more likely to make a mistake or miss something if you are suffering from ill health or injury and more likely to be off for longer overall if your condition gets worse. I am not encouraging you to take a day off work for a mild head cold or an ingrowing toenail, but look after your own health and do not be a martyr.

Take care of your back and make sure you are standing with a good posture when you are consulting and especially when you are operating. If you speak to older vets, you will find a significant number of them suffer with a bad back, especially the large animal vets. Adjust the height of the table when you are operating so that you are standing upright and not stooping over the patient. In consulting rooms, use any available hydraulic lifting apparatus to make sure you are not lifting too many squirming, heavy dogs and ask someone else to help lift the big ones and the chubby ones.

In large animal practice, the days have gone where it was considered macho for gentlemen to display their physical strength at the expense of their lower back, so use the calving aid and preserve your health and fitness. Ask the farmers to help and observe that it is usually the one who groans the most and the loudest who is having the least effect when doing any physical work such as pulling on a rope.

Cat bites and deep scratches on your hands can quickly become infected; if you get bitten, irrigate the wound as soon as you can and get your hands into warm water and thoroughly soak and irrigate for some time. It is not enough just to run it under the tap, but really soak it and repeat this whenever possible, but if the bite is deep or looks at all infected, seek medical attention. Human doctors may not be aware of the potential risk from the bacteria in cats' mouths so take a copy of the advice provided by the VDS as an inexperienced doctor may be reluctant to prescribe the necessary antibiotics unless prompted.

I have mentioned this previously, but when you start out in your first job you will not be thinking that personal finances are of high priority as long as you have enough money to pay your bills every month. Do take out some sort of sickness and injury insurance now, just in case the unexpected happens and you are unable to work. It is all too common to feel invincible and immortal when you are young, but if you are ill or injured it helps if the bills are being paid while you recover.

Dark times

I hope you never need to read this section because I hope you never feel in the depths of despair and find yourself questioning your happiness in your life and your ability to be a good vet. Unfortunately, something may have happened in your professional or your private life which has made you feel that you are in a very dark place and you cannot see a way out. It might not be a sudden event but a gradual feeling that life has been going wrong for a while and you haven't been able to do anything about it. At the very least, you may feel you might want to stop being a vet and at the very worst, perhaps you feel that life itself is not worth living.

You may think that no one else can understand how you feel or has ever felt the same way that you do now. You may think that you are alone with these emotions and that everyone else is doing fine but, actually, there will be a number of people out there who you know well, and who you think are so happy and confident in their lives, but who have been feeling just as you are feeling now.

I have been in that situation myself and have questioned my ability as a vet and also my worth as a human being. I have made mistakes at work and in my home life and lost people I love and felt that life has dealt me insurmountable problems. I know at first hand just how low you can feel but please believe me when I say that there is help for you out there and there are people who understand and who can help you.

If you cannot reach out to your doctor or to friends or family then phone this number – just put down this book and phone it now. It is a number specifically for people in veterinary practice who understand just what it is like to be a vet and you will find they will listen to you and they can help you.

> Vetlife phone number: 0303 040 2551 and website: vetlife.org.uk

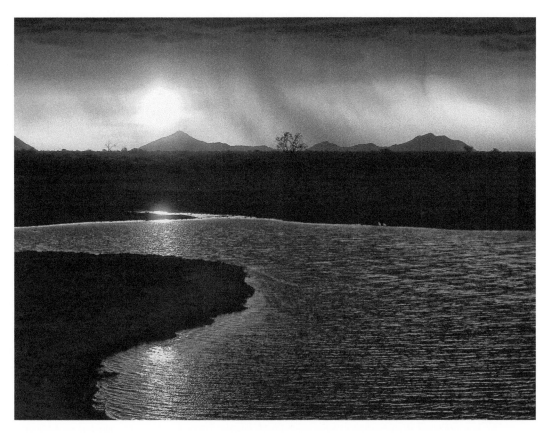

Every vet experiences dark times when the pressure of life and work becomes overwhelming and it is hard to see if the clouds will ever lift. The stress of being a vet and caring for the health of our patients and coping with the needs of our clients can take its toll on our mental health.

Depression and anxiety

You might be reading this and thinking that things are not that bad but that you are just not very happy with life. Perhaps you have reached a point where you are not enjoying your work as much as you should and your enjoyment of life generally is not what you expected. Every day seems the same, flat and uninteresting and you cannot raise any enthusiasm for anything either at work or at home. If you do nothing, then there is a considerable chance that you will gradually feel worse and worse, so do not wait but seek help now. The deeper into depression you sink, the harder it is to summon the energy to seek help and part of the condition is to feel that you do not need or deserve help. If you are feeling like this, look at the resources mentioned above and others which are available which may help, and take action now because help is out there.

Quite often, it is tempting to blame the practice you are in and to keep moving on, looking for the perfect job. The incidence of depression and anxiety in vets is high relative to other professions for a variety of reasons, both because of the nature of the work and also our personality profiles. There used to be very little recognition of this and any mental health issue used to carry a stigma and be perceived as a weakness and hidden away, with vets suffering in silence and not asking for help from anyone. There is much more awareness and openness about mental health nowadays and, although we still have some way to go in being as open and honest about these illnesses, there is much more recognition and support available than there used to be, and more and more people are talking about their experiences.

You are part of a much more understanding veterinary community now and there are people who understand what you are going through and who can support you while you make the changes which will bring you out of this dark place, so please ask for help from the relevant professionals and do not soldier on indefinitely, suffering alone.

Nowadays there must be very few practices that are not aware of the importance of mental health and you should not continue to work in a practice where you feel that you cannot ask for help if you feel unwell either in body or in mind. Your health is far too important to stay in such a practice and you will find it hard to recover in an environment like that.

I have been a veterinary surgeon for many years now and was a practice owner of a rapidly expanding small animal practice which grew from a two-vet practice to one with five branches and a central hospital employing 13 veterinary surgeons and 30 support staff. Over the years, I have employed numerous new graduates and mentored and coached vets in my practice to achieve further qualifications and enhance their careers. I have been an elected member of the RCVS Council and some would say that I have had a very successful career as a veterinary surgeon and led a charmed life.

What many of my colleagues and employees did not know is that during that time I have also suffered from severe clinical depression when I was also working full-time. I was a practice owner working days, weekends and nights and caring for my two young sons who were diagnosed with learning difficulties and autism from the age of 18 months. I was managing to turn up for work and function, but I constantly felt very anxious and as if I was just managing to keep my head above water. The smallest setback or problem took on enormous proportions and I was probably not an easy person to be around, but I could not recognise that I was in need of help, nor did I know where to seek it.

I was reluctant to accept that there was anything wrong until the day I found I was crying more than the owners of the old dog who I had just had to put to sleep. I realised the owners were comforting me rather than the other way round. Thanks to my supportive family, friends and very understanding veterinary partner, I went to the doctor and I received the help I needed. I was shocked by how vulnerable I felt in admitting my illness and it made me question many assumptions I had made about others in the past. I am sharing this with you to illustrate that there will be many people whose lives appear to be successful and sorted and who you would never guess are suffering, because there is still a great reluctance to talk about it.

This was not that long ago, in the 1990s, when there was far less understanding of mental health, and suffering from depression was considered to be a sign of weakness by many people. Over the years, I had heard many negative comments about vets and nurses who could not cope with life in practice and who had breakdowns. I felt I was a strong woman who had worked hard to become a vet and had felt driven to prove that I was as good as any male vet if not better. I thought I was logical, balanced and tough and it was a complete surprise to find out that I was not infallible after all.

I never experienced suicidal thoughts but sadly, suicide can seem to be the first time a vet demonstrates just how ill they are, and there have been too many tragic losses of young vets with everything to live for and who needed help.

Suffering a mental health problem does not mean that you cannot have a long, happy and successful career as a vet. I managed my anxiety and depression and regained my enjoyment of working as a vet and indeed I felt that working helped by giving me confidence and self-worth. When I was concentrating on problem-solving and performing difficult procedures there was no time to dwell on my own problems.

I have shared this here because I believe that the more that people talk about their experiences, the less stigma will be attached to these illnesses.

Reach out for the help available and speak to people about it as this is the first step to recovery.

Looking out for your colleagues

Our profession attracts intelligent people who have proven that they are hard-working by qualifying with a highly respected degree after five years or more of intense study. We enter a workplace where we do not know what each day is going to bring in terms of difficulty and intensity of work or how emotional a consultation may turn out to be. Each day we do not know if we will be performing four new procedures or if we are going to be sworn at or have to put an animal to sleep because the owner requests it. Working as a vet in practice requires resilience and every day, we vets face multiple challenges that the average person does not.

Even if you are fine and have no concept of needing support and are full of enthusiasm and enjoyment in your job, do take the time to find out what resources are available, because you may never need it yourself, but it is highly likely that at some time in your veterinary career you will work with a colleague who is struggling. The small teams that comprise the veterinary workplace mean that you may well be on the front line in identifying and helping someone who you work with and you might even be instrumental in saving someone from a breakdown or even suicide. It might be another new graduate who is a friend of yours or a veterinary nurse or even your boss. No one is invincible and as a profession we are very good at keeping quiet and being reluctant to ask for help or even recognising ourselves that all is not well.

We all have a responsibility to help a colleague who is suffering and just as we would not walk past if they were struggling to breathe or bleeding, if we see them struggling mentally then we should offer help.

CHAPTER 14

Challenges you may encounter in practice

It is never boring being a vet in general practice and the fascinating variety of the work presented also means that you will be constantly facing new challenges. When you first start work as a new graduate, there will be some potential hazards waiting to trip you up but most of them are manageable if you know what to expect and you will soon be adept in handling these situations. Every vet starting out in practice has faced these hurdles and although it is not possible to cover every possible challenge that you may face, a little advance warning and some coping techniques can help when you start out.

One of the most important tasks in practice is making the clients happy and keeping their trust and confidence. It is not enough just to make the sick animals well and perform excellent surgery on them without acknowledging that ours is a service industry; to a successful practice, the clients' needs and desires and appreciation of their experience are paramount. Sometimes you can feel as if you are giving your all for the clients and working your hardest but they still seem to want more and more from you and the practice you work in. Some of this will be outside your control, such as convenient parking and low prices, but as the veterinary surgeon, you do have a significant effect on how happy the clients are with the practice in many different ways.

When our practice surveyed the views of our clients, they rated the professional skills of the veterinary team as the first priority, which is what we would hope and expect, and the next most important thing for them was to have vets and nurses who handled their pets well and who listened and explained. These were recorded as being of far more importance to the clients than reasonable fees and value for money and illustrates just how important your role is in a practice, along with the rest of the veterinary team.

Clients often complain about fees when really they are unhappy with the experience they have received and it can all be based on a very trivial mishandling of client expectations or from a client feeling that they have had an offhand reception when they phoned for an appointment.

You will identify with this as you will often be a client or customer yourself in a restaurant or a retail outlet and you know if you would be happy to return there or if you would recommend it to your friends. No one minds paying for quality service and just as you may be willing to pay very well for a good meal in a smart restaurant, you will resent the bill if they do not give you what you ordered and you have to wait a long time before it arrives. You might still be a little put out if the food is perfect but the waiter slaps it down in front of you without a smile.

You have a fundamental influence on the experience of the clients when they entrust the health of their animals to you and there is more to being a good veterinary surgeon than just having the essential skills and knowledge. Challenges arise when clients do not get what they want and expect and there is a great deal that you can do to make their visit to the practice match their expectations.

The client is not the enemy

There is a false perception which can insidiously penetrate the culture of a practice in which the client becomes 'the enemy'. The client phones to ask to speak to you just as you are bringing the coffee cup to your lips (sigh), or calls in to the surgery when you are having your lunch break (sigh), or demands repeat prescriptions or flea control without phoning first (tut, sigh). They turn up on the wrong day for an appointment adamant that they have not made a mistake (trying it on) or may fail to follow your advice but blame you when the patient is no better (gormless idiots).

Every week in most practices there are a few clients who just seem to go out of their way to be awkward and ignore the usual protocols and procedures. Everyone is busy rushing round and working hard and these pesky clients are making demands on our precious time and not doing as they are told. How well the surgery would run if only all these annoying clients did not keep coming in upsetting the smooth running of the practice with their selfish demands (the inconsiderate twits).

It is important that we recognise that these time-consuming and irritating clients are just human beings and we humans can be really annoying at times, especially when a little worried and stressed and out of our comfort zone. We have to remind ourselves that as service providers we should do our best to match or preferably exceed their expectations and were it not for these clients and their funny ways, we would have no revenue and no jobs.

Reading this, you may think this is blindingly obvious, but just look around and you may see a receptionist casting their eyes to heaven when speaking to a client on the phone, or a veterinary nurse refusing an old lady's request for a worming tablet just because she had called in on a busy day without telephoning first. We vets can be just as bad, and when we are asked to phone a client back and explain something we resent the time we will have to give up in the middle of our busy day, so we might prevaricate and complain about the client being inconsiderate. It is easy to get sucked in to this culture of having a dismissive approach to clients and it is a very destructive attitude for any veterinary professional.

There will be times when it is simply not possible to accommodate someone without an appointment and it may be impossible to dispense four repeat prescriptions to someone who just popped in on the off chance in the middle of an evening consulting session but, as a general rule, if you can help a client, then do so. By all means, remind them that next time it would ensure that they didn't risk disappointment if they phoned first, but try to get into the mindset that you are on their side and will help them if you possibly can. There are more clients lost to a practice because of an offhand phone call or an encounter with an unhelpful member of staff than are lost due to misdiagnosis or a mistake which has been rectified.

Clients are just people, like you or your brother or your mum or your grandma, so treat them with the same consideration and respect that you would want for your family and friends. Give them the benefit of the doubt and go out of your way to make sure that they feel you want to help them. Smile as you speak to them, even when you are on the phone as they can hear the smile in your voice and the very act of smiling makes you feel better and more relaxed.

I was advised by a colleague that 'there are no such things as difficult clients but only clients who have not had their expectations met'. I am not convinced that I agree with this because, although the majority of clients are a pleasure to see, I have come across clients who really are very unreasonable and generally difficult and who I suspect actually enjoy being difficult. I expect that the same clients are also on the 'heart-sink' lists of the local doctor's surgery and the dentist's list and are the parents who the school teachers dread seeing on parents evening. Some people seem to thrive on combat in all their interactions with the world and will always delight in being a thorn in everyone's side. Some clients have unreasonable expectations of the service we provide and are on occasion disappointed, when they may exhibit behaviour which is marginally unpleasant, but some are simply the spawn of the devil, completely unreasonable and not manageable. It has always been this way because of the glorious diversity of the human personality and I expect it always will be.

In the average practice, these clients from hell are few and far between, but we can choose whether to let them get to us or not. The only thing we can change is how we ourselves deal with the people we meet and how far we allow a negative experience with a client to disturb us. I have found that it has helped me to try to influence change and attempt to transform a bad interaction with a client like this into a good one. It makes me feel better because then I am sure that I have done my best and it often results in a better outcome for my patients and in the long run, they are my primary concern.

Clients' complaints and concerns

Vets tend to be caring people who set themselves very high standards and when someone complains we can find it very hurtful and take it personally, especially if we perceive the complaint to be unjustified. There are many resources available for how to handle client complaints and the following are just my own thoughts on how to handle a client who is not happy and is complaining to you in person. Clients may complain by letter, email, telephone, Facebook and website reviews or tweets, but each of these methods allows you time to think about how to respond. However, when you are face to face with Mr or Mrs Angry in the consulting room, it is a different matter. You may be able to defuse the situation there and then if you use all your communication skills to try to resolve the problem to the satisfaction of all parties. Few people complain for fun and there is usually some reason or misunderstanding which can be sorted out before it escalates. It may be an unjustified complaint, but the client usually genuinely believes they are in the right and they need you to convince them otherwise.

Fight or flight

In response to a complaint, try to neither fight nor take flight, as neither position helps the situation. Often the immediate response to a client who is unhappy and complaining is to be defensive, especially if you are taken by surprise and you did not see it coming. We all tend to react in a similar way when we feel under attack and may attempt to defend ourselves with a counter attack, but do try to resist this knee-jerk reaction. It takes two to argue, so if you do not enter the ring in a defensive and combative manner but stay calm and listen quietly, then usually they will run out of steam relatively quickly. You can then invite them to a private space to discuss the problem – it is never a good idea to have an argument with a client in public and with an audience, such as in the waiting room.

Clients sometimes fear that they will not be listened to when things go wrong and that they will be ignored, so it really helps to acknowledge their complaint and assure them that you are going to be looking into the problem. Do not feel you have to resolve the problem there and then. It may be that they do have a valid complaint and you may be able to resolve the issue on the spot, but in some cases this is just not possible. You might not have all the facts and you might need to collect more information before you can help them; most reasonable people will accept this and be reassured that you are taking their problem seriously.

If the problem is more complex, you may need to seek assistance from someone else, but in the first instance you have removed the unhappy client from the public space and accorded them the courtesy of listening to them. Your swift action may well prevent the escalation of a trivial matter into a major one and the client will be impressed by the care and concern you show.

Never think that complaints are just not your problem and give in to the temptation to run away. An unhappy client is a problem for everyone in the practice and if you are the first person to encounter their concern, then do your best to handle it at least until you can safely transfer it to the relevant member of staff. Scuttling into the back of the surgery like a scalded cat, leaving the reception staff to deal with it, is not a reasonable or mature and professional thing to do.

If there has been some minor misunderstanding, such as a client waiting for over half an hour because their arrival was overlooked, or they have been charged for something twice and it is indeed an error made by the practice, then it may be that all they need is an apology and for things to be made right. In my experience, once the client appreciates that the practice has recognised that a mistake has been made and said sorry, then the client will also often apologise for becoming angry in the first place.

And so, my personal golden rules when faced with an aggrieved client would be:

- Invite them to go somewhere private to discuss it, such as a consulting room, unless you think there is any element of threat to you.
- Allow them to speak without interruption until they run out of steam.
- Express concern for the way they feel and give them your full attention.
- Never match their level of anger but speak calmly and courteously.
- Adopt a look of concern on your face as well as in your words.
- Summarise their concerns and repeat the information back to them.
- Stay very calm, even in the face of unpleasant accusations.
- If possible and appropriate, deal with it yourself and do not offload them on to another member of staff; if the problem is significant and you cannot handle it yourself, tell the client that you are going to contact the relevant people who can help.
- If this is going to take some time, tell the client when they can expect to hear from the practice and by what means and ensure you have their correct contact details.
- If a client is persistently abusive or uses foul language, say that you are not prepared to listen and leave the room.

Some golden rules with clients when a consultation seems to be going badly

When people are asked to rate vets against other professionals, we come out relatively high in their estimation, so most of your clients already think you are a dedicated, caring person who is honest and trustworthy and who likes animals. That is such a significant and advantageous head start when compared to other professionals, to know that people want and expect to like you. As an old vet once said to a vet I know, 'clients are much less likely to sue you if they like you' and blunt though this may seem, it is in fact true.

The fact remains that not everyone will like us and there will be times when it is very clear that things are going wrong. We all have consultations where things just don't seem to be going well and you and the client are just not getting along. The dog doesn't like you and the owner thinks his dog is right!

Every suggestion you make seems to be rebuffed and you are getting one-word answers to every question and every suggestion you make is being met with opposition. Your instinctive reaction after several unpleasant exchanges is to be just as surly and unhelpful in return, but this is, in fact, the moment when you need to take control of the consultation and start a charm offensive to turn it around.

Give the owner the benefit of the doubt and assume that the majority of people have their pet's interest at heart and that any resistance or difficulty within the consultation is not deliberate but may be due to some underlying cause. Use a different approach and be sympathetic even if you feel annoyed with the client for being terse with you or for not bringing the poor animal in sooner. Go out of your way to try to make him or her feel that you are both on the same side, working together for the good of their animal.

It has been said that empathy cannot be learned but you can certainly learn techniques to cope with certain situations where you feel at odds with a client in a consultation. First of all, be honest with yourself and ask yourself if it is you who have started this consult poorly. Have you been welcoming and greeted the client and the patient as you normally would or are you irritated because they have left it for several days before bringing their dog in late on a Friday evening, or have you got off on the wrong foot because you are rushed off your feet and aware of a waiting room full of people? It is not your client's problem if you have had a busy surgery and there may be valid reasons for their apparent lack of concern for their pet. If you can remain calm and not judgemental, but compose yourself and try starting again with a positive viewpoint, you may be able to change the tenor of the consultation.

Ask yourself if you have listened to them properly and I mean really listened, giving them eye contact and not with your back half turned to them while you fiddle with the computer. It is so easy to unintentionally appear offhand, so ignore everything else and give them your full attention until you can establish a rapport. There is far more to communication than simple words, and your body language and facial expression will convey to the client that you are listening to them.

Try to confirm what they are actually trying to tell you by asking them if you have understood their concerns and repeating back to them your understanding of what they wish to gain from their visit. Of all the skills that are the most important, it is this active listening that will help you in this situation and it is so easy for either party to misunderstand one another and create tension.

It may be that you cannot change the tone of the consultation and the client is just having a bad day. More commonly, they feel worried that you have misunderstood why they have come and they may think that there is something seriously wrong with their animal that is going undiagnosed. They may be feeling guilty at not coming sooner and be angry with themselves as much as they are with you. Clients often need reassuring that you are taking them seriously and doing everything you can to come to a diagnosis and that there will be positive actions that can be taken. Fear and worry can make people appear angry and uncooperative and some people have other things going on in their lives about which we know nothing, and which spill out into the rest of their lives. You do not have to spend any longer with them than the length of time a consultation takes so you can afford to take the strain for that long.

When clients need help with animal handling

Some clients find it surprisingly hard to handle their own animals in the surgery and do not know how to hold a cat or a dog securely for examination. It may seem obvious to us to continue to hold the dog when it is on the consulting table, because if they let go it will jump off, but that is because we know that is what is going to happen because we see it time and time again. The owner may prefer you to ask a nurse to hold their pet and they may also be squeamish about blood or faeces or not want to be part of an uncomfortable procedure by being the one restraining the animal. They may be concerned that we are judging them for their competence or incompetence in handling their own animal. Showing empathy and understanding towards the client and how they may be feeling is a really useful way to ensure a consultation goes well, because they feel cared for and part of the process.

> *I was once in a consultation with a Yorkshire miner who was about six foot six and built like a brick outhouse. His friendly springer spaniel had a cut foot and his wife was delayed outside in the car park phoning their daughter at the time when he was called in to the consulting room. The dog had a bandage on its paw and he seemed really troubled by my suggestion that he should hold the dog so that I could take the bandage off to have a look and see if it needed stitching. He was jiggling about from foot to foot and walking up and down the room and sweating and telling me to 'just get on with it' in a really agitated way. Eventually, I asked the nurse to come in and hold the dog and I took the blood-soaked bandage off. There was an almighty crash and we turned round to see him lying full length on the floor having fainted and fallen like a felled oak tree. His wife then charged in, took one look at him and said,*
>
> *'Daft bugger can't stand the sight of blood, he always does that, didn't he warn you?'*
>
> *The poor man was very sheepish after he had come round and was a very pleasant client whenever we saw him from that moment on, though he was much happier when he didn't see the red stuff.*

Dealing with deliberate animal abuse and ignorance

In the worst-case scenarios, during the course of our work we may be faced with evidence of deliberate animal cruelty. The incidence of cruelty to animals has been allied to a significantly increased likelihood of child abuse and domestic violence occurring in the same household. If you see a case where you suspect animal cruelty, speak to a more senior member of staff to discuss the actions you ought to take. You need to be sure of your facts and this is not a situation that you should handle alone, so speak to others and seek help and advice from organisations such as the BVA, the RCVS and the VDS.

Ignorance is often the cause of inadvertent ill-use of animals which, although not deliberate, can be very distressing for the vet who sees the results. It is harrowing to see an animal who has been left to suffer with an untreated condition and is in pain, or is being overfed to the point of pathological obesity and subsequent suffering. It is very difficult to resist berating the ignorant owner from your moral high ground, but you should consider the potential outcome of a knee-jerk reaction like this. It is far better to keep the animal under the supervision of a veterinary surgeon than to give them a tongue lashing, which makes them leave the surgery in a rage with their animal in tow still untreated and seriously reduces the chances of them ever consulting a vet again. Make sure your response is measured and that your emotions do not divert you from the best course of action to make that animal's quality of life better.

Clients with a disability

There are clients with whom consultations are more challenging because they have a disability or an infirmity which may or may not be obvious. You probably have experience of friends or family members facing difficulties of one sort or another and there is an infinite variety of major and minor barriers which disabled people face when they interact with others.

You may be completely unaware that the client you are speaking to is illiterate when you ask them to sign a form, or you may be trying to explain diabetes to someone and be unaware that they are struggling to hear what you are saying because they are profoundly deaf.

This is where you learn to develop your communication skills as a vet and it brings it home that despite having become a vet because you like working with animals, you now have to become adept at communicating with people. You will need to be sensitive, understanding and patient, and the best vets are the ones who are willing to go the extra mile for their clients as well as their patients. Often, animals belonging to owners with a disability are a hugely important part of their lives and it is an immense privilege to be the vet for a guide dog for a blind person, a hearing dog for the deaf or a support dog for an autistic individual.

I would recommend that you always address your questions to the disabled person and not just to the carer if they are present. The carer will know if they can communicate or if they need to speak for them, but it is courteous to address them and include them.

Ask them how you can help them to make it easier to administer medication in a direct way without avoiding the issue, as an injection may be necessary instead of a course of tablets, or you might need to check to see if they have anyone to help them with topical applications. Little things can make all the difference to your clients and they may need a little extra help and thoughtfulness.

Aggressive animals

In the course of your work, you will meet the challenge of being presented with some animals showing aggressive behaviour of varying degrees and no matter what the needs of a patient, the health and safety of human beings takes priority in this situation.

There will always be a way to handle a situation that does not involve you being a hero and risking injury for the sake of the patient. It is tempting to rush into hasty, ill-considered decisions when dealing with an emergency with an animal and you may well act in haste and regret at leisure if you become injured and unable to work either temporarily or permanently.

Always warn the owner if you suspect an animal of being a potential biter to be careful that their own pet does not bite them while they are at the surgery. You are responsible for the damage their dog might cause them while in the practice. This might seem unfair since the dog is theirs, but if you don't warn them and they are bitten, then you might be held liable. The assumption is that as the professional, you are in charge. I also warn the owner to be careful generally if I think their dog has the potential to bite as, if a timely warning can prevent a child being bitten, or indeed anyone being bitten by the dog, then even if my opinion is unwelcome I feel better for having delivered it.

Never ask your work colleagues to put themselves at risk of being injured by taking any shortcuts when handling animals. It can be tempting when there is a busy op list to take what might seem a very minor risk, but you must take care of yourself and each other.

Feisty cats

There are cats who loathe being handled and this is not confined to feral farm cats. My sister-in-law's cat, who has been raised from a small kitten in the lap of luxury, is a scheming psychopath when handled. I have also experienced a pet Bengal cat attack me by flying horizontally through the air straight at my face like a missile as soon as I opened the door of the bedroom she was in with her newborn kittens. Many vets now advocate minimal restraint with cats who are used to being handled, although this greatly depends on the individual cat and you must know your patient. In my opinion, there are occasions when this is not possible and other means of restraint are necessary, such as gauntlets or securely wrapping them in a towel or confining in a wire cat basket where an injection can be administered through the mesh without opening the box.

Most vet nurses are brilliant at this and if you are working with a good cat handler, then watch in awe and count yourself lucky because you are much less likely to get scratched or bitten and you will be learning from an expert. Most vets showing their war wounds will tell you that their scars are from injuries delivered by cats.

Experienced vets may boast of collecting blood samples single-handed though this is a skill that takes a long time to learn and still carries an element of risk of the 'exploding cat syndrome', when they seem to have far more teeth and claws than they should have and are using them all at once at lightning speed.

Being injured at work

It is vitally important that you look after your own welfare when working as a vet, because there are undoubtedly risks which present themselves and which should be assessed and addressed. There is never a time when your safety or the safety of your colleagues or an owner takes second place in any situation you may find yourself in. Vets are frequently injured in practice by dog and cat bites and scratches, cuts from scalpels, needle-stick injuries, and crushes and kicks and worse from large animals. A relatively minor cat bite that becomes infected can have serious implications and an injured hand may mean that you are unable to work for a significant length of time.

Adopt safe practices with the handling of needles and syringes and be tidy, so instead of putting a used syringe down on the side, put the needle straight in the sharps bin and the syringe in the bin. It is all too easy to cover it up with something else in the course of your work and then someone picks it up and gets stabbed by a hidden needle lurking under a piece of blue towel or some cotton wool. Recapping a needle after drawing up a drug is best avoided if possible, but if necessary, lay the needle cap on a flat surface and push the needle into the cap, only then using your other hand to clip the cap on.

In the past the veterinary profession has been too accepting of a relatively high incidence of injury in the course of doing our job, and there is much more awareness now and recognition of how important it is to take appropriate action to protect ourselves.

There were situations early in my career when I was handling a difficult animal and I told myself that I just 'had to get on and do it', putting myself at risk. Sometimes I got away with it and on some occasions I didn't, but, in retrospect, I should not have proceeded with anything where I could have been injured; in time, I came to realise that there is almost always a better way of doing things if you take a step back and think. If you are in danger of being bitten then the chances are that the animal is also frightened and distressed and there is likely to be an alternative solution, such as another pair of hands to help restrain the patient, or sedation or a general anaesthetic, making handling more acceptable and safer for both the vet and the patient.

Escapologists

It is a terrible experience for all concerned if a patient manages to escape from the practice premises. It must be terrifying for the animal itself and inevitably causes a great deal of distress to the owner. It also causes embarrassment to the veterinary team who may have allowed that to happen and bad publicity which can damage the reputation of the practice.

On a warm day in a stuffy surgery, it is not unusual for some bright spark to decide it would be a really good idea to let some air circulate and to prop open an internal door, perhaps between the prep room and the corridor or even wedge open the exit door of the practice. I used to go completely ballistic if I saw someone had done this and had thoughtlessly and carelessly undermined the safety of the animals on the premises.

Escaping is naturally a talent that many cats and some dogs have got down to a fine art, so be really careful of having an animal on the loose. It is worrying and distressing to have to go hunting for an escapee even if it is the owner who has let it escape from the car in the car park, as one can only imagine the fear the animal is experiencing being at large in an unfamiliar environment. Most vets will tell you their own horror stories of escaping animals and sometimes the story ends without a tragedy and the pet is safely recaptured or arrives at the owner's door under its own steam, but sometimes they are never recovered and get injured and even killed.

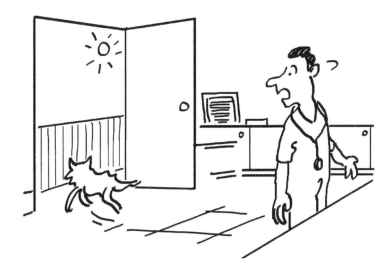

Clients are often relatively inexperienced in transporting their animals, especially cats and small furries and birds. They do not realise the need for a secure cat carrier or bird transporter until they actually need one in an emergency.

> *A client of mine brought a chipmunk into a branch surgery in a bird nesting box but neglected to close off the exit hole in the side of the box. He took the top off the box, the chipmunk shot out of the side door and then did several circuits of the consulting room without apparently touching a surface at all. It then managed to get through a gap under a door and was at large in the back rooms of the surgery. Those little devils are really speedy and extremely difficult to catch, I can assure you.*

Dogs have escaped from surgeries while waiting to be admitted to be examined and they can slip their leads or collars in an instant and be off out of the door before you know it. Clients often have their dog's collar fastened quite loosely, because they rarely ask their dog to go anywhere they are not keen to go anyway. This is not the case when you are trying to get an uncooperative patient into a kennel and if they pull back from you they can slip their collars over their heads and be free. Some dogs seem to have no neck, or necks which are the same width as their heads, so be vigilant or you can be left holding an empty collar at the end of a lead with a dog on the loose.

I have mentioned cat baskets elsewhere, but cannot stress too strongly how brilliant and skilful cats are at devising methods of escaping from cat carriers or cages, especially when you are trying to transfer them from the carrier to the cage in the ward. Always make sure the door to the cat ward is closed, even on a very hot day, and beware someone opening the door and coming into the ward behind you. If a cat escapes in the ward, secure the door first and foremost and do not let anyone else open it before you have secured the cat, whatever foul language they hear from you as you try to catch the miscreant who is doing the equivalent of the motorcycle wall of death round the walls. Beware the scenario where the cat escapes possibly by biting or scratching you and is loose in the cat ward with you swearing and cursing, which someone else hears and opens the door to see what the commotion is. The escapee then sprints past them like a streak of furry lightning looking for the nearest exit.

Escaped cats at large outside the premises are best caught by their owners as they are far more likely to eventually come to them and be rescued if they have not managed to find their own way home. There are various resources from the BVA and the VDS for how to cope with the aftermath of an escape incident and the main thing is to show just how concerned you are and the efforts you are going to put in to help to try to relocate the animal. Contact the owner immediately as they may be able to come and try to catch them, and also, they should never find out that their pet has escaped by him or her appearing on the front doorstep. Do not be tempted to try to keep it to yourself while you try to catch it – honesty is the best policy.

> When I was a new graduate, we used to transport animals for routine surgery from a lock-up branch surgery to a central practice by car. A Cavalier King Charles spaniel had come in for castration and he clearly disagreed with the decision, so he broke free in the back of my car and waited for me to open the door, whereupon he took off, using my head as an elevating trampoline, and was last seen hurtling round the corner at speed. Frantic pursuit and phone calls to the owner followed, but he made his own way home unscathed and the very understanding owner brought him back for the operation the next day, much to the dog's disgust. I was always much more careful after that incident to double check that every animal was secure before I opened the vehicle door.

As a footnote, never take a budgie out of a cage if the window is open or the extractor fan is uncovered and on, for obvious reasons. It may be an urban myth but sometimes these horror stories are true.

Clients who bully vets

Some clients will try to bully vets, especially young vets who are new to the practice and give off any whiff of vulnerability. This bullying can be quite subtle and if challenged, these clients would be outraged at such an accusation, but trying to coerce a vet into doing what they want, or undermining their confidence with misinformation, is indeed a form of bullying.

A common technique used by a manipulative client is to say that a previous vet has agreed to do something which you are currently refusing to do, such as dispense a course of antibiotics or analgesic medication without having seen the patient. You have been told the practice protocol and you know your responsibilities for prescribing, but a client can put a great deal of pressure on you in order to achieve their own ends. In a situation like this, you must politely stand your ground and steadfastly refuse. You do not need to engage in an argument but you must politely state the facts and the reasons for not doing as they want. You may need to repeat this more than once, but you do not have to apologise for doing the right thing.

It may be that another vet, possibly your employer, did break with protocol on a previous occasion but more often you will find that the client is giving you a false version of the facts or being economical with the truth. It may be charitable to believe they have been mistaken, but sometimes it is a deliberate attempt to coerce you into doing something you should not. Maintaining your professional integrity is paramount and you are a professional who must make your own decisions. Breaking the rules in such a situation, or even just bending them, can result in significant and unfortunate repercussions for you, so be stalwart in the face of any attempts to intimidate you.

> *Our small Pennine town is rather notorious for its ageing hippy population and a rather generous supply of recreational drugs locally. A client who kept budgerigars arrived at the surgery demanding antibiotics 'just in case' because he had always kept a supply in from another practice which he usually consulted but which was currently closed. I repeatedly explained that this was not possible and I could not prescribe for a patient who was not under my care. He retorted in exasperation that he could buy crack cocaine in the local pub more easily than get antibiotics for his birds out of me!*

Sometimes you will be asked to undercharge for an item or knock something off the bill because a client alleges that your boss did so last time. I have heard many vets say how it is the discounts by the practice owner that can make it really difficult for an employed assistant to charge correctly on a subsequent occasion. This is very true, and ideally the practice owner would never waive fees or discount medication but he is entitled to give his own money away, whereas you, as an employee, are not. If the client challenges you about this and says they were charged less last time, then tell them you are not allowed to alter the price of anything because you are an employee and leave it at that.

Bullying can also take the form of a constant low-level criticism of you or continual questioning of what you are doing by a client during a consultation or a course of treatment. I am afraid there is not an easy answer to this as you may be caught between a choice of confronting one of the practice's clients or just putting up with it. My advice would be to resist rising to the bait and responding unless they make a false and insulting remark, and even then to challenge it calmly and without losing your temper.

The F-word

Just as none of us like being told we are overweight even by our nearest and dearest, the task of telling owners that their pet is fat can be a minefield. I have friends of mine who have asked me to tell them honestly if I think their dog is heavier than it should be and have been quite offended when I have said yes. Never use the F-word and tell them their dog or cat is fat as the chances are they will take it as a personal insult.

'Wow, what a fat bitch' or 'what a porker' are terms probably best avoided unless you really feel the owner is ready to hear them and has a sense of humour. Phrases and words such as 'overweight', 'heavier than he should be', 'a bit broad in the beam', 'chubby' or 'well-covered' are better received and any other slightly friendlier terminology is usually better accepted by the owners than cold-sounding terms such as morbidly obese. As always, you should use the wording and approach best suited to your audience and in some cases with owners who appreciate a scientific approach, it is appropriate to use professional language, but always remember that telling an owner that their dog is fat is like telling them to their face that their child is fat.

I know that some slim, sporty young vets may not agree with me and believe that it is our duty to leave the client in no doubt whatsoever that they have overfed their pet to the extent that it is clinically obese and to then lecture them about the risk of the many diseases caused by obesity. There is no doubt about the risks and we need the client to understand that their pet is having too much food and not enough exercise, but this has to be done in a helpful and not a judgemental way. The reality in practice is that this news, when unsympathetically delivered, does not go down well and it creates major feelings of guilt in the client who usually is in denial and resents handing over money to be told their pet is fat and that it is all their fault.

In addition, it is often the case that the owner is overweight themselves and when you look round and see their enormous children standing there with their bellies hanging over their trousers, you are in danger of not only appearing to insult the dog but the whole family. You may think that as a result of your pronouncement the client will see the light and change their ways, possibly buying a bag of suitable food from you and from that day forth

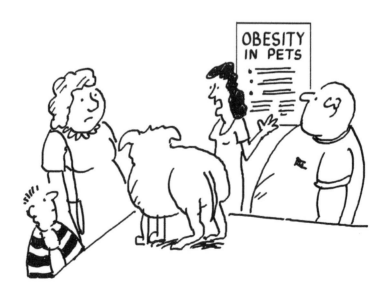

will follow your instructions and cut out high-calorie treats. The whole family will take up hiking and the next time they come to the surgery they will be full of gratitude as their healthy animal is lean and lithe and they will love you forever.

Unfortunately, the most likely outcome if you hit them with the bald truth straight between the eyes is that they will be embarrassed and offended and say very defensively that the animal only has one or two small meals a day. When they get home, they will decide that they do not like you or your advice and that you do not really appreciate just how big-boned and gorgeous their voluptuous Beyoncé Basset is. They will probably tell the receptionist that they do not want to see you again as you were very rude to Beyoncé and will ask to see another vet to see if they are more appreciative of their pet's curvaceous attributes. They may even change practices rather than face being told that Beyoncé is a porker and that she needs to lose a third of her body weight or she is heading for an early grave.

I believe it is far better to empathise with the client about the difficulty in not overfeeding the dog they love so much, and to discuss the weight problem and how to tackle it as sympathetically and sensitively as you can. Tell the client that you are going to help them to help their pet and that it is going to take time but it is achievable, and that the aim is for Beyoncé to live a longer and happier active life. Most clients will have heard about the risks of diabetes and they probably already know that they need to do something but do not know where to start. They don't want their pet to feel hungry and they need help to achieve the weight loss, so offer support in the form of nurse clinics if they are available and explain about the low-calorie diets and the benefits of exercise and alternative healthier treats in a helpful and sympathetic way.

The C-word

Mention of the word 'castration' in relation to dogs and cats and any discussion of the details of the surgery is often surprisingly unpopular with some clients. Some owners seem to think that their dog looks down at his testicles and thinks 'yeah, right, heck I am one hell of a stud and I know exactly what these beauties are for. Bring on the girls, it's time to party.'

They seem to think their dog is proudly aware of their own testicles and those of other dogs and that they will feel less of a real male if they are removed. There is a lot of anthropomorphism going on here which those more qualified than I could explain to you in detail, but the blunt use of the word 'castration' can definitely cause a sharp intake of breath. Use of the term 'neutering' may be more palatable for the client to hear, but just make sure they know exactly what you mean by it and that it is removal of the testicles and not a vasectomy which is being proposed. Never assume a client knows the fundamentals of anatomy and reproduction or understands medical terminology, because in some cases you have to spell it out in short, succinct phrases.

Clients often need to know why male cats are usually castrated and many are not aware of the marking behaviour of unneutered tom cats and the fact that they are more likely to fight, get abscesses and transfer diseases such as FIV and FeLV.

The myth that a female cat or dog has to have a litter

Some clients feel that their animal has missed out in some fundamental way if they have not had the chance to reproduce. This is another area where human emotions are attributed to an animal who does not have a concept of feeling unfulfilled if they do not reproduce, and is certainly not going to watch fondly while their offspring grow up and pursue all their hopes and dreams. We have to do some tactful education for the sake of animal welfare and to save people breeding from their dogs and cats when they have not really thought about all the ramifications and responsibilities of having a litter of pups or kittens and finding homes.

Clients are often surprised by the fact that a cat can have a litter at such a young age and can be completely unaware of when bitches come into season and when they are fertile, so take the opportunity to educate the clients at the time of vaccination.

Myths about vaccination

Some animal owners think that annual vaccination is not necessary and that vets only do it to make money out of them. Vaccination has been such a success story that preventable diseases such as distemper are rarely seen and we have forgotten the ravages of some of the diseases that have been successfully controlled by vaccination in both human and animal populations.

Over the years, I would agree that there have been more vaccine boosters given than has now been proven necessary, but I also remember the harrowing days when dogs were regularly presented with distemper and how my heart would sink when I saw a young dog with diarrhoea, a hacking cough and mucopurulent discharge from the eyes and nose come in to the surgery. When parvovirus first emerged, it killed large numbers of dogs, young and old, and the smell of the haemorrhagic diarrhoea pervaded the surgery. Young cats regularly died of FeLV-related illnesses and the 'cat flu' viruses were widespread amongst the pet cat population.

When you discuss vaccination with clients, give them the facts and take the time to explain why they should have their animal vaccinated against these preventable diseases and about the risk of leptospirosis as a zoonosis. Scare stories about vaccines abound on the Internet and 'My dog died six weeks after a booster' makes a far better news story and sells more papers than 'Vaccines continue to keep pets well'. We need to continue to fight to give evidence-based advice on vaccination and its benefits and do our best to counteract Misguided Malcolm the homeopath with his nosodes and Loopy Linda and her crazy views which abound on the web.

When to act and when to wait

If you are not sure about doing a non-urgent procedure that is new to you or challenging, then do not dive in full of enthusiasm and ill-prepared, but wait until you are in the right circumstances and with the right support.

There are very few genuine emergencies which have to be acted on there and then, but there will be many situations where you will feel manipulated by others into doing something immediately against your better judgement. Clients may put pressure on you by saying that they do not want to leave their animal with you and they do not want to have to come back another time and they want it doing there and then. It is so tempting to comply and do something that deep down you think might not be the right course of action. If it goes wrong for any reason, you can be sure that the client will then say it is all your fault, so make sure that it is you who is in charge of making clinical decisions and not the owner.

If it is possible, then admit a tricky case like that for observation or for a second opinion at no extra charge to the client and make them aware that they are getting a bargain, because two vets are going to give them the benefit of their knowledge. They will usually appreciate the care you are taking in ensuring that their pet receives the correct treatment and feel reassured. Most owners just want what is best for their animal and though they may appear irritated that you are not going to wave that magic wand and act immediately, they will usually realise that you have their animal's best interests at heart and that that is all that matters.

If you do admit a case for observation and time to think and weigh up all the options, be clear to the owner about what you are going to do and when you are going to contact them. Keep your word and contact them at the time you have promised them.

If you are presented with a case with a serious life-threatening condition and you are on your own with no other alternatives available, then you may have to pluck up your courage and act there and then. You may have to just get in there and do something scary for the first time ever because otherwise you would be standing there and watching your patient die and you are the only person present who is potentially able to save its life. This is a situation where you have to stay calm and trust yourself and even if the patient dies, you know you took responsibility as a trained professional and you tried your best and were their only hope. If a dog has a ball obstructing its airway so that breathing is seriously compromised, then you need to take a deep breath and do something without dithering and delaying. If you are in a situation like this, you are not operating on a healthy animal but one in dire need and some critical cases will die and would die anyway, however experienced the veterinary surgeon treating them was. It is always traumatic to lose a patient, but far worse to have stood by and let it happen because of a reluctance to take action when no other course of action was available.

This does not apply to many other conditions presented as emergencies but which can be stabilised for a time while you weigh up the facts and decide what the best plan of action is, seeking help if necessary. Most practices will have some sort of support in place for you as a new graduate and even experienced vets will call for help when they need to.

If a more experienced vet does come and help you out with something tricky such as a gastric torsion, then make sure that you are completely involved and watching and learning so that next time you can handle it yourself if you need to. Do not think, 'Phew, great, Brilliant Bob is here and this is no longer my problem. I can sit back and let someone else sort it out.' Do whatever you can by getting scrubbed up and assisting and let Bob show you what a twisted stomach looks and feels like. Help by keeping the owner informed and stay there until the procedure is complete, even though another vet has taken over the surgery. One day when you are an experienced vet and about to leave the building and a new graduate asks for your help with a GDV, remember this occasion and return the favour.

There will continue to be cases which challenge and surprise throughout your years as a vet and it is important to remember that, although you may be seeing something for the first time, you have the training and skills which can be applied to most situations, however novel and unusual.

Once when I was away on a flotilla sailing holiday in Greece, we were having a barbecue on an uninhabited island a long way from the mainland. A fellow holidaymaker fell down a 30-foot drop while collecting wood for the fire and staggered back to the boats where he sat down and, although initially talking normally, he became incoherent and showed all the signs of concussion or a possible subdural haemorrhage. He had broken his radius and ulna and clearly suffered a significant head injury and the only people around were a retired ENT consultant and me. We had a brief case conference and between us we splinted the arm with a snorkel while others organised a way to get him back on to a boat as soon as possible to get him to a hospital. We located the first-aid kit and managed to get an intravenous cannula in to administer fluids, while we motored as quickly as possible to the mainland and the hospital. Fortunately, the man made a full recovery, and I have never been so glad to reach dry land and hand a patient over to those better qualified than myself; with no other option at the time, I could not just stand by and say it was not my problem and potentially let him die. There is a difference between being an overconfident, have-a-go hero taking an unnecessary risk with an animal, and being the only vet on the premises when a severely injured road accident comes in. You have the training and you are the best option available until another vet arrives.

Identification of inpatients

One black and white cat in a kennel or a cat basket can look very like another black and white cat on a busy day, and there could be more than one black and white cat on the operating list. It is important to ensure that all animals are identified at all times as most vets will tell you of horrific repercussions from misidentification.

If two cats are out of their cages or baskets at the same time and are of similar appearance, it is all too easy on a busy day to mix them up. I have heard tales of cats being anaesthetised and opened up for a cat spay when they came in for a blood sample, and male cats clipped up for a spay. It is not as rare an event as you might think for the wrong cat to be handed back to an owner in the wrong basket, and the worst horror story of all is of the wrong cat being put to sleep due to misidentification.

Make sure this never happens to you by making sure you play your part in ensuring each animal is always identified correctly, and by making sure you know exactly what you are doing and to whom. You may be working with inexperienced members of support staff and even though, theoretically, it may be their job to make sure they have the right animal, it will be you who has to explain and apologise to an owner and that is not a pleasant experience.

Always check the consent form to see what procedures the client has agreed to, as there may be a request on admission for a dental scale or a wart removal in addition to a routine procedure. You might have booked the case in originally, but some additional issue may have arisen of which you may be unaware. It might not even be on the clinical history, so always check the consent form and double check against the history.

Knowing your right from your left and making sure it is the correct lump

Make sure you remove the correct offending, potentially malignant, lump as many older dogs have multiple lumps, some of which may be benign fatty ones, which the owner has not agreed to have removed. It is a difficult conversation to have when a client comes back asking why the wrong mass has been removed and the offending one is still there.

Make sure it is the correct leg or eye you are operating on and ensure the right and left markers are correct when you position an animal for an X-ray. This may seem obvious advice, but amputation of the wrong limb or enucleation of the wrong eye has happened and it should not happen to you if you take care.

Postoperative care

It is tempting to think that once the abdomen has been closed and the patient has recovered from the anaesthetic, your job is done but if you have ever had any surgery yourself, you will be very aware of the importance of postoperative pain relief and nursing.

Ovario hysterectomy in the bitch is major surgery and we regularly send these patients home a few hours later on the same day to be cared for by their owners. We blithely hand out a postoperative care letter in a rush during evening surgery, but we should really pay considerable attention when owners collect them to make sure that our patients do receive the correct level of care when they go home. Do not assume that clients will be sensible about this, because I have seen a client encouraging their bitch to jump into the back of the car in the surgery car park after being spayed, all the while clutching the postoperative information letter in their hands. They may not register the importance of restricting exercise and ignore your advice to keep the patient on a lead unless you explain why it is so important. The practice may have a system where the nurses discharge the patients and explain to the owners how they should look after their pet, but if they are not available then make sure you look after your patients' well-being at this crucial time and give comprehensive advice.

Clients are often so happy to see their animals that they do not really grasp the importance of their role in aftercare and may need some facts reinforcing. They let their cats go out the same evening after surgery and allow dogs with bandaged paws to jump in muddy ditches and forget to bring them back for dressing changes. They do not have the same level of knowledge and what may seem simple common sense to you may not be obvious to someone with little or no experience.

Owners may not recognise when their pet is showing signs of pain, so you may need to spell out when and how much medication they must give and that they need to provide a safe and comfortable environment for their pet to recover. Even the logistics of needing to provide a litter tray for a convalescent cat and keeping it away from other cats at home might not occur to them and you will be doing them a kindness if you gently point out the preparations they may need to put in place.

> *If, like me, you have ever had to look after a young, healthy dog after an ovario-hysterectomy, you might have some sympathy for the owner the next time you tell them to restrict exercise after surgery. If you are a very good surgeon, the wound is small and the level of pain relief is optimum, then the patient is not aware that she is not meant to do anything athletic when she gets home. It is really hard to make sure that they do not run up the stairs when other family members leave the door open, and despite restricted exercise they keep bouncing around encouraging you to play with them when they should be resting and following post-op orders. They might need to be confined in an indoor kennel or kept on the lead in the house and this was the only solution for me when my Labrador bitch Nelly was spayed recently. She would have climbed the Matterhorn the next day if I had allowed her to, and it was a very long week or two of restricted exercise for both of us.*

Owners apparently behaving oddly

It is surprising how many owners, when given some worrying news about their pet which necessitates them changing their plans, will refer to a seemingly trivial thing such as a hair appointment or a social event. Even though you have just informed them of a life-changing diagnosis threatening their animal, they may say they cannot come back the next day because they are taking their daughter to a party. It sounds incredible to you when you have just told them how important it is for them to come back, but it does not mean that they do not care. People who have received worrying news do think aloud on occasion, and they focus on minutiae and insignificant topics when they are shocked or surprised by a turn of events. They will frequently go on to correct themselves and say that of course their plans can be changed and that nothing else matters, so do not be quick to judge them if they rabbit on about the window cleaner coming when you have just diagnosed lymphoma in their dog.

Some owners cope well with a crisis and some do not, and your focus of attention needs to be the well-being of your patient. If a client is deflecting your attention by having hysterics or is getting in the way when you are trying to do your job, then you may have to kindly but firmly ask them to leave so that you can concentrate on what you are doing. Ask a member of support staff to take them into another room and comfort them and calm them down away from the patient. It is impossible to think and work with someone who is really dramatically inclined, and is weeping and wailing and throwing themselves all over your patient; believe me, I have been in situations where I could not hear myself speak let alone listen to a heart. Be polite and try to make them stay and be quiet, or ask them to wait outside until you have news for them. You can even resort to telling them they are upsetting their own pet by their actions but if they have gone the full Lady Macbeth, then they must leave the scene.

There may be times when owners have beliefs which you may not share but which are very important to them. I have been asked to put a cat to sleep slowly so that a ritual could be held during her passing to ease her through some portal or other, the details of which I cannot remember. This was clearly very important to the owner and once the cat became unconscious it was not making any difference to her, so I administered an anaesthetic dose initially and waited. The owner made many strange incantations round the elderly little cat and as the soul left the body, I gradually gave the remaining amount of pentobarbitone all the while carefully avoiding catching the eye of my veterinary nurse as the sound of wailing and the incense drifted around us. It was all very peaceful and although I did not share her beliefs, it made the owner feel better and apparently she liked my aura!

We were once called out on a visit to euthanise an old dog who was off his legs and when we arrived, they had set up a table in a field on a warm summer night with candles around and all the friends and relatives gathered to say goodbye. It was rather heartwarming, although the pressure of performing well under such circumstances was quite intimidating, as you can imagine. Fortunately, my patient was a very cooperative, gentle soul who was reassured by the presence of his family and he slipped peacefully away in the company of all those who loved him. Once they had laid him to rest they all had a wake in his honour which was a lovely send-off for an old gentleman.

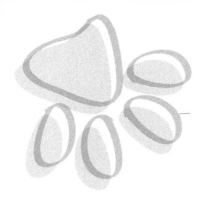

CHAPTER 15

Being a vet in real life

First opinion practice

I have heard vets say of themselves and of others that they are 'only in first opinion practice' as if this was a lesser status than a vet working in a referral centre or a university small animal hospital specialising in a particular discipline. A good vet in first opinion practice is providing a vital service for society, and we should be proud to be one of the thousands of vets seeing the animals owned by the general public and keeping them healthy and well cared for.

Animals and humans need and bring out the best in one another and I believe that this is becoming increasingly more evident as society changes. Pet ownership fulfils a need in society and as people have progressively more diverse family arrangements the stability and simplicity of the bond between humans and companion animals becomes ever more important and so does our role in caring for these increasingly valued members of the family. It is a highly skilled job and the training you receive at vet school is only the beginning of a lifelong process of adding to your knowledge and skills.

Veterinary knowledge and available treatment options have developed so far over the past 20 years that it was logical that some disciplines would be better served by having dedicated vets focusing on a particular organ system, such as cardiology, or on developing skills specifically for orthopaedic surgery, and so referral centres were the inevitable result.

The opportunity to refer a case to a colleague who has extensive experience of similar cases and who has invested in the necessary equipment to deal with diagnosing and rectifying a specific problem, is a huge benefit to vets in first opinion practice. It provides much better outcomes for our patients than the days when we had to perform procedures for the first time with a book open to guide us because we were the only option available. Vets did achieve excellent results, but there were also some failures and some poor outcomes and it is good that those days are past.

Even though we now refer some cases and do not attempt to treat everything ourselves, this should not be seen as a dumbing down of first opinion practice where advances have made it possible to achieve far more than was ever possible in the past. First opinion practice is a different discipline requiring different skills and approaches and the work is of equal importance to that of the vets in the referral centres. They may be pushing the boundaries of what is achievable surgically, where equipment is state of the art and cost is not an issue, but they still rely on the first opinion vet for those referrals and for the continued care of their patients after they have discharged them. Never say, 'I am just a small animal vet' or 'I am just a mixed practice vet' but be proud because these are vital services and require special individuals, and you achieve positive outcomes for animals every single day.

I believe that true job satisfaction for a first opinion vet comes from the small daily triumphs which may sometimes appear insignificant but have the capacity to resolve problems for animals and make a massive difference to their lives and that of their owners. The diagnosis of a complex medical case such as a pituitary tumour or a puzzling horse lameness is really rewarding in itself, and even if there is no one to give you a round of applause and tell you that you are brilliant, the fact remains that you have done a good job and you should be proud.

Every year that goes by, your experience will increase and you can constantly expand your knowledge and ability; this will always be the case if you keep your mind open and responsive to new information. You already know more when you qualify than many older vets such as I did years ago, and the quality of the veterinary services are far more advanced than they were when I first graduated. The vets who have been qualified for 20 years have had to change with the new technology and have had to keep learning or be left behind as things moved on. I have no doubt that you will also have to embrace ever more advanced technology and react to a different world as you continue to work and there will be many changes to come, both in first opinion practice and in referral practices.

It is impossible to know for certain just what the future holds for the graduates of today, but there will always be a place for a good first opinion vet while ever a human owns an animal. Many children benefit from the presence of the family pet who can provide unconditional love and company and a daily lesson in caring for them which cannot be taught in school. The benefits of pet ownership for older people has been well documented and there are increasing numbers of charities training support and assistance dogs. The use of guide dogs for the blind has been around since 1934 but there are now also support dogs for the disabled, for autistic children, for veterans suffering from post-traumatic stress disorder, and horses for heroes for veterans who have lost limbs or have mental health issues where working with horses can make a huge difference. Children with disabilities are helped by the Riding for the Disabled Association and therapy horses have helped children with learning difficulties and people who have suffered abuse.

The role of the first opinion veterinary surgeon is pivotal in looking after these animals owned by society and we should not underestimate the influence we have and the potential we have to make a difference.

Vets in the community

You can choose to be as involved as much or as little as you want to be in your local area but there are a few considerations to be aware of. If you live in the area in which you work, then people will get to know that you are the local vet and this can have its good points and its drawbacks.

I have learned the hard way never to try to do any veterinary work from my front door-step because it is doomed to failure. I never keep any veterinary instruments or medicines at home and if someone comes knocking on my door with a sick or injured animal, I never try to treat it beyond basic first aid if essential, because at best I will be doing an inadequate job and I know I will regret it. I always advise them to go to the vet and will help organise a taxi or even give them a lift there, but unless something is bleeding to death for want of a pressure bandage, I do not treat them at my home. You can be sure that if you do it once, then it will definitely happen again and will encourage others as word gets around. It is usually the clients who have the least respect for you and your free time who are the ones who will pop round to your house on your day off and abuse your goodwill. Acquaintances may also try this, but true friends care enough about you to respect your need for time off and will rarely ask you to examine their animal unless they are forced to through exceptional circumstances.

I once made the mistake of doing a few favours for the owner of my local pub who had retrievers by foolishly agreeing to give boosters to them on my day off because they were so busy behind the bar! This kindness was followed up by requests to check their ears once or twice and to take stitches out after a spay and each time it seemed rather churlish to refuse. One day I went in and the publican announced that he was changing to a different practice, because when he had called in for some flea treatment for a cat I had never seen and which had never been to the surgery, our nurse had followed practice policy and quite rightly refused to dispense a prescription medicine without authorisation. He had been round to another practice and they had happily broken the rules and given him what he wanted. All my grovelling on the pub carpet taking stitches out as a favour to him had counted for nothing; it was a salutary lesson in the fickleness of some clients and you live and learn.

Local agricultural and pet shows

It is not uncommon to be asked to attend the local country show and judge the dog classes and children's pet shows and, although this can be great fun, it can also be a poisoned chalice. Take care before you agree to anything to find out exactly what it is they are asking you to do and consider if your involvement can also be seen as an endorsement for something you may not agree with. I do not like to see any companion animals except dogs at shows, as I am not comfortable seeing cats sitting in baskets looking miserable and stressed, or small furries at risk of overheating and escaping in some flimsy tent on a hot day. I used to be moderately happy to judge the dog with the waggiest tail and the prettiest bitch, although this can also be a minefield for causing offence where you least anticipate it.

> *Never underestimate how competitive the parents of small children can be and how much they want their little precious darling to win the prize. Once, as a very young, foolish and trusting vet I was invited to judge the local children's pet show and afterwards I vowed never to do it again. In trotted a beautifully clipped standard poodle who could have qualified for Crufts with a smug-looking mother and child, and next up was a boy with knobbly knees with a stick insect in a tank. There was a fat corgi towing a girl dressed as a princess completely out of control, and a Shetland pony with a pimply youth who looked as if he wanted to be anywhere but at the end of a lead rein but had been press-ganged into it by his mother. In the end, I gave the prize to a lad with a guinea pig as he seemed to be knowledgeable about how to feed and look after it, whereas the other children did not seem to have much involvement in the care of their animals. This decision resulted in outraged huffing and puffing from the Crufts champion poodle owner with her wailing child who she had obviously assured of winning the prize, and the situation was even worse when I found out that the guinea pig owner was my vet nurse's nephew. Accusations of a fix were made very audibly in my hearing and the atmosphere surrounding what was intended to be a light-hearted event turned quite sour.*

If ever you do get roped in to judge a pet show, prepare in advance and have some questions ready to ask each child. At the end of the day, be prepared to be treated like a leper by everyone but the winner and their family! Good luck!

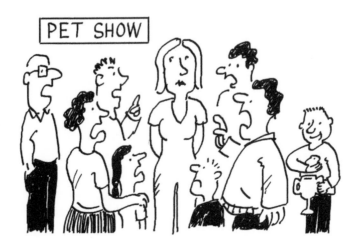

Giving advice about their animals to friends and family

I do not know why, but people always love to ask you about their animal and ask for your opinion when they have already asked another vet for theirs. Beware the friend of a friend who asks what you would advise for a dog with a skin condition or when to worm a litter of puppies or restart a lapsed vaccination, because half the time they will then quote a different vet who gave different advice. People will also insist on asking you what sort of dog they should have and then disagree with your recommendation.

My sister's friend owned a hyperactive Dobermann with spinal problems which very sadly managed to kill itself by running into a tree in the dark and breaking its own neck. Neither she nor her husband had the time and patience to train a big dog and she asked me at a wedding what sort of dog I advised she should get as a replacement, because she wanted a quiet dog with no problems. I mentioned a few easy breeds with good conformation but laughingly said to avoid Dalmatians and dachshunds, only to meet her six months later with one of each! The Dalmatian dog was ricocheting around the room like a bucking bronco and the dachshund looked unfeasibly long in the back and, from an engineering perspective, if it had been a bridge it would have been condemned.

It's a vet's life

- Always scoop the poop of your own pet as you can guarantee that if you miss it once some beady-eyed local will spot the offending pile and you are always a vulnerable target because you are the vet who should know better.
- If you have small children and you take the classroom hamster home, it will die in your care. Try to avoid the responsibility at all costs. On average, school hamsters live to over ten years of age. This is because if they die during the holidays, someone always replaces them with a younger model of the same appearance.
- If you own a cat, then it will crap in the beautiful tilled soil of the flower beds of your next door neighbour who is the local gardening fanatic. There is nothing you can do about it, but they will expect you to prevent it happening because you are a vet!
- If you are on call, the phone will ring about an hour after you go to sleep, whatever time of the evening or night you lay down your head on the pillow. You might as well go to bed at the usual time and get some sleep, so do not delay going to bed in case the phone rings. It will get you even if you wait until after midnight!
- If you spay the nurse's bitch, it will be fraught with complications, will bleed like a pig and will hold its breath under the anaesthetic, resulting in you gaining several grey hairs.
- If you are ever feeling pressured into saying roughly how many pups a pregnant bitch is going to have and are about to open your mouth, then go and bang your head repeatedly on the wall. Do not on any account give a definite number without any caveats, because

either one is hiding from the scanner or you will count the same puppy twice. The client will always remember that you said eight when it was seven.

- Never say how long an old animal has to live even if it looks terminal, because you will meet the owner a year later and he will tell you it has never looked better and you were wrong.
- The law of 'it will only take five minutes' means that if you try to do anything in a hurry just before evening surgery, it will always take you three times as long as expected and will not be straightforward.
- If you go away on holiday to get away from the pressures of work, there will happen to be a client in the airport departure lounge who wants to discuss his dog's diarrhoea, even though you are clearly uninterested and wearing shorts.

I once went on a package holiday and a demanding client was on the same tour, so I spent the whole week hiding from her in various bars while she tried to talk to me about her elderly poodle. I had come on holiday to escape talking about sick animals so I kept my occupation a secret. I enjoyed inventing the most uninteresting occupation I could think of when people asked me what I did for a living. My favourite was to tell them I was a tax inspector but this usually resulted in being shunned by my fellow travellers for the rest of the holiday.

- If you get a circular lesion on your arm or a persistent itch, you may have to tell the doctor that you have ringworm or cheyletiella that you have acquired in the course of your work because they may not recognise it as such.
- You will need to learn to keep your mouth closed when expressing an anal gland or an abscess and you will inadvertently go out in public with arterial blood on your face or collar.
- I once had to nonchalantly catch a cat flea that was meandering around on my son's face in the doctor's consulting room. This can be an occupational hazard of being a vet's child.
- There will be clients who live locally and who swore to you on their mother's grave that they would pay their bill and who will have subsequently become bad debtors. They will not be bothered in the slightest when they see you, but you will seethe inwardly.
- The incidence of three-legged adopted cats in your immediate circle of family and friends will be higher than average and at least one will be called Stumpy.
- You will forget to worm and deflea your own dog, despite advising other people what to do every single day.
- You will be in the pub celebrating your birthday, relaxing and acting the fool when you will suddenly catch the eye of your most demanding client.
- You will feel quite bereaved when other members of the team leave the practice and move on. You have shared significant events and experiences and you will miss them.
- You will eat junk food such as cake and biscuits because clients like to show how much they appreciate you going the extra mile for their animals.

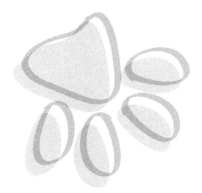

CHAPTER 16

End of life care
and euthanasia

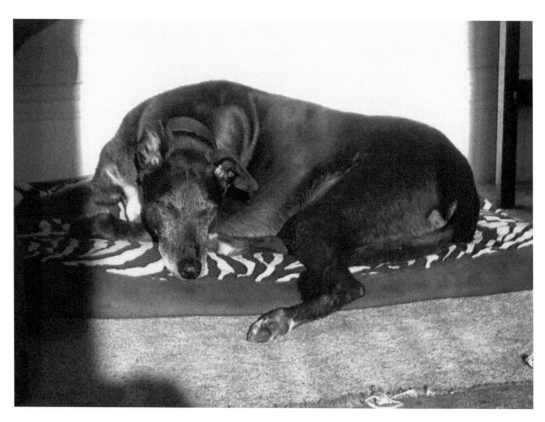

Every animal deserves a good life and a good death. This is Gnasher the lurcher, who I rescued as a puppy from a very bad start in life and who lived 11 happy years with us before she was diagnosed with a cardiac-based neoplasia. When her quality of life deteriorated, I took her for euthanasia and I still miss her but have no regrets. One of the most important services that vets provide is easing distress and relieving suffering by the practice of euthanasia.

When I first qualified many years ago in the late 1970s, the attitude of the general public to their ageing, sick and injured animals was very different to nowadays. Although people cared about their pets, it was much less common to consider them as family members or on a par with children and certainly there was no use of the nauseating term 'fur baby'!

There were not as many medical treatments available for animals and the techniques for anaesthesia and surgery were far less advanced, so there was more acceptance that on average animals had a relatively short expected lifespan compared to now. There was less demand for complex surgery and expensive treatments for an animal that the owners perceived to be nearing a natural end to their expected lifespan. Chemotherapy was not available and life stage diets were unheard of, the majority of dogs being fed on tinned food and very cheap processed food and biscuits or just leftovers and household scraps.

Cats were only just becoming sufficiently valued for some owners to agree to the very simple repair of a broken leg but very often owners refused any treatment at all for cats and opted for euthanasia. The older generation would find it incomprehensible that anyone would pay for an injured cat to be treated at all when you could just go and get another one, and owners were much more likely to opt for euthanasia when their pet became old and infirm.

Times have changed over the years and a growing number of people are now looking for good-quality veterinary care for their pets as they age and want to keep them as healthy as possible for as long as they can. They are seeing improvements in the end of life care for humans, where there is a much more enlightened approach to ageing and palliative care and the hospice movement has made it possible to die without being in pain and to have a good, peaceful death with dignity.

There are currently facilities opening up in the United States providing hospice care for pet animals, and while some consider this may be going too far, it may be a sign of things to come. I do believe that we could do much more to improve the quality of life for many of our elderly pets towards the end of their all too short lives and to ease their passing.

Many clients come to us when their dogs and cats are getting old and infirm, looking for help and advice because they do not possess the knowledge of how best to look after an elderly animal and they want to do the right thing. We are uniquely well placed to offer them this advice and have the opportunity to make a real difference to their pet's last few precious months of life; we should place more importance on this amelioration of effects of the ageing process in addition to the diagnosis of disease and necessary surgical interventions. The care of the ageing but reasonably well pet could be much improved in many instances and we should be advocating small and simple lifestyle changes and preventative measures to help owners make the right choices with their senior companions.

The relatively short lifespan of cats and dogs compared to humans means that the speed of the ageing process in the last year or two of life comes as a surprise to some owners. There is a wealth of advice for owners of young dogs and cats about diet and training and toys, and naturally everyone loves a cute puppy or a kitten. There are millions of posts and photos on social media and advice is ubiquitous for young animals but rather more scarce for the older pet who is slowing down and may have bad breath and dandruff and the odd weird lump.

You may have nursed an ageing pet of your own through this end of life stage, but when I first became a vet I had had no experience at all of looking after the elderly, neither human nor animal.

It is an area of veterinary medicine which I believe is not emphasised nearly enough to the general public for various reasons, and we should be much more proactive and make our clients more aware of what is available and possible for these older animals. The skill of the first opinion veterinary practitioner in caring for ageing animals and supporting their owners should be considered as important as performing heroic cutting-edge surgery. It might not make such good television, but when you put an elderly spaniel on cardiac medication, it can be like a miracle to the dog and their owner.

Practical advice

We may think that making small management modifications are simply common sense but this is not always obvious to owners and is part of the pastoral care we should provide as general practitioners.

Clients may need to be told to feed several smaller meals a day rather than one or two larger meals and you may think that is obvious, but dogs and owners are creatures of habit and if Bouncer has been fed once or twice a day for the last nine years they may need to be prompted to try a change to their routine. They may need to gradually change the content of the diet to one better suited to the nutritional needs of that older individual and the results can be marked and may prevent the digestive upsets which may seem trivial to us but not to the owner of a cream carpet and an old dog with a sensitive stomach.

Owners may be asking too much of an old dog in terms of exercise, and may not recognise that the pet may appear willing to undertake the exercise but may suffer for it afterwards. They may still be expecting their ageing, arthritic pet to go for a ten-mile hike over rough terrain every weekend rather than several short, easy walks a day over softer ground.

Increased water intake due to reduced renal function and a reduction in bladder control in older dogs can mean that the owners may need to work out some system for letting their pet out more frequently if they want to avoid them urinating in the house. We accept that old people need to get up during the night, but we expect old dogs to cross their legs for ten hours or suffer the stress of worrying about having soiled in the house.

Cats may need to start urinating in the house for the first time and need to be provided with a litter tray, because they feel vulnerable going outside and can no longer defend themselves against the neighbour's cat.

When a client requests euthanasia for an old animal, their decisions may be influenced by a breakdown in house training which they have been struggling with. They may even exaggerate other symptoms to justify their decision such as loss of enjoyment of life or loss of appetite, simply because they are too embarrassed to give the real reason for asking for euthanasia, which may be that they have reached the end of their tolerance of coming down to a puddle and a pile to clean up every morning before they go to work. This can reach crisis point if they have small children and they are struggling to cope to keep the house clean and hygienic with an incontinent old dog.

Owners often find it difficult to assess how much pain their pet is experiencing and, because an old, arthritic dog in dull pain with aching joints does not actually cry out, they may fail to recognise signs of pain and discomfort. You have learned about the indicators of pain and the scoring of different levels of pain, but an owner faced with the gradual onset of symptoms may not recognise that their dog or cat is suffering. Old animals experiencing a slow decline become stoic in the face of considerable pain and discomfort and you may need to convince an owner that their pet is no longer comfortable and needs pain relief. Some owners think that once you start giving medication for arthritis, it has to be continuous and they wait too long before seeking veterinary attention, or think that the side-effects of pain-killers will shorten the life of their animals. I still drive along the roads and wince when I see an elderly dog hobbling along beside an owner and feel like screeching to a halt and jumping out to cross-examine them or haul them off to the vet.

In the early stages of an animal's decline into old age, simple changes such as a comfortable, draught-free, well-padded bed and some analgesia can make a marked difference to creaky joints, and when an owner says their dog has taken to getting onto the sofa, it may not be because the dog is becoming disobedient, but it may just be very uncomfortable sleeping on a hard floor in a draught.

Loss of vision and hearing can make an old dog or cat feel very insecure and reduced cognitive ability generally can make them panic in unfamiliar surroundings. When you see an elderly dog in reasonable physical health, do not forget to ask the owner about any changes in behaviour such as increased nervousness or intolerance of situations in which they were previously relaxed. Old cats can gradually lose more and more vision, especially if they have retinal problems caused by undiagnosed renal disease or hyperthyroidism, for example, and they can function so well in familiar surroundings that the owner has no idea that they may have reduced vision.

I have owned dogs all my life, most of whom who I have adopted during the course of my work. I had an old whippet who became gradually more blind and deaf in her last year and I was not aware how blind she had become because she used to follow me closely everywhere. I took her for a walk beside the local canal and she was startled by a cyclist, and because she was not able to see where I was, she panicked and went hurtling off, blind as a bat, in the wrong direction down the tow path. This episode made me realise that the time had come to keep her on a lead for her own safety and reminded me how animals adapt to slow, insidious loss of a sensory function. As animals become older and more vulnerable, we need to advise our clients of modifications such as this to keep them safe.

I had a client who only realised his dog was virtually blind when he was refurbishing a bedroom and took the old bed to the tip for disposal. The dog strolled into the empty bedroom that afternoon and jumped up as normal as if the bed was still there, landing in a surprised heap on the floor. He had gradually become completely blind but because he was in a familiar environment he had coped with his loss of sight, as long as the furniture was not moved from its usual place.

Gradual loss of cognitive function is well known in humans and also occurs to some extent in dogs and cats; owners may be unaware that this can be connected with underlying disease which may be treatable and that there are drugs which can help. When these are prescribed, owners often come in jokingly requesting them for themselves or their spouses because the difference can be so marked. I have even heard them being recommended by one client to another in the hairdresser's, which made me smile.

When animals become older, it is advisable to ask the owner to bring them for health checks at more frequent intervals and this is well received if the client understands how the signs of ageing progress rapidly in the older animal. Timely treatment of conditions because of prompt diagnosis has a significant influence on the progression of diseases in the ageing population, and the year between annual health checks may be too long an interval to allow undiagnosed disease to go unchecked.

End of life care

End of life care and death of human beings is addressed much more sensitively nowadays and the concept of a good death after a happy and healthy life is also very important to clients. They may need considerable help from us to ensure that their care of their pet in the final days and weeks is as good as it can possibly be. Some clients ask for their pet to be put to sleep as soon as they know they are significantly declining, whereas others cling on to every day that they have left. It is important to monitor these patients and make appropriate repeat appointments to ensure the client has support and knows what they can do to make them comfortable; we need to be the advocate for that animal and ensure that they have as good a quality of life as possible. It helps a great deal if the vet and the client are working together at this stage of life and it makes it easier for the client to make the right decision at the right time if they have maintained close contact with the vet.

Vets receive more thank-you letters and gifts of appreciation for putting animals to sleep than they ever get for diagnosing and treating a life-threatening disease or performing brilliant surgery. The euthanasia consultation is a unique event and the experience for the owner in how their pet is treated, and how they themselves are treated at this time has continued and immeasurable effects long afterwards.

Euthanasia and its effect on us as vets

Part of our job as vets is to end the life of the animals in our care, and because we care about animals this can be very hard on us emotionally. There are times when we have to experience this more than once in a day and an experienced friend of mine recently had six euthanasia consultations to perform in one day and felt that he had reached the point where he just could not handle another one. We all have our own limits when it comes to emotional resilience and if you have reached a point where you feel it is causing you harm, then do speak to your colleagues and enlist their help. Above all, make sure you talk to people about how you are feeling because the support of your veterinary team colleagues can make all the difference in these harrowing situations.

You may have experienced a significant bereavement in your life, possibly of a close relative or a pet of your own, but there will be new graduates who have never experienced a bereavement of any sort. You may have some understanding of how the client might be feeling but every individual's experience of grief is unique and their reactions as they go through such an emotionally charged experience can be many and varied. During your life as a vet, you will have to perform euthanasia many times and you will see very many different reactions from different people and the emotions you experience during and after these consultations will vary too.

There are many books and articles written about the grieving process and we are becoming much more aware of the need for bereavement counselling for animal owners. Although many vets provide this service on an unofficial basis in the course of their work, it may be that a client has deep and specific issues that overlap with this and other areas of their lives and they may need to be referred to a trained bereavement counsellor. The loss of an animal can trigger the memory of other unresolved emotional issues and in some cases, it is professional help that is needed, not just the ear of a sympathetic, untrained amateur, so do direct people to the necessary support resources and do not take too much upon yourself.

Performing euthanasia well

If a client sees or perceives their beloved companion to have suffered or to have been treated with anything other than gentleness and kindness during euthanasia, they will always remember it. Grief and feelings of helplessness and guilt after the loss of a pet can also manifest themselves in anger and a euthanasia consultation which goes badly wrong is highly likely to result in a complaint which can be very difficult to resolve. A bereaved and angry client is unlikely to be reasonable and we need to do everything we can to ensure that we actually make the experience as painless and peaceful as possible for all concerned, and take the time and trouble to comfort the owner as much as we can.

I am sure you will have seen euthanasia performed many times during EMS and rotations and seen both good and bad euthanasia consultations. You have probably been asked to leave the consulting room on some occasions as this is a very personal and emotionally charged time and clients often prefer not to have an audience for their grief. You will have had some opportunity to observe how the best consultations were handled and this experience helps you to choose and use the most effective techniques to perfect your own style now that you are the vet who is performing the euthanasia.

Everyone has their own unique approach to the euthanasia consultation and it is an occasion where you will indeed 'perform' a euthanasia because the spotlight will most definitely be on you. You will find that it helps if you have a basic framework or routine to guide you in orchestrating proceedings to ensure maximum efficiency and minimum drama. If you follow a certain sequence in the way you approach the consultation, including how you organise the owner and those assisting you, it means you are in control of proceedings.

Making the decision

I have spent many hours of my life talking to clients about euthanasia in all manner of situations, such as on the phone, in consultations and even in the street or in the pub. I am not in practice at the moment, but I still received a phone call last night from a friend in this dilemma who wanted to talk it over. The question of when is the right time, and when is too soon, and when is too late, tax clients and vets alike and this is because there is no right answer to this question.

There are not many occasions when an ageing or sick animal goes straight from not being a candidate for euthanasia one hour, to a patient who should be urgently relieved from suffering the next. Usually, there is a day, a week or even months of being in a twilight time when it is not the wrong thing to put a geriatric patient to sleep, nor is it unreasonable to give them a little longer. This is the time when you will be called upon to listen to your clients going through the stress of making that final decision and you need to demonstrate understanding and offer guidance.

Although most clients do recognise when the right time has arrived, we also owe it to our patients to help our clients make the right decision on those occasions where we can see that an animal is suffering and that it is time to let them go. There is rarely another occasion in the life of a human being when you are obliged to request and authorise the death of an individual who you love. Most vets themselves find this decision really difficult with their own animals and, speaking from experience, there have been occasions when the answer has not been clear to me and I have had to ask a colleague for their help in making that choice.

Your communication skills are so important during this conversation and though it may become a daily occurrence for you, it is an exceptional and emotional event for the owner. You have to give the client your full and undivided attention at this time and listen carefully to what they are saying. You can help them to feel better and reassure them that they are making the right decision.

There have been times where I have felt that an owner was acting in haste in requesting euthanasia because they felt pressurised by certain circumstances, and I have encouraged them to go away and think about it again before going through with it. It really depends on what has triggered the decision and because I had the privilege of being a practice owner, I have even taken an animal in to give an owner a chance to go and think about it calmly and rationally, rather than acting in haste and regretting it when it is too late.

Dogs which have bitten people can cause an owner to immediately rush in and demand euthanasia because they are understandably distraught and feeling guilty for this having happened. This is a difficult situation to deal with, and ultimately you may have to euthanise a healthy animal if that is the right thing for all concerned. A decision like this should never be made in haste, however, and it may be that once the owner has calmed down, and the circumstances in which the incident happened have been fully considered, there may be a different solution to the situation. Do be careful of forcefully recommending a second chance for a dog which has bitten, because you may be assuming some degree of responsibility should that dog bite again. Make sure you advise about adequate controls and inform the owner that the decision for keeping the dog is theirs and not yours to make.

Reaching the end

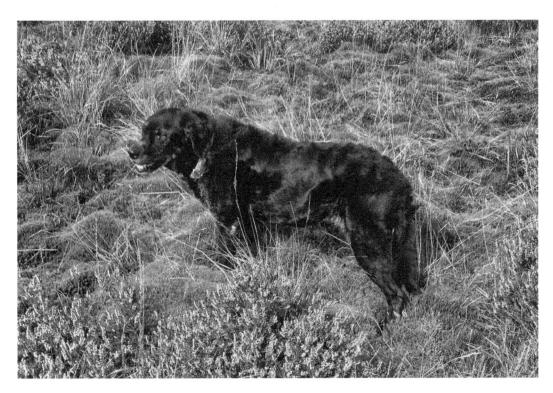

Baggy the Labrador enjoying her last walk up on the moors in the heather, 'reading the news' with her nose. Bagheera had a wonderful life, was loved by children and enjoyed a long life free from illness and injury until her old legs, despite treatment, finally gave out. We can treat disease and repair trauma but there comes a time when all we can do to prevent prolonged suffering is to offer them a pain-free death.

If you are regularly seeing an old dog or cat who is reaching the latter stages of life then do, if possible, prepare the client well in advance. However hard a conversation it may be, I think that, as vets, we have a duty to our patients to make sure that owners are aware of the seriousness of their pet's condition, and if possible give them some idea as to the timescale and likely progression. This will depend on a number of factors and many elderly animals present with multiple problems which grumble on for a long time, but I think there has been a reluctance to discuss the subject of the approaching death of our patients with their owners. It might be easier for us to avoid awkward and upsetting conversations, but I think we should accept this as part of our responsibility to the pet and their owner, especially when it is obvious to us but not to them.

Consultations to discuss pain relief and alleviation of other symptoms with medication at this stage of life gives you the chance to prepare the owner for the inevitable loss of their companion and gives you time to gently explain and answer any questions they may have. You will need to be sensitive to their wishes and some clients do not want to think about it or discuss it until the time arises, but others will wish to be forewarned and prepare themselves.

You may open the discussion by suggesting that if your patient should be taken ill out of hours then your client should not hesitate to call the surgery if they are worried and to inform them of the emergency service arrangements. This can open up the discussion as to how likely this is to happen in the near future and what action should be taken out of hours. Some people will have been through this before with a previous pet and others may want to have more information, but at least the subject has been brought into the conversation. It is a kindness to make sure that they know what arrangements have been made for times when the surgery is closed as they do not want to have to find this out at two in the morning with a pet in extremis. It is far more common nowadays to have a separate out of hours service and your clients need to know where the out of hours service is located and how to contact them in an emergency. If they have no transport, then make sure they have the contact details of an animal ambulance should they need one, and to know what they need to do. In this way, you may play your part in some way in helping to minimise delay and ease distress for both your patient and their owners.

Euthanasia

Your practice support staff should make sure, if at all possible, that a client awaiting a euthanasia appointment is not sitting in the middle of a busy waiting room surrounded by other clients with lively, healthy animals while they are spending the last precious minutes with their pet. If it is possible, then schedule the appointment for a quiet time and invite them to wait in an unoccupied room or even in their car until you are ready to see them.

🐾 Make sure you know the name and sex of your patient because it does not go down at all well if you use the name of their other dog, which is two years old and in rude health.

- Have the necessary consent forms filled in in advance, giving you permission and instructions for disposal of the body.
- If the animal has been under treatment, read the clinical notes so that you are able to answer any last-minute questions and can confirm the appropriateness of the decision if it is a clinical one.
- Have a pen ready for their signature.
- Be prepared with everything you might need for the euthanasia ready to hand.
- Have a box of tissues handy.
- Turn your phone off (obvious I know but . . .).
- Make sure you look professional and are not covered in bloodstains or hair.
- Inform other members of staff in the building so that they can keep the background noise down.
- Make sure you are not going to be disturbed by another member of staff asking you if you want a coffee halfway through the procedure.
- Do not have the syringe of pentobarbitone and a black disposal bag visible as the first thing the client sees when they walk in.

Informed consent

Once a decision has been reached, it is advisable to obtain written permission for euthanasia and this permission needs to be clearly understood by the client. This needs to be informed consent and not just a quick scrawl on a piece of paper and you need to be reasonably sure that they do have the authority to make that decision.

Insisting on completing paperwork at an emotive time like this can be awkward and resented by the client, but is essential. Many owners hate signing the form that allows euthanasia, especially if they are long-established clients who have known you for a while and they may particularly resent the mention of payment at what they consider an inappropriate moment.

It is also an opportunity to agree in writing as to whether they want to bury their pet at home or have them cremated with all the relevant costs that are involved. It is not an easy conversation at the best of times, but it can be even more difficult discussing costs of individual cremation with a distressed owner just after euthanasia over the body of their departed pet.

Your boss, however, will tell you that a significant proportion of bad debts come from unpaid euthanasia consultations and most practices will have a custom or protocol for dealing with the fees and payments. It's always difficult asking for money at this time, but assess the situation and with tact and good support staff, it is often possible to propose to the client that signing the consent form and paying in advance before the euthanasia will mean that they will not be upset by an invoice arriving in the post a few days afterwards. I suggest you follow practice protocols, but there may be occasions when you need to use your own judgement on whether to press the point or not. Our practice used to take a more lenient approach to regular clients and send the invoice a few days later, but be more stringent with new clients. Some prefer to get the payment out of the way beforehand and others find the mention of money like a red rag to a bull. Always, always get the consent form signed as a failure to pay is one thing, but in a very small number of cases failure to obtain written consent could turn out to be much more serious.

Be prepared

Avoid rushing in and out of the room, having forgotten your scissors or the paperwork, and giving any indication that you are in any way ill-prepared or in a hurry. Have everything ready and prepared before the client comes in so that the atmosphere is calm and drama-free which reassures the owner and helps to minimise stress for their animal.

Before you perform your first euthanasia, find out what the usual procedure is in that practice. Every practice will have their own ways of doing things which will be familiar to the support staff and possibly the clients. Some practices have a quiet consult room or even a dedicated room solely for euthanasia which offers a private place for the client to sit with their animal before and afterwards. This is not always possible in a surgery with limited space but there are usually ways in which privacy and consideration can be provided for these special circumstances.

Make sure that all other members of staff in the building know what you are in the process of doing. There is nothing worse than hearing guffaws of laughter outside the door of the consulting room or someone whistling happily as they mop the waiting room while you are giving the final injection with a devastated owner. These consultations are often scheduled at the end of surgery when the rest of the staff may think everyone has gone and it can inadvertently appear crass and uncaring.

Bring the client into the consulting room and show an appreciation of how they must be feeling. Your client expects you to be sympathetic but professional and while they do not expect you to be in floods of tears, they do want to feel that you care about them and their pet. They are often looking for understanding, warmth and support at this time and reassurance about what is about to happen, and they want you to be strong for them and to help them through the ordeal.

As discussed previously, there may be occasions when you do not entirely agree with the timing of their decision and you may feel that they are acting too soon or have left things too long, but this is not the time to be judgemental. If it has come this far, then it is your job to respect their decision once it has been made and to make it as easy as possible for your patient and indeed your client.

It is tempting to be critical of another person's views and wishes if they are different to your own, but you never know exactly what is going on in another person's life. That client may be unable to cope with an old dog with urinary incontinence because they have other demands in their home life, such as a disabled child. The client who appears to have waited too long may have done so because the dog belonged to their deceased husband and they could not face bringing them to you and severing that link. Never be too quick to judge at the time of a euthanasia whatever state the animal is in; this is not the appropriate time to criticise the owner or make them feel even worse than they do already and you will achieve nothing.

Many clients will still ask you to examine their animal before you perform the euthanasia even though they have asked for it to be done, because they want reassurance that they are making the right decision. Even though they have requested a euthanasia appointment, when it comes to the moment of reality they may experience a wobble in that certainty and want you to confirm that they are doing the right thing.

This can be a very difficult moment and it can make you inadvertently seem impatient because you thought the decision had already been made. The decision must ultimately be theirs, but you can help them by confirming the problems their pet is facing and with a case that has been under treatment you must make sure you are aware of the details before they come in.

Never show any sign of impatience at this hesitation on their part, but if you genuinely feel the time has come for that patient then there are phrases which can really help that client. A few well-chosen words which, to be honest, may seem like clichés but are sincere and appropriate all the same can ease their pain.

Phrases such as 'having had a good innings' and needing to be 'allowed to go peacefully' are all appropriate in different circumstances:

> 'You've given Gnasher a really good life and now it's time to let her go.'
> 'Quality of life is the important thing here.'
> 'I understand how you must be feeling, but Gnasher doesn't know that life ever ends.'
> 'I can see how much you love him, but it's time to let him go to sleep now.'

Ask the owner if they really want to stay if you feel they are struggling with the situation because some clients think that they have to be there and that they will be judged as heartless if they do not stay. Help them to make the right decision for them and their pet and do not judge them if they choose to leave the room. Not everyone has the same degree of tolerance for situations such as this and some people simply cannot cope with being there. Their pet does not know what is going to happen of course but may be very agitated by a distressed owner, so it can be easier for all concerned if they leave, although it is best not to appear to be putting any pressure on them to do so.

Many clients want to be able to hold their pet in their arms as they go to sleep, and the use of an intravenous catheter and an extension line can make this possible. The placement of the catheter before the final injection is administered can also help ensure that any difficulty finding the vein is not at the actual time of euthanasia and this is less distressing for the owner. Old, sick and moribund dogs can have veins which collapse really easily and it may be necessary to use the saphenous vein in the hind limb. You can gently and calmly ensure that you have a line in by using such a catheter and it is less problematic than searching for a vein at the actual time of the final injection.

You may need to decide whether you insert this with the owner present or if they are happy to let you take the pet into the back room beforehand. There are some clients who will not want this and will be upset if you suggest it and you must use your own judgement and knowledge of the client and the patient. It may be less traumatic for the client with a fractious cat and if you explain exactly what it is that you want to do and why, then they may readily agree.

Tell the owner exactly what you are going to do at every stage of the process so that they know what is going to happen. Do not rush into it but ask them if they are ready for you to proceed.

Warn the owner about terminal breathing before you proceed because, although some combinations of drugs make terminal breathing less likely, there will be the odd case in which the dog or cat appears to be gasping for breath in a distressed and conscious manner. This can be really traumatic for an owner to see if not forewarned and seems to be much more likely to occur if you have not mentioned that it might happen in advance.

Some animals will remain immobile for what seems like quite a long time before suddenly taking intermittent breaths for a moment or two and of course this usually happens just after you have pronounced life extinct. For many owners this will be their first time being present at a death and it is really frightening for them as they do not know what to expect and their only idea of what it may be like comes from horror films.

Be prepared for the animal to urinate or defaecate just as the client cradles them in their arms so put something absorbent such as disposable bedding or a towel underneath and perhaps warn the owner.

Clients often want you to close their pet's eyes and you may warn them in advance that this is not the same as in the human. I usually gently arrange the body to make them look as if they are curled up asleep and I close the eyes as best I can by stroking the forehead skin forwards which apposes the eyelids to some extent. I reassure them that they have 'really gone now' and tell them that they can touch them if they want to. I stroke the head and say what a great companion he or she has been and generally reassure the owner that their pet has had a good life and a peaceful death and then I step back to allow them space to say goodbye.

I sometimes put my hand gently on their shoulder as a comfort depending on the circumstances and if they want to hug me then I let them, and I hand them tissues and support them as best I can, as I would for anyone in distress. You will have to choose your own way of comforting people with which you feel comfortable and naturally this varies from person to person and with different clients. This is a very sad moment and clients often apologise for their tears and for being upset and you can really help them at this time of grieving by just being there and being kind and reassuring.

Some owners want to keep the collar and some appreciate the offer of a little bit of hair clipped off and put in a little bag as a keepsake to take away with them, whereas others do not want to take anything tangible away. You just have to play it by ear and listen to them and be attentive and supportive and you will not go far wrong.

Clients who are hard to like at this time

Some clients will bring an animal for euthanasia and you may feel that they have done it far too soon or for the wrong reasons and not feel any warmth or sympathy towards them. On some occasions, these are also the clients who put in an Oscar winning performance of desperate grief and demand your sympathy and attention.

One of my less tolerant friends told me that when he had been subjected to a prima donna having hysterics after insisting on the euthanasia of a dog with a treatable condition, he felt an overwhelming desire to give her a round of applause and sarcastically compliment her on her acting skills.

Whatever you may feel about a decision, the fact is that you are a professional and this would obviously not be appropriate behaviour and would have serious repercussions while achieving very little. There might be circumstances in your clients' lives about which you know nothing so try to give them the benefit of the doubt. I know that this can be very hard when a client is asking you to endorse a decision you disagree with after the event, but you can be civil and polite without actually going against your principles by concurring.

The body

Let an owner stay and say their goodbyes for as long as they want to, preferably uninterrupted and in private and as long as is reasonably possible in a busy surgery. Having left them for a little while, do go back to check that they are all right as it may be that they are standing there waiting for you to come back because they do not know how long they should stay. They may never have been in this situation before and feel that they might be considered uncaring if they leave too soon but they may have said all their goodbyes already and appreciate being escorted away from the room.

Assure the owner that you will look after their beloved pet now and treat him or her with dignity and respect. This is a concern that clients often have, and they worry that once they leave the room their pet will be handled roughly and shoved into a body bag in an offhand and undignified manner. It comforts them if you assure them that you will treat their pet as if they were your own.

Discussing what happens with the body can be a bit of a minefield, especially in the choice of words you use and it is really difficult to avoid saying the wrong thing. Some people will not feel comfortable about using the word 'body' or 'death' and so all sorts of softer terms are used such as 'passed away' and 'the remains'.

Clients need to know what a communal cremation is, but they don't want to hear you actually say that 'they all get incinerated together' even though that is what happens. You may ultimately have to say exactly that if it is apparent that they have not really grasped what you mean by communal cremation. You cannot lie to the client and say something other than the truth about the disposal of their pet but there are ways of putting it which are less harsh than others. Don't tell them half-truths just to make them feel better, such as saying that their ashes are scattered in a memorial garden unless you are absolutely sure that is the case. If they all go into a landfill site and the client asks you directly about where they go, then that is what you must say. Every so often there will be headlines in the newspapers or on social media about what happens to the bodies and you must not deviate from the truth, however comforting you wish to be. It is important that you are truthful and clear, and using simple language to state the facts is often the best option.

You will find your own way to talk to clients about this, but I find clear, comprehensible language in a respectful tone is preferable to flowery, unctuous, oblique references which may be misinterpreted.

> Do not go too far the other way of course and do what a young Antipodean locum did in my practice. He said cheerily, after putting a cat to sleep:
> 'OK mate, so you want Fluffy to go up in smoke?'
> The client did see the funny side of it, but he made sure I knew for the benefit of our other more sensitive clients and I gave the vet a little advice in how to rephrase the question.

You need to make sure that you do know exactly what the client wants to do with the body, because if Fluffy is wrongly marked for communal cremation when the owner thought you knew telepathically that they always wanted individual cremation for him, then this will cause all sorts of problems later on. They may think that just because their last pet was individually cremated then you know this is what they want for this one, so do make sure there are no misunderstandings.

There is a considerable extra cost to private cremation which many clients are completely unaware of and their natural desire to do what is best for their animal may be impossible within their finances. The discussion about costs of caskets and weights of bodies is never an easy conversation but it has to be done, and human funeral directors make no bones about the cost of cremating your nearest and dearest, believe me!

Make sure clients know exactly how much it is going to cost because once the grief has eased they might regret agreeing to pay for individual cremation. Unfortunately, bad debts incurred for individual cremations are fairly common in practice and most practices have a small collection of uncollected ashes in a cupboard somewhere where the owner has not come back because they do not want to pay the final bill.

> I learned not to discuss funeral arrangements in front of children because one father found himself agreeing under pressure from his two teenage daughters to have Hammy the pet hamster individually cremated in a top-of-the-range coffin, the cost of which was eye-watering. I received a phone call once he had arrived home cancelling all the arrangements before the cremation service had collected Hammy. I have no idea how he explained this to his children and only hope he did not blame us for losing the body.

If a client wishes to bury their pet at home, it is wise to give them some advice about the depth necessary to inter a body as the cadaver now contains barbiturates and also because if they are dug up by a fox the following morning, then the owner may well blame you for not warning them, unfair though that may seem.

Sympathy cards

Sympathy cards are very much appreciated by clients who have lost an animal and they are better written by you yourself, especially for clients who you have been seeing regularly. A generic one written by a member of staff who the client does not know is not as well received, especially if you get a detail wrong such as the name or the sex of the pet. If you can, include a few words about the pet who they have lost and which makes the client know that it is a personal message of sympathy and not a computer-generated card. Sometimes my nurses signed the card too, especially if they had been involved with the client and the animal and I believe it can help the practice team come to terms with the feelings they experience after euthanasia of cases where an animal has been a regular visitor to the practice.

I have heard that some clients will choose to go to another practice after a pet has been put to sleep, just because they find the memories too painful. It is likely to be inconvenient for them to change practices as well as being bad for the practice in losing a client, despite your having done a really good job for them over the years. If the client feels supported by the practice by a small gesture such as a card, they are more likely to come back to you with a new puppy and will be a truly bonded client.

House call euthanasia

If a client asks for a non-urgent home visit for euthanasia, always try to determine the size of the animal before you go out to the house, and ask about the temperament. Some breeds today are really heavy, and you will need to ascertain in advance exactly what the client intends to do with the body afterwards. The request for a house call is sometimes made expressly because they cannot lift the dog, but they may then expect you and a six-stone nurse to remove the body. It may be necessary to warn the client that they will need to organise home collection by a cremation service if they are too big to manage and you need to be sure that you are not committing yourself and, indeed, your support staff to lifting unmanageably heavy weights. It is far better to be aware of this before you go and not have to have the discussion when everyone is upset and emotional and you are standing over the enormous body of a St Bernard or a mastiff.

You will usually have a nurse to help you to raise a vein, but there may be the rare occasion where you have to put an animal to sleep either on your own or with the owner. A useful way to raise a cephalic vein if you are ever in exceptional circumstances and on your own, is to use a rubber tourniquet designed for this purpose. If one is not available, then use the old method of a pair of artery forceps and a rubber band and clamp the rubber band so that it forms a tourniquet just above the elbow. Make sure the skin is slightly swept laterally making it less mobile across the cephalic vein. Once you have the catheter or needle in the vein you can quickly release the forceps and administer the pentobarbitone. This used to be necessary much more commonly in the past when vets were often out on call single-handed to put animals to sleep; practices nowadays have a policy of not sending a vet out unaccompanied, but this may come in handy one day in a crisis, so always carry a tourniquet and a pair of curved scissors, and maybe a pair of artery forceps and a sturdy elastic band on a house call.

If you are taking the body away with you then take the stretcher with you and perhaps an old sheet or a towel to wrap the body in and not just a black plastic bag. I often ask the owner if they would like to provide a favourite blanket as this can be quite comforting for them as a memory afterwards. Remember to have something absorbent under the animal's rear end before you put them to sleep as the clients may not be aware of the fact that they may release the contents of their bladder afterwards. Nobody wants the last memory of their pet's existence to be the cleaning of urine and faeces off the living room carpet. Some clients prefer to have their pet euthanised at home and then to bury them in the garden and may appreciate it if you offer to help move the body from the centre of the living room and outside until they can organise the burial.

I have been in the situation where a client demands a house call because their dog is aggressive and they cannot handle it, and you need to be prepared for this in advance. You may need to advise the client about sedation beforehand and there will be other considerations necessary to keep everyone safe.

Euthanasia of healthy animals

Your obligation under the oath you took is to protect animal welfare and it is generally accepted that the appropriate and timely performance of euthanasia does ensure the welfare of an animal by prevention of any further suffering, even though you are preventing that suffering by ending that animal's life.

Our oath states: 'my constant endeavour will be to ensure the health and welfare of animals committed to my care' and you may find this difficult to square with the euthanasia of a healthy animal.

Over the years, I have had to put healthy animals down for a variety of reasons and I have had to come to terms with this, despite feeling very emotionally invested in animals in general. I have lost count of the times when people have said, 'I couldn't do your job because you have to put animals down', implying that being a vet is a job for the cold-hearted killer of innocent animals. Nothing could be further from the truth and the majority of vets I have met over my career are following their vocation to relieve suffering in animals wherever they possibly can. They care enough about animals to see that there is a need to end the life of an animal to relieve distress and they perform euthanasia because they care very deeply about their patients' quality of life and frequently do so at no small cost to themselves emotionally.

For a person who becomes a vet because we are so appreciative of animals and value their lives and want to heal them, euthanasia is a very difficult part of our job, and there is increasing evidence of how traumatic this is for us emotionally. It is a fact, however, that in this country, healthy farm animals are slaughtered every day for food and we have agreed to train as vets able to treat every species of animal, and so we could argue that we are part of the food production industry.

Some vets will state that they will never put a healthy pet animal down and that the decision and responsibility for solving the problems for the owner of an unwanted pet is not their problem. They do usually agree that if a dog is proven to be dangerous then they would see the need for euthanasia of an otherwise healthy animal. When the subject is debated, they will sometimes agree that in extremely unusual sets of circumstances they might consider it, and these qualifications as to what is and is not acceptable in different situations illustrate just how complex this subject is.

There are no easy answers to this moral dilemma and I would advise you to approach each case on its merits and if appropriate, offer information on rehoming and other treatment options such as behavioural therapy, but ultimately you will have to reach your own decision as to what you believe is the best option for the animal and for you.

At the time of writing, the BVA has a decision tree for guidance on euthanasia available on their website. If a vet does not agree with a client's request to euthanise a healthy animal, then they are advised to seek support by asking for a second opinion from another vet and the presumption appears to be that if both vets agree then the request can be refused.

This does not, however, address the concern that a client might seek other means to bring about the animal's demise and that the animal might suffer in the process. There have been times when I have strongly disagreed with the decision an owner has made but, despite looking for other solutions to save the life of that animal, none have been practical or agreed to by the owner. I have then reluctantly, but professionally and considerately, performed euthanasia and I have comforted myself by making sure that the end of that animal's life was as peaceful and pain-free as possible. I do believe that animals have no concept that life ever comes to an end and that it is freedom from pain and fear at the present moment of time which matters to them. I would certainly rather perform pain-free euthanasia than suspect that the client has taken matters into their own hands and killed them inhumanely. I know that others cannot perhaps reconcile this viewpoint with the death of healthy animals, but this is how I have handled this painful aspect of being a vet and though I cannot tolerate an animal suffering, I can live with the decision of an owner and agree to take the life of the animal they own. I believe the decision and the moral responsibility and the guilt is theirs, however, and do not allow them to attempt to make it mine. If they are signing the permission form, then the responsibility for that decision is on their shoulders and not on yours and you can make this clear and not allow the client to absolve themselves by blaming everyone but themselves.

The fact remains that, in practice, we do sometimes have the unpleasant task of putting animals to sleep for varying reasons and it is part of the job for us. Performing it well so that the animal and the owner are not unnecessarily distressed will certainly help you feel better about it; a peaceful, pain-free death can be one of the greatest gifts we can bestow on an animal and one which is often not yet accorded to us as human beings.

CHAPTER 17

Paperwork and procedures: do it or weep!

Dry and dusty record-keeping and other boring stuff

This might not be the most exciting topic but keep reading – it is important and keeps the practice operating smoothly!

Most practices nowadays will have a sophisticated practice management software system and the days of handwritten record cards and book-keeping have gone. This should make keeping clinical and financial records much more accurate and user-friendly, but there is still the weakest link in the recording chain and that link is us, the human beings.

Accurate record-keeping is of vital importance for the practice clinically, financially and legally and your role in this is pivotal. Failure to keep precise and comprehensive clinical records is contrary to the RCVS Code of Conduct because, as a medical professional, you have a duty to record significant facts accurately. In the case of a complaint to the RCVS, they will want to examine these records in their entirety to confirm that you acted professionally, so make sure you write up your records correctly and fully every single time. It will be poorly perceived if records are entered at a much later date and especially if they are altered some time later after a problem has arisen, so always take the time and trouble to make sure that what you are writing is a true account of what you have done.

All vets are understandably worried about complaints brought by clients and it is surprising how much the memories of the vet and the client can vary and how different their recollections of an event can be after a relatively short space of time. Veterinary indemnity insurers such as the Veterinary Defence Society in the UK (VDS) defend vets when things go wrong or when they are accused of making mistakes and it delights them if they receive full and comprehensive clinical records containing the evidence of the true facts of a case. It enables them to provide evidence to an aggrieved client who has forgotten or neglected to disclose all the facts, such as the vet recording that they advised a scan or blood tests which the client refused at the time and conveniently forgot to include. The worst-case scenario is where no clinical records of a case which is under dispute exist at all and it is extremely problematic to defend a vet who has forgotten to write up a consultation or a procedure or has written such minimal notes that they are no help at all.

It is very frustrating for a vet to take over a case where a colleague has not written up the clinical records properly and it makes your job much harder if you have to turn detective to try to surreptitiously find out what has been diagnosed and what treatment has been dispensed. Poor record-keeping makes both the practice and your colleague look incompetent in front of the client and will not endear you to your workmates.

Poor record-keeping can have quite serious ramifications.

- Subsequent loss of helpful information for diagnosis and treatment which could result in inadequate treatment.
- Loss of revenue for the practice by inaccurate charging.
- Loss of supportive evidence which could help if concerns are raised about the handling of a case.
- Loss of records of base-line parameters such as weight and relevant symptoms such as temperature and heart rate, resulting in misdiagnosis or delayed diagnosis.
- Conflicting medicines being prescribed or a drug being administered twice in error.

In the middle of a busy consulting session it is very tempting to concentrate on the examination and the owner and to scrimp on the time and attention needed to enter the history, treatment and recommendations on the computer. The same applies when you have performed an operation and are either in a hurry to move on to the next patient on the list or if you become distracted in the aftermath of a complex op.

If you defer writing up a consultation or an inpatient procedure until later, then the chances are you will forget to record something. In a consultation, this might be part of the history or a clinical sign, such as the rectal temperature or the colour of mucous membranes or a suggestion of a blood test which was refused by the owner. There are many times when it is appropriate to record a normal finding such as 'heart sounds normal' or an absence of vomiting, and this can also be useful because it can be as important to have a record of what was normal or absent as it is to record a positive or abnormal finding.

If, for any reason, you cannot record information on the computer, such as those occasions when the system crashes, record everything on paper because however good your memory may be, it is highly likely that you will forget something.

Clinical records should be complete and accurate and as concise as possible, using abbreviations which are easily understood by your colleagues and with correct spelling and with no personal comments about the owners.

> *There have been stories of clients seeing derogatory comments about themselves or their animals in the clinical history that they were never intended to see. This can be very embarrassing and is the veterinary equivalent of a*

politician leaving his microphone on when on the campaign trail. Personal comments about how attractive a client is or is not should never be recorded in the records, nor should any reference to their intelligence level, degree of obesity or personality. I was not happy when a vet once recorded TATSP against a client record because he considered them to be 'thick as two short planks' and he was also fond of writing SOD on the records of those aggressive patients who tried to bite him. I once had to do some quick thinking when challenged about this by the client who glimpsed it on the computer screen, and I reassuringly said it meant 'Symptoms of Dyspepsia', though I am not sure from his expression that I got away with it.

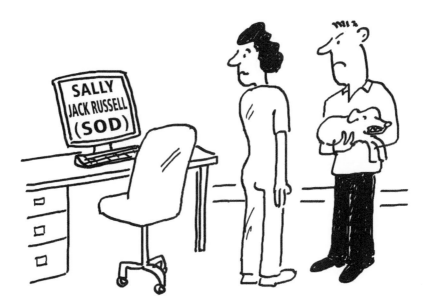

It is important to charge for all fees incurred on the day because it is not well accepted by a client if they think they have paid their bill in full and days or weeks later are asked to pay for some laboratory test that you forgot to write up at the time.

When recording clinical records and history, do make a conscious decision to think about how much insignificant detail you should include, for example one single soft motion in a puppy should not be recorded as diarrhoea which is a symptom of a gastrointestinal disturbance and could create problems with subsequently insuring a cat or dog. Never deliberately conceal a significant finding, but use your clinical judgement as to what is an abnormality and what is, in fact, a variation of the normal.

Protocols and health and safety

Protocols are there for a reason and not simply as a means of decorating the surgery wall with multiple laminated artworks. It may seem that at every turn you are faced with a notice nagging you to do this and do that, but they are not there solely to fulfil the obligations of the Practice Management Scheme inspection. They are there to make sure that procedures are followed for certain tasks and to safeguard the animals and the people in the practice. Human nature being what it is, however, if you show me a protocol then I can show you three people who have found a way to ignore it or gone to some trouble to circumvent it. We all know that we should not prop open the fire doors in the surgery or fail to replace something in the fridge, but we are all rebels at heart and the boss is often the worst offender, as usual.

On a busy day, we vets can become a little bit casual about the protocols for handling the drugs we use and it can be tempting to try to save time by cutting corners and not following good practice. It is not good practice, for example, to draw up a syringe for a premed for the induction of a patient and then leave it lying around without a label on the side, somewhere in the prep room or the pharmacy. This is how mistakes are made as another member of staff may administer it to the wrong animal thinking it is something else.

Whenever you draw up an injection, concentrate on what you are doing and take care that you are accurate with your dosages and are aware of exactly what it is you have in your hand. It is all too easy to pick up the wrong bottle when you are under pressure or to miscalculate a dose if you are not careful and you should get into the habit of following the protocols religiously. Always update the records promptly when you have administered an injection to an inpatient so that a duplicate dose is not given accidentally.

I may seem to be concentrating on and reiterating very obvious and basic advice, but this is because I have witnessed the aftermath of these mistakes and they can have detrimental and even fatal consequences. Getting the decimal point in the wrong place and overdosing an animal is not as rare as it should be in veterinary medicine, or in human medicine for that matter, and it usually happens when someone is distracted or not concentrating, or when protocols have been ignored. After a while, you will develop an inbuilt awareness of what looks visually 'normal' in a syringe for a particular dose for the average patient, but as a new graduate you do not yet have that imprinted on your brain and you are more likely to make a mistake at this stage of your career. It is harrowing to know that you have unintentionally caused a problem for an animal in your care and is an experience that I do not want to happen to you.

Inpatient records

If you are in charge of a patient who has been admitted, then follow the practice protocols and if you are required to record TPR at intervals, be diligent and record them whatever hour of the day or night. At risk of repeating myself, do write up each inpatient record as soon as you reasonably can, including any extra disposables used, such as catheters and intravenous fluids, and hospitalisation fees and prescription diets.

Complete and up-to-date clinical records are so important when handing over a case to a colleague and for informing the owner about the progress of treatment so that they are reassured that their animal is not sitting alone and ignored in a kennel. It can be exasperating taking over a case where no one has recorded food intake, urination or total fluids and the nurses hate answering the phone to a client and being unable to say whether an animal has improved and eaten or passed urine.

Money, money, money

When people decide to be a vet, they do not think of the multiple times a day that they are going to have to discuss money with a client or price up the cost of treatment. Discussing costs of veterinary treatment with clients and advising them to agree to costly investigations is one of the most difficult parts of the job for many vets in private practice. It has been cited as one of the positive aspects of working for a charity where, in the interaction between the client and the vet, there does not have to be any discussion about money and affordability. Most vets do not set out to be involved in sales and marketing, but this is a part of life in practice where you know the value and necessity of investigative diagnostics and you have to inform the client in such a way that they give their permission for you to spend their hard-earned money.

A successful practice relies on good record-keeping to ensure that the revenue received from clients is sufficient to continually reinvest in the staff and the equipment of the practice. If you do not accurately record all the procedures you perform and all the medicines you dispense then the practice will not perform as well financially, and ultimately the pay and conditions of the staff and the practice may well suffer. Every year, practices lose a considerable amount of money due to careless or occasionally deliberate failure to record all services and medication on the practice management system.

It is very tempting to underprice a procedure or omit to charge for something, especially when you are a new graduate lacking in confidence about your skills. It does become easier with time as your confidence grows, but older vets are often equally guilty of a tendency to undercharge and the worst offender of all is not infrequently the boss.

When it comes to the costs of running a practice, the disposables we use in the course of our work really add up to a significant amount. With a surgical procedure, we can easily forget to record the administration of a drug or the use of a special dressing or bandage, the cost of which may seem trivial in a single instance but adds up over time to a considerable amount. It may also have an effect on efficient stock control, when an item that has gone from the shelf but not been recorded is not automatically reordered by the system.

Charging accurately for your time is important too, and recording ten minutes for a dental procedure on a dog instead of the 30 minutes it actually took you to remove a tooth may make you feel you have been very generous towards a client. You may feel you have been very kind, but they will probably be oblivious and might even wonder how thorough you have been if you did it so quickly and cheaply. They will forget about your generosity anyway in a very short time and most likely feel ripped off if they are charged the correct amount at a later date or with another animal. Undercharging devalues your own work, and variability in the amount charged for the same procedure undermines confidence in the perception of the client who does not want it to be a lottery but a fair price for a good job done.

Your employer will have a pricing structure to which you must adhere and any underpricing or giving away a free consultation is fundamentally giving away someone else's money. The practice owner may be the worst culprit for not charging correctly, but it is his profit he is giving away and his decision if he wants to be magnanimous with his own cash.

Subconsciously, I think we may feel that if we charge the client less then we may avoid any conflict and they might like us more, or be happier with the service, but in reality clients just want to feel they have received value for money. Clients are confident they have received value for money if they feel they had your undivided attention and the best treatment for their animal and this is not achieved by a rushed free-of-charge consultation or a catheter that has not been charged for. They might thank you for that free consultation but it does not mean they like you any better or think you a wonderful vet half an hour later when they get home. They might even wonder why they were charged the full amount the time before, and will certainly expect more free consultations in the future.

Even if you, as an employee, are not directly involved in the finances of the practice, do keep an awareness and a respect for how much things cost to replace and restock. If someone accidentally or carelessly leaves the fridge door open overnight, it can cost thousands of pounds in wasted vaccine, and if the endoscope is balanced precariously on a surface and falls on the floor and breaks, it costs a great deal of money to repair or replace.

Some drugs are extremely expensive, so just be aware that if you carelessly draw an excessive amount up into the syringe you are squirting money down the drain. Some drugs are really cheap, but get into the habit of avoiding unnecessary waste and being careful with the practice property. You may have your own practice to manage one day and be directly involved in the running of a business, so be curious and careful about financial matters even if they do not directly affect you at the moment.

I heard a nurse laughing at a new graduate who was putting an injured pigeon to sleep by an injection of pentobarbitone. It was the new graduate's first month in practice and she had weighed the pigeon and was working out how much pentobarbitone it was going to need for euthanasia. The nurse found this hilarious as most vets just drew up a full syringe of pentobarbitone knowing that it costs very little. The new graduate did not know the cost per ml and did not have the experience of knowing roughly how much to give and was painstakingly working it out. I pointed out that if that injection had been metomidine, then the cost would have been significant and that the new graduate had my respect for the care she was taking with the practice resources.

Estimates

Working to an estimate can be a real challenge for a vet and it would be much easier if we were always able to perform our work without giving a second thought to the costs involved. We would prefer to use all the skills we have learned and access all the investigative resources available, and knowing we may be forced to do a less than perfect job because of financial constraints may contribute to our stress levels.

There is a difference between a quote where you are guaranteeing the precise cost for a specified undertaking such as a neutering operation, and an estimate, which is an indication of the likely cost but which can vary in response to circumstances and is not binding. You really need to have a crystal ball or be a psychic to give an accurate estimate in some cases and you may feel a certain amount of resentment at being asked to make such a prediction when presented with a complex case. There can be so many variables and possible complications that you cannot give an accurate estimate and, in a case like this, you have to do the best you can to inform the owner of the possible range of costs.

If you look at it from the client's point of view, it is unreasonable to expect them to allow you free access to all of their disposable income. The client must be able to make a decision based on as much information as you can give them and be able to give their informed consent before you embark on any work for them; this includes the likely cost in addition to the potential risks to their animal.

It is very tempting to give a really low estimate and an overly optimistic prognosis in order to encourage the owner to agree to the treatment plan you wish to pursue. If you knowingly underestimate, then you are very likely to have a disappointed and dissatisfied client further down the line who feels that they were not warned of how much it was all potentially going to cost. If something does not go exactly according to plan and you did not warn them at all, they will resent being asked to pay more than your original estimate. Eventually, that client loses their trust in your estimates and thinks that the bill will always be higher than the one you quoted, making them far less likely to agree to your proposals in the future.

I found my clients were accepting if I gave an estimate that included a lower figure for a case where all goes according to plan, and a higher figure to allow for reasonable complications should they arise. There were no nasty surprises for the client, and if it came in at the lower fee, which was often the case, then they were pleasantly surprised and it gave them confidence that they were being treated fairly. As you gain experience, you will find it easier to be able to give a more accurate estimate but always give yourself some wriggle room for the unexpected.

Sometimes it is impossible to give an estimate beyond the first 24 hours of treatment, such as in the case of an acute emergency. You may need to inform the client of the likely costs of stabilising a case after a road accident and further estimates may have to be given at the end of that initial period when you have more information about the full extent of the injuries. The client is fully informed of their initial financial commitment and no promises have been made about the total treatment costs until more information is available. It is essential that the client is given the promised revised estimate the next day and for the following days so that they know by how much the costs may be escalating on a day-by-day basis. They will be understandably shocked and probably quite angry if they are presented with a massive bill after ten days of treatment during which time money has not been mentioned.

X-raying a client's wallet

Always resist the temptation to try to guess the financial status of the client in front of you when you are discussing a treatment plan for an animal. It is your professional duty to discuss the available treatments which might potentially help your patient and then you and the client together agree to a suitable plan which will depend on their personal wishes and on their willingness and ability to pay.

A client may turn up in a top-of-the-range car but not want to spend any money at all on their animal, begrudging even the bare minimum of treatment options; they may even opt for euthanasia on grounds of cost. Another seemingly penniless individual who has come on the bus might want to pay for anything and everything that might possibly be of benefit to their pet and be fully able and willing to pay for state-of-the-art treatment. It is for each individual to choose where to spend their disposable income and it is for you to advise on the options available that, in your opinion, would be beneficial for their animal. This is their prerogative and it is not for us to judge from appearances and be tempted to offer a treatment plan that we believe they might choose, but rather to fully inform each and every client of what we recommend for their animal.

> I have a friend who owned a large publishing company in London and bought a beautiful property locally which was the size of a small stately home. During the week, he commuted to London but at weekends he loved to get down and dirty and work on his land where he kept some chickens, hives of bees and a pig. One day he arrived at the surgery in his vintage, mud-spattered Land Rover, smelling quite pervasively of pig, and wearing wellies and grubby, torn overalls with an equally filthy springer spaniel called Wooffles in his arms. He had inadvertently run Wooffles over and the dog had suffered a badly broken leg, so we whisked him through and after administering initial analgesia and fluids, I went to ring his owner to discuss further treatment for fixation.
>
> My nurse said worriedly in passing:
>
> 'I don't think he will be able to afford to have it referred, he was driving an old banger and I don't think he's got much money. He looked really worried, poor man.'
>
> His old banger was a vintage Land Rover Defender and his worried face was caused not by cash flow concerns but worry about what his family were going to say when they found out what had happened. Our nurses definitely had no need to worry about his financial situation at all and fortunately Wooffles made a full recovery, though he still had very little road sense.

Debt

Debt control is very important for a practice and, because a significant proportion of the work performed is caused by unforeseen events and may not have been budgeted for by the client, there will be occasions where clients do not pay the bill at the time of treatment. Practices may have different approaches to payment of veterinary bills and some are stricter than others about payment at the time of treatment. Vets are obliged to provide emergency treatment to an animal to ensure the relief of suffering, but it is also important that the client appreciates that there will be a cost involved and that there is no national health service for pets.

You may be fortunate to work in a practice where you never have to be involved in the collection of money from clients, and think that the sordid collection of money is nothing at all to do with you, but in actual fact, your actions are likely to be very important in preventing bad debt in the practice.

Clients should be given information about the costs of treatment wherever possible, both in the estimate at the onset of treatment, as mentioned previously, and on an ongoing basis. It is very tempting when you have a complex case requiring several consultations to shy away from discussing potential costs because you wish to concentrate solely on what you can do for your patient and you want to continue the treatment and provide the best available care. You might think that the next vet who takes over the case can deal with the question of money or that the client will ask the receptionist when they make the follow-up appointment, but all vets should involve themselves in keeping the client informed.

Clients often have no idea at all how much veterinary treatment can cost and this may be especially true where people have only ever used the NHS for their medical and dental treatment. Your reticence to discuss an escalating bill can mean that it is quite a long time down the line before they realise quite how large it has become. Some clients are on very low incomes and may qualify for free treatment by a charity such as the PDSA, so it is very important that you speak to them early on about money and discuss the options. You are not doing them any favours at all in allowing them to build up a considerable debt for treatment which they may be unable to pay, because this could lead them into real financial problems and repercussions in the future which could, of course, affect the well-being of their animals too.

Some clients can afford to pay but choose not to, and may employ many and various means of not paying the bill which is very frustrating for the practice owner. You will be surprised how many times these clients forget to bring their wallet or purse to the surgery and promise you on the lives of their loved ones that they will come back and pay, only to leave the surgery never to be seen again. Clients who are skilled and experienced in avoiding paying for treatment will employ all sorts of ruses and techniques, such as sending their children, who have no means of paying, to the practice to collect an animal after surgery. I once brought a dog which had had a wound stitched back to a branch surgery in the animal ambulance and while I was unlocking the surgery door, two young men liberated the dog from the van and left at speed with the patient running along behind them. There may be times when you have to be quite assertive and hold on to a bottle of ear drops or a flea treatment and say firmly that they can collect the medication when they return with the forgotten credit card.

The responsibility of accurate certification

You will need to sign certificates in your role as a veterinary surgeon and the signature of a vet is used in many official documents as a means of legal authorisation. You will have received training about the importance of certification during your time at vet college and I would urge you to ensure that you take a great deal of care over this, because veterinary certification carries serious responsibilities. You are a guardian of public health, and the safeguarding of communal health of both humans and animals may rely on safe certification, so follow the official guidelines accurately and never allow anyone to talk you into signing anything if you are unsure that you should. This includes resisting your employer telling you to sign something you know is not right or encouraging you to be creative with information such as dates on a certificate. It is your personal signature and your reputation as a veterinary surgeon and you should resist any such request because you will be the one who bears the responsibility for inaccurate certification.

The RCVS has guidelines about certification in the supporting guidance for the Code of Conduct which sets out the 12 principles of certification.

Pet passports and import licences

Clients requiring pet passports and export licences for their animals will often leave things far too late before they plan to travel and will then expect you to know all the regulations for every country they may choose to travel to. Your practice should have protocols about pet passports and any necessary vaccinations and export certificates, with which you should make yourself familiar even before you become a veterinary inspector.

You may be asked for advice about animals travelling abroad, but try to avoid the pitfall of trying to be helpful and inadvertently giving the clients the wrong advice. Direct them towards someone more knowledgeable who might be another member of staff, but more likely DEFRA, and make sure the client knows from the outset when you are not certain of the facts.

Export certificates are different for virtually every country and they frequently change, so be aware that what they were asking for last month may not be the same next month. It is the responsibility of the owner to find out what that country is demanding at the time of export and it is impossible to be sure that you know what all these regulations are, so do not take it upon yourself to give information which might turn out to be wrong. The process of issuing pet passports, export certificates and the timing of rabies boosters present great potential for mistakes and the repercussions can be serious as the VDS newsletters illustrate all too frequently.

Take great care when filling in any form of certificate associated with pet passports as it is so easy to make a mistake with a date when you are distracted and under time pressure. Owners always seem to leave things until the last minute then come rushing in in a hurry, wanting to make their problem into your problem, and they may put pressure on you to rush through the paperwork.

It is not unheard of for owners to ask you to backdate a rabies vaccination date but clearly, as a professional, you will not agree to anything like this because your livelihood as a working veterinary surgeon is at stake and it relies on your integrity and honesty. It is fine to be helpful and for the practice to send a reminder or prompt a client to remember their rabies booster is coming up but the responsibility to comply is theirs and not yours.

There are few experiences worse than answering the phone to an irate client standing in Calais with a dog who has been refused travel because the passport is not valid, especially if it is because you have made a mistake. The client will be stressed and angry and will be looking for someone to take the blame and they love to blame the vets and not themselves. They do not want to take responsibility for anything while their children are wailing in the car and their spouse is looking daggers at them as the ferry is about to leave for home. The worst-case scenario when you have made a mistake can mean expensive quarantine which is not good for the pet, the owner or the practice. Your professional indemnity insurer will be able to advise you if a problem arises and they have useful guidance for keeping yourself out of trouble, as do other organisations such as the BVA.

Filling in all those practice forms and reports

Most well-run practices will have numerous internal forms and reports for their employees to fill in about health and safety compliance in taking online courses for fire hazard awareness and first aid, expenses forms, holiday request forms, feedback forms and progress reports. You should have genuine sympathy for the staff in the office who have the unenviable task of chivvying all the staff into filling in all these forms because it really is like herding chickens, not quite as uncooperative as cats but very nearly so!

Form filling is boring and not half as interesting or exciting as the veterinary work, so it is all too tempting to put it on one side and forget all about it as it piles up in your inbox. Filling in accident reports and questionnaires, health and safety protocols and feedback forms is, however, all part of your job, and if you look at your contract of employment this responsibility will most likely be included. It enables the practice to comply with legislation and also allows them to produce management figures and forecasts which assist in planning for the future more efficiently, which is in your best interests too. Insurance forms should be filled in promptly and accurately also so that the client or the practice is reimbursed for the work done without the form sitting in an inbox for days on end.

Don't have Flo nipping at your heels, fill in your paperwork promptly.

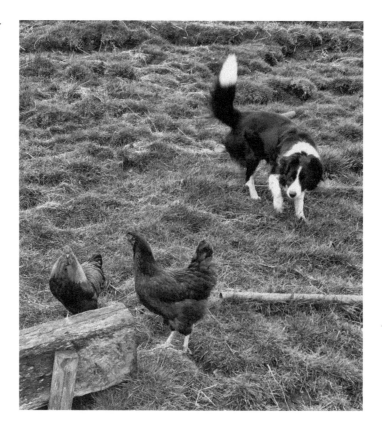

This may all sound very obvious, but in the hectic life vets lead it is all too easy to think that paperwork can be left to another time when you are not busy. Usually that time never arrives and you end up with an intimidating pile of paperwork with something really important lost in the depths and someone in the office ranting at you and pulling their hair out. Why not surprise the office staff by being the one member of the practice that they can rely on to make their job easier by doing your paperwork without needing to be nagged. Often the more senior vets are the worst offenders for prevaricating and this includes your employer or line manager, so be different and make your office staff smile.

Following health and safety protocols

The practice has to protect the health and safety of the people who work there so follow the correct procedures and ensure that the people you are working with comply too. It is sometimes tempting to push the boundaries and cut a few corners to save time here or there, but the rules are there for a reason. You do not want a colleague's injury on your conscience or to be injured yourself, possibly resulting in you being unable to work. Take care of students and children seeing practice as they may not be as aware of what might appear obvious risk, such as sticking their fingers through the kennel bars and attempting to stroke feral cats.

Recording the treatment of your own animals

If you own a pet yourself who requires goods such as pet food or services such as treatment, then do follow the practice protocol for pricing for your own animals. It can help if you ask a colleague to price up the work for your animals so that there can be no doubts about the accuracy, and certainly this may be advisable with certifying the forms when you have an insured animal. If you take a bag of food from the shelves or a flea treatment from the dispensary for your own animals, write it up there and then and do not leave it till later. The costs charged for animals owned by staff depends on the rules of the practice in which you work so be careful not to simply follow the behaviour of other members of staff. You may see other members of staff taking items without paying for them and even though this behaviour may be prevalent, do not blindly copy a light-fingered member of staff and think that it is fine. It is not because of the value of the item that has been taken but because of the lack of honesty and the damage that is done to the trust that should exist between employer and employee. Disgruntled employees who feel undervalued and underpaid may feel that the practice stock is fair game, but theft is always inexcusable and dishonest.

Lab results

When a sample is taken from an animal for testing in an external lab, it should be sent off promptly and with the correct labelling and paperwork for the tests you want performed. Take care that it is taken correctly and in the right container and that you fulfil your part of the process by labelling and storing it correctly and putting it in the right place to be processed or sent off. The loss or delay of a blood sample, resulting in a client having to return for a repeat sample to be taken, does not go down at all well and you can be sure it will be Fang, the vicious security dog, whose sample gets left on the windowsill in the sun because you thought someone else was dealing with it and they thought that you were.

Think clearly about exactly what parameters you really want to test for and don't use the scattergun approach to analysis but think about how and why you are spending your clients' money. Laboratory work should be targeted and used as an assistance to diagnosis and it can significantly increase costs. If a lab test is necessary for accurate diagnosis, then of course you should recommend it, but not simply as defensive medicine where there is a temptation to test for everything to make sure you are not missing anything. Your clinical skill as a veterinary surgeon should help you to select the appropriate tests and evidence-based medicine should influence your decisions about which diagnostic tests should be made.

Lab results should be recorded on the client records and interpreted as soon as possible and, while there should be a system in place to inform the vet when the results come back, you might have to be proactive in going and looking for them. Contact the owner to give them the results as soon as you reasonably can because they will be concerned about their animal, and if they have been delayed, contact the owner and say so without leaving them in limbo wondering what is happening.

If you speak to veterinary nurses and receptionists, they will say that they hate having to be the ones who have to chase vets to look at lab results and phone owners. It is a waste of their time and they are the ones fielding multiple phone calls from worried owners and having their ears bent, while the results languish in your intray. Vets are notoriously bad for prevaricating about phoning owners back about anything at all and, if you promise a return call to a client to give them the results of a lab test at a certain time, then do call them back even if it is just to say that you are still waiting for the results. It does help if you tell the owner roughly when to expect the results back so that they know that there is no point in phoning in the next hour or all the next day for some results which you know are going to take 48 hours.

Clients are sometimes very surprising in their reaction to those laboratory results which do not show any abnormalities and which say that the beloved pet is not a diabetic or suffering from hypoadrenocorticism after all. Owners may appear somewhat disappointed and certainly not very happy about paying for lab results which contain the good news that no abnormalities have been revealed by the tests carried out. Although they should be pleased that their animal is not desperately ill, they have an illogical resentment that they should then have to pay for something which does not show anything wrong. When you communicate that lab results are 'negative', for example those which do not show kidney disease when the dog was showing symptoms at the time of sampling but has now miraculously recovered, do not just baldly announce 'it's all normal'. Announce with great pleasure and positivity that the news is good and their animal has completely normal kidney function and so you are able to rule out renal disease. Never, ever, apologise for advising taking those blood samples in the first place and in running those tests, because at the time you made a valid clinical decision based on your training as a vet and you felt it was the right thing to do, so make that announcement of good news with positivity and a smile.

Membership of professional bodies and societies

Make sure that you are registered to practice with your professional body which is the Royal College of Veterinary Surgeons (RCVS) in the United Kingdom. The fees may or may not be paid for by your practice depending on your contract with your employer, but in any event do check yourself that your registration is renewed annually. Inform the college promptly if you move practices halfway through a year and remember to follow it up so that you never attempt to work without being on the register.

Keep up to date with recording your Professional Development Record (PDR) during the Professional Development Phase (PDP) for the Royal College scheme, and log all your CPD as you go along so that it is a less arduous task than trying to do it all in one go for a deadline. Do not defer recording it until it becomes a major, time-consuming piece of work to fill it in and make sure you have everything checked and signed off by your PDP Dean. The scheme was devised to help you to record your progress and to support you in achieving competence in your first year or so in practice, and it can also be helpful in reassuring you by showing just how much experience you have gained as the weeks go by. Your employer should support you in completing the PDP and you can use the information in your record at the time of an appraisal, perhaps asking for opportunities and assistance in ensuring you have covered the majority of the year one competencies.

Make sure you check the paperwork and are covered by professional indemnity insurance which is provided by several companies in the United Kingdom, the largest of which is the Veterinary Defence Society (VDS), a non-profit-making organisation run by vets and for vets. If the practice is paying for cover for you, still double check and also make sure you have your membership number and the phone number to hand in case you need to contact them if things go wrong or you need advice.

The majority of vets do have their indemnity cover with the VDS and personally, I have only ever had cover from them and in all my experience of dealing with them they have always been extremely helpful. Over the years, I have had to consult them when a client has made a complaint about a case that I or one of my employed vets have been handling, and I can honestly say that whenever I have felt I have been in a tricky situation, they have never failed to reassure me and give excellent advice and support. Do not hesitate for one moment to contact them if ever you feel you may have made a mistake or can see a difficult situation looming on the horizon. They will advise you and support you even if you are at fault, and they will usually have heard of the same predicament before so know exactly what to do and will understand just how you are feeling too.

CHAPTER 18

Being a professional

During your time at university you will have received advice about how you should behave as a veterinary student and what is expected of you by your university and the RCVS in order to maintain your fitness to practice. You should already be familiar with the Royal College of Veterinary Surgeons Code of Conduct for veterinary surgeons, which sets out the principles by which vets registered to practice in the UK are expected to conduct themselves.

The RCVS also provides comprehensive supporting guidance for various situations in which you may find yourself and it is well worth reading the guidance relevant to the area in which you are working as it is wide-reaching and can be really helpful. If you are unsure how to respond in a set of circumstances, whether in relation to client confidentiality, a request for information by the police or in signing a certificate, then do nothing until you have checked that you are doing the right thing according to the Code of Conduct and supporting guidance. The Code and its guidance is online on the RCVS website and you can also contact the Professional Conduct Department of the RCVS to ask for advice by phone or email if you are unsure. There is a wealth of useful information from the indemnity insurer, the VDS, which will be available to you when you are first registered with them so take some time to read it.

Always trust your instincts and if you think something sounds as if it might possibly be the wrong thing to do, or if what you are being asked to do is very out of the ordinary, then the chances are you are right to refuse at least until you have checked it out.

There are fundamental privileges which we enjoy as professional people and we hold a position of trust and respect which is valued by the general public. We have been granted the right to prescribe prescription drugs because we are trusted to exercise diligence and appropriate control, and to perform acts of veterinary surgery on animals because we have received the appropriate training. As a result of the good standing we enjoy as professional people, more is expected of us as individuals in terms of our behaviour than is expected from other members of the public.

We are trusted to behave honestly and with integrity in all public areas of our lives and not just at work, and to uphold the high standards that protect animal welfare and the public regard for our profession and its reputation at all times. We are expected to be people of high moral standing in the community and to be incorruptible, and this is why our signature is trusted in signing certificates and countersigning passport photographs or firearms licence applications.

You don't have to be a paragon of virtue all the time and what you choose to do in your private life is still your own affair as long as it is legal and doesn't impinge on you and your responsibilities as a professional. We all have our own quirks and preferences and you will see this in all aspects of the veterinary community, but rather more is expected of you by society because of the profession of which you have chosen to be a member.

As a professional and in a position of responsibility as a professional, you should also look out for the well-being of others in the workplace and do your best to behave professionally towards them.

Make sure that in all your dealings with animals you behave as a professional should. Make sure, of course, that your own animals are always well cared for and that you always treat those who are your patients with care, never treating them harshly even when handling them is proving challenging.

The RCVS does ask that you disclose any convictions you may have and so, for example, you will have to report any drink-driving offences and any other criminal convictions. There are some spectacular transgressions which vets have been guilty of in the past, including drug smuggling and murder with prescription drugs, but also less dramatic ones which have resulted in vets being struck off because they have brought the profession into disrepute.

Honesty is essential for a professional person and as a veterinary surgeon you need to hold to that principle throughout your working life. It is quite possible that you will come under pressure to behave dishonestly at some time by your clients, possibly even your colleagues and your friends and family. What may appear a fairly innocuous request for a pack of flea product or some antibiotics 'under the counter' without your employer's permission, is actually a threat to your integrity and honesty. I cannot stress enough how important it is that you refuse any such request and explain to the person asking that you cannot and will not comply because, however close you are to that person and however much you trust them, it is against the code of conduct expected of veterinary surgeons and is of more potential significance than they are likely to realise. Most reasonable people who care about you will completely understand this once you explain and will not ask again.

I once overheard a woman at a horse show boasting to her friend that she had a 'tame vet' who supplied her with phenylbutazone and antibiotics for her horses without examining them because she had the vet 'in her pocket'. She was dismissive of the abilities of vets generally and highly disparaging when speaking of young vets, holding forth about how she knew more than they did about horses anyway. She was not speaking about the vet who was risking his career with gratitude but with disdain, and his actions were potentially damaging both for him if he was found out and also for the horses she was supposedly caring for. She was not risking anything at all and would most likely have hung him out to dry without a second thought if it suited her purpose.

There will also be occasions during the course of your work when people you know will ask you to bend the rules for them and ask you to help them save a bit of money by not charging correctly or filling in a certificate for insurance incorrectly. At the start of your career you may be lacking in confidence and more vulnerable to requests such as this. Some people are very clever and try to manipulate you by saying that your boss has done this before or that no one will know. It is just not worth the risk: just keep saying no without feeling any need to apologise or elaborate further.

A friend of mine sarcastically retorted to a farmer who had asked him to falsify a certificate that he would do it if the farmer agreed to pay him an amount equivalent to his annual salary every year for the rest of his life, because that was what he was asking him to risk in complying with his request.

Beware the client who asks you not to record a significant clinical finding such as a lump because they are going to get their animal insured and come back after two weeks have passed. They are asking you to be complicit in defrauding an insurance company which, as you know, is an offence.

Social media

Read your contract and ensure you comply with the practice rules on social media but do use your own common sense too in looking after your own personal reputation.

As you embark on your career, you may want to have a good look at what information about you is out there and perhaps take some steps to remove anything you now feel is not appropriate for all to see in the future. It is not a great idea to have drunk, semi-naked photos of you available for a disgruntled client to find online, so just be aware of how you want to appear publicly, both socially and as a professional, now and in the years to come.

Never post photos of clients and their animals without their consent or post a clip of something at work which might seem hilarious at the time but which should not be in the public domain. Think twice before you recount any snippets of information about your colleagues or clients.

There are forums and groups online which are for veterinary surgeons and which can be an excellent source of information and peer support. Most societies have some form of discussion group or forum and will have other vets contributing and you will be able to access a large resource of experience and advice on a myriad of topics, both clinical and professional.

Some, for example VetSurgeon.org, SPVS and the BSAVA and BVA specialism forums, have specialists and certificate holders who will give their advice on management of cases and there are invaluable sources of knowledge on wildlife and exotics, in addition to job adverts; there is usually a healthy discussion of off-duty topics of conversation too.

Always treat your colleagues online with respect and never criticise another vet or a client to anyone else in your discussions online because, although these forums are closed, there is still the chance that a derogatory remark could be reported outside of the intended audience. There will be occasions when you might strongly disagree with a diagnosis or a treatment, but do try to discuss it civilly with the colleague concerned even though you are not face to face.

Continuing professional development (CPD)

CPD is an essential part of being a professional veterinary surgeon and your whole career should include lifelong learning. It is humbling to think how little each of us know of veterinary medicine and surgery compared to all the knowledge that is out there and this is probably increasingly true for today's graduates as science and knowledge progresses so quickly.

You have to continue to read and learn and keep up to date with developments, especially in the field in which you have chosen to work, or you will become out of date and unskilled – this has never been more true than nowadays when the rate of innovation and change is so swift. You will be constantly presented with advances in surgical techniques and with new drugs and the discovery of emerging diseases. Even if you are taking a career break, parental leave or travelling, I do recommend that you keep up to date as much as you can by continually reading and attending courses online or in person, because a year or two away is a long time when you are out of general practice.

If you are a skilled prevaricator like me, then do try to discipline yourself to schedule the CPD into your diary and do small chunks at a time, but regularly and often. This is often easier when you are at work than at home with all the distractions that exist so, if you are working out of hours and there is a quiet time when you are in the practice, you may find that you are in the right place and in the right frame of mind to do some background reading or research.

There are many resources now such as online courses and webinars to enable vets to study in their own home or workplace, but I would recommend that you also attend some courses and events in person if you can. There is something irreplaceable about meeting your fellow professionals face to face and sharing time together enjoying that common bond which unites you and inspires you. Ours is a small profession and it is a pleasure to meet up with colleagues who share our interest in all things related to veterinary medicine and surgery. Discussions with colleagues are a rich source both of information and reflection, and the shared experience and comradeship provide important emotional support. Other vets uniquely understand just what the reality of your life as a vet is like and in the majority of cases there is a willingness to share triumphs and disasters and support colleagues, which you may not find in other, larger professions or online.

The cost of courses and the investment in terms of paid hours both for the attendee and the vet covering their work back at the practice, means that employers like to see a definite benefit to the practice or company. Make sure your choice of CPD improves your veterinary skills and expands your knowledge pertinent to the work of the practice and is not just the pursuit of your hobby interests and the areas in which you already excel. It makes more sense in the early years of your career to seek CPD in areas where you feel you are not as competent and may feel uncomfortable tackling, rather than on topics that you enjoy but will be of little use to you.

I used to feel that I was a bit poor at ophthalmology and this feeling of uncertainty and lack of competence caused me concern so, although the last thing I wanted to do was spend a whole day immersed in looking at retinas and becoming handier with the equipment, I made myself sign up when I would have much preferred to go to a course on feline medicine which sounded far more attractive. My hesitancy and reluctance to see eye cases was much reduced after the course and I felt much more confident about ophthalmology in general and the sense of achievement was considerable.

CPD does not have to be entirely clinical and topics such as different techniques and means of communication and client management skills can be highly valuable to you and the practice. Learning about well-being and leadership skills is also useful at any stage in practice and it can be great fun to learn about and very illuminating if you are interested in people and enjoy improving your interpersonal skills. There are often courses about practice management, human resources and practice finance which are interesting and informative, not just for potential practice owners but for clinical directors and branch managers.

If you are really lucky, you may be able to do your CPD in combination with various enjoyable activities such as skiing or cycling; they may be in pleasant venues and offer the opportunity to meet your fellow vets. Your employer may be happy to pay for you to use your allowance on the registration and accommodation costs of a CPD course in the Alps with opportunities to ski or travel overseas.

Some contracts will have a clause relating to CPD with some form of a commitment from you to ensure the practice recoups some of the benefit of the cost of a course; the practice may require some repayment from you if you leave immediately after attending a course.

You may need to show some justification of why your allowance should be spent on investment in your particular interest in animal behaviour or acupuncture and how it will also benefit the practice. Your employer might well prefer you to have an interest in dermatology or dentistry because this is likely to be helpful and more profitable for the practice, and I am sure you can understand this point of view. The cost of CPD for a practice is considerable, but if you do your research and can justify it, you may find your employer is amenable to investing in a course on a subject which you are interested in and which will also further your career.

Do not take everything you hear during CPD courses as gospel but keep an open mind and evaluate the information you hear. There is a tendency for vets to go on a course and perhaps hear that something completely new is being advocated, and they rush to put it into practice without considering it carefully. The Internet is an amazing source of knowledge but also an amazing source of hypothetical nonsense stated as fact on occasion. As a trained professional, you need to use your knowledge skills and training to differentiate the good from the bad and check the sources and references carefully.

A colleague of mine and I once returned from a BSAVA congress with a new anaesthetic premedication regime we had heard about in a lecture and which sounded brilliant. Because we had heard about it in a lecture from an eminent professor, we used it the next day and it resulted in severe adverse reactions in our first two patients. It taught me a painful lesson not to believe everything I heard however eminent the source. Some 'experts' extrapolate their findings outside their realm of expertise and it transpired that the protocol had only been used once or twice in practice and was more experimental than tried and tested.

It is not acceptable to rely on the qualification with which you leave vet school and just potter on through your veterinary career without continually challenging your knowledge and beliefs; vets must continually adapt and learn throughout their careers. Over the years, different methods of treatment do come in and out of favour and some new treatment supersedes an old one only for it to become fashionable again later. Using honey in wound dressings was an old-established remedy a hundred years and more ago, which went out of fashion as new wound dressings were developed, but has recently come back in again. Groundbreaking developments which have been hailed with enthusiasm have then been superseded by even better or safer techniques or drugs. Keep an open mind and remain receptive while ensuring that you challenge new advances and look for evidence which is based on reliable respected research.

The olden days

When I was a student in Wales I observed dogs and cats anaesthetised using ether-soaked cotton wool in a jam jar, and as a young graduate we used halothane in a very basic vaporiser. We have now progressed in general practice to the current sophisticated anaesthetic agents and the use of the complex anaesthetic machines and blood gas analysis.

Immobilon (etorphine) and its reversing agent, Revivon (diprenorphine), was hailed as a wonder drug when it came out many years ago, because of its reversibility, rapid onset and duration, especially for equine procedures in the field such as castration. Immobilon was in regular use when I was a young graduate and in addition to revolutionising anaesthesia in horses, it was also used in small animal practice, especially with dogs which were hard to handle. It was a huge risk to vets because of the perils of accidental self-injection and was also used as a means of some vets taking their own life. I considered it a happy day when its routine use in practice fell into disfavour, although a similar drug is still used when darting wild animals on game reserves. It is not an exaggeration to say that I was absolutely terrified of using Immobilon and now when I look back, I find it hard to believe that I actually risked my life in that way. At the time, the job demanded it and I survived, but there were accidents and vets died from accidental self-injection.

Vets regularly used to put themselves in danger by wrestling with aggressive dogs and injecting them with Immobilon into the muscle of a hind leg from behind the surgery door while a brave nurse hung onto the end of the lead. We were all aware that even a scratch or contamination of a cut with a drop of the drug could result in death and were advised to keep Narcan, which was then considered to be a safe antidote for humans, close to hand and ready-loaded in a syringe.

I had conversations with farmers and horse owners in Yorkshire which went as follows:

'If I inject myself by mistake, I want you to take this syringe and inject me in my buttock.'

'You what, love?'

'If I inject myself by accident or it squirts in my face, you'll have to inject me or I will die. Don't mess about, just stab me in the backside with it if I ask you to and don't take too long about it.'

'Eh love, I can't wait!' was the reply.

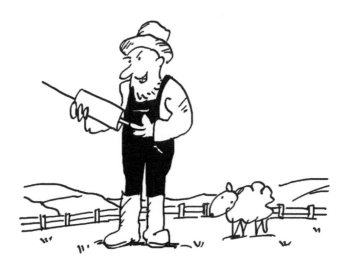

Veterinary politics

People often confuse the roles of the two major veterinary bodies which are so important for veterinary surgeons in the United Kingdom.

The Royal College of Veterinary Surgeons (RCVS) is the regulatory body of our profession and holds the register of vets who are allowed to work in the UK. Its Code of Conduct sets out the ways in which a veterinary professional is expected to behave to uphold the respect the general public hold for the profession. Its role is different to that of the British Veterinary Association (BVA) which is the representative body for veterinary surgeons and supports and champions the UK veterinary profession in all interfaces, such as with government and other official bodies, and with other animal-related topics of interest.

The Royal College of Veterinary Surgeons

The RCVS currently states 'We aim to enhance society through improved animal health and welfare. We do this by setting, upholding and advancing the educational, ethical and clinical standards of veterinary surgeons and veterinary nurses.'

Sometimes, there appears to be resentment that the RCVS does not appear to support individual vets but that is not the role of the college according to its royal charter. It is there to regulate the profession and provide a way for the general public to raise and voice concerns about veterinary surgeons.

Concerns raised by the public are received by the college but are considered by two independent committees, the Preliminary Investigation Committee which considers all concerns raised and the Disciplinary Committee which adjudicates over the cases which are considered to warrant an official hearing over matters which may have brought the profession into disrepute. There has been a great deal of work done in recent years to try to communicate more openly and effectively with the profession.

The RCVS is taking a more proactive role in promoting well-being in the profession with its Vetlife initiative in association with the Veterinary Benevolent Fund, the British Veterinary Association, the British Veterinary Nursing Association, the Veterinary Practice Management Association, the Veterinary Schools Council, the Veterinary Defence Society and the Association of Veterinary Students.

The British Veterinary Association

The BVA is our representative body and is governed by vets and for vets. There is a great deal of support for young graduates offered by the BVA Young Vet Network (YVN) which is for final-year students and qualified vets for the eight years after graduation. I would strongly recommend that you become a member and visit their website for current information.

At present, members are offered:

- Free personal accident insurance with an option for a discount on income protection cover in case of injury or accidents
- A helpful handbook for new graduates
- Face to face meetings in your region of the country
- Graduate representation
- Free professional guidance
- Free and discounted continuing professional development
- Guidance for completing the PDP
- Discounted recorded webinars from the Royal Vet College
- YVN, a forum for private online discussions with other young vets
- Career coaching by email or phone on a one-to-one basis at discounted rates.

There are other subgroups, societies and professional bodies accommodating various interests, such as the British Small Animal Veterinary Association (BSAVA), the Veterinary Hospitals Association (VHA), British Association of Veterinary Emergency & Critical Care (BAVECC), and the Society of Practising Veterinary Surgeons (SPVS) and you will find in each an excellent way to meet vets who share your particular interests.

You might eventually consider becoming involved in the running of a society or in representing a region for one of the associations such as the BVA or being involved in running a BVA Young Vet Network regional scheme.

Being part of a society or standing for a veterinary organisation means that you can be instrumental in the way your profession moves forwards in the coming years and it can open opportunities to meet interesting individuals and to be a part of the future. Never feel that your voice is not as valuable or worthy of an audience as any other vet out there, however young you are or however few your years of experience, because your opinion matters. You will find that you have much in common with many of your older colleagues and you will have the chance to learn and grow as a vet and a person. The best veterinary politicians I have met have always been willing to listen more than they speak and to maintain an open mind, willing to change.

CHAPTER 19

Six months in practice

Your first six months in practice will have been full of new experiences and you should have the satisfaction of a sense of achievement and a fulfilment of the ambition you have worked towards since you first decided to be a vet. The first days and weeks are often exhilarating but also exhausting and the time passes so quickly that there is barely a moment to reflect on how far you have come. New graduates usually arrive into the practice full of knowledge and enthusiasm, refreshingly keen to gain experience and I have always felt that they inject fresh life into the practice and bring many tangible and intangible positives to the veterinary team.

Now you are six months qualified you are no longer the 'newbie' but are now fully contributing as a working vet and more and more independent. At this stage of your career, you will still be experiencing situations for the first time and learning and increasing your skill levels and hopefully you are still full of passion for your career and enjoying life as a vet.

The first six months can also be a time during which your confidence may have been severely challenged because although you graduated with the competences required for your first day in practice, it does not necessarily mean that you were very good at them. It may have been the first time in your life when you were presented with so many demands of a practical nature and you will have achieved varying degrees of success. Things will probably have gone wrong on occasion, and minor mistakes will have been made or narrowly averted, and there will have been times when someone had to come and bail you out. This can be hard for a high achiever who is used to doing well in everything they have faced before but do not let any self-doubts creep in now, because you will become better and better as you become more experienced.

If you consciously decide that you are going to find being a vet interesting and enjoyable despite it being hard work, and you nurture that mindset and approach, then it probably will be so. Your attitude to life and work has a big influence on the people around you, and both your clients and the people you work with will respond to your positivity in a way which helps to make it happen. If you enter practice expecting it to be awful and anticipating the worst of every situation, then you will probably find that this becomes reality and the negativity can eat away at you and make you difficult to work with and help. I know this can be easier said than done, but the fact remains that becoming a good vet is not an easy path and the right approach and a good sense of humour can make all the difference.

Your employer should have given you a supportive introduction to veterinary work with a reasonable caseload to handle, and should have nurtured you and looked after you by not allocating tasks that are beyond your capabilities, and by giving you help when you needed it. You should feel much more comfortable and relaxed about being a vet and be experiencing some very positive achievements as you progress: those successes are the rewards of your hard work.

I know this will not have been the case for everyone and that some practices still exist where new graduates are thrown in at the deep end without the necessary support and left to sink or swim. Some employers still have the view that, because they had a baptism of fire as a new graduate, then why not you, but I do hope you have been treated well and received good mentorship and, above all, are still enjoying being a vet.

Most vets over a certain age will tell you horror stories of their first months in practice and mine was not much better when I look back, and to a great extent I think luck had a lot to do with my coming through that time relatively unscathed. I was the first female full-time vet in the first two practices I worked for and I felt there was a certain need to prove myself to be as capable as a male graduate, if not more so.

In my first six months in practice, I had some wonderful highs and some terrible, soul-destroying lows but I picked myself up and with the help of everyone around me, I still enjoyed those exciting months doing the job I had trained for.

I had some good experiences, such as performing my first few bitch caesarians and splenectomies and experienced the challenge of being involved in emergency vaccination programmes and treatments for parvovirus when it first emerged as a new disease. I calved cows and lambed ewes successfully and won some of the farmers over so that they even asked for me by name, especially for lambings.

I had some bad experiences, such as seeing cases of animal neglect and hearing clients say they did not want to see that new vet because she looked too young to know what she was doing. I had to put young dogs with distemper to sleep simply because their owners had not had them vaccinated and I saw young dogs die after road accidents because they were running loose on the streets all day. I had to accept that people would choose to have cats with broken legs put to sleep because they could 'easily get another one'.

I was once sent on a house call by my employer with instructions to euthanise a litter of newborn puppies and was incensed at being told by the owner who had requested it that she couldn't do my job because she thought it was 'evil to take life like that'.

*I had to work over Christmas and be alone and away from friends and fam-
ily for the first time over New Year's Eve in a strange city where I did not know
anyone. I was already feeling quite sad and sorry for myself when my sister
thought it would be hilariously funny to ring me with a bogus emergency call.
She had had a few drinks at a party and laughed hilariously at my struggle to
make sense of the phone call and my attempts to persuade her to bring her
rat down to the surgery. She was laughing like a drain when I finally rumbled
her but by this stage I was not laughing at all and had a complete sense of
humour bypass!*

*I worked with some wonderful nurses who were so generous with their time
and patience, even though it took me twice as long to do a cat spay or a bitch
spay or couldn't find a vein. They nudged me in the right direction when I needed
help, with suggestions to place an extra suture here or there, or with hints as
to what to do next with a difficult case and they looked out for me with general
encouragement and kindness.*

*There were occasions when I felt I was just managing to cope and that I was
an imposter as a vet and just avoiding disaster. There are so many emotions
that can run through your mind when you are doing a demanding and unpredictable job and you feel you might be found wanting at any moment, like flying
a plane with only one engine and no parachute. I had to learn how to pause
and collect my thoughts, and how to take a step back, make a practical plan
and use my training rationally, and to swallow my pride and ask for help when
I needed to. I also learned that 99 percent of the things we worry about never
actually happen, and that in order to carry on I had to forgive myself if I made
a mistake or when I was not able to manage something without assistance.*

I would like to think we live in a more enlightened age now and I hope that you will not
have had the six months of terror and apprehension that vets of a former era sometimes
appear to wear as a badge of honour. It is not necessary nowadays to be subjected to a testing
six months of sleeplessness and stress to prove yourself fit to join the crusty, old, battle-
scarred vets in practice. I hope that you have reached the end of your first six months still
enjoying seeing the patients and meeting their owners and that each new day is approached
with interest and enthusiasm and not dread and exhaustion.

Although we can protect ourselves to some extent, there will be times throughout our
veterinary career when, in order to progress and achieve, we need to stretch ourselves and
risk our dignity by pushing ourselves out of our comfort zone. It is natural and indeed desirable to feel that you have been stretched and tested in your first six months in practice, but
you should not feel that you are completely out of your depth, chaotic and exhausted. If
this is the case, then review the demands of the job you are in and discuss it with a suitable
person, perhaps someone outside the practice if this seems the best option, but if possible
with your immediate superior at work. Make sure that they are aware of how you are feeling

and give them the opportunity to make things better for you. They may not have recognised that all is not well unless you tell them clearly and unambiguously. Do not assume that they will pick up on how difficult you are finding things through dropping hints or exhibiting low-level 'martyr-ish' behaviour and complaining to everyone you work with. Most employers really do care about your health and well-being, so if things are really bad and you are not happy then do not just put up with it, but speak out.

It is not always the first six months in practice that is the greatest challenge but the year which follows, because gradually more will be expected of you in terms of working independently and you can expect to be allocated more complex work.

At the end of the first six months, it can feel as if you have reached the crest of a wave and are now surfing down the other side rather faster than you would choose. The novelty of actually being a vet at last wears off a little bit and the intense support which you were given as a completely new graduate in the first few weeks may gradually have reduced. You will be expected to start to push the boundaries of your confidence more and more, and to deal with more unpredictable and challenging situations where you have to think on your feet.

You may now be expected to cope with a busy consulting session completely on your own with no extra time on a regular basis for example, and be expected to perform simple operations without another vet assisting. You may still be allocated some backup, but the supporting vets will be expecting you to call on them only when you really need it, and not as a psychological prop for work you are now capable of doing on your own. It is still relatively early in your career, so you will inevitably still have times when you need help, but these occasions should be becoming less frequent than they used to be. The safety net is still there, but the body harness has been removed and you are relying on yourself much more to work through your cases and make decisions.

Use your holiday allocation

You will have been given a number of days of paid holiday which will be written into your contract and although it is easy to carry on without taking a break in the first few months, you will have been working very hard and concentrating very intensely and it is mentally and physically exhausting. It is important to take your holidays at regular intervals to recharge your batteries and to have a complete break from work. Holidays are an essential resource for your mental well-being so do not squander them by staying at home and doing something boring, but go away and invest some time and money on yourself. You are no longer a student but are now earning money and you can afford to have some time away.

Many contracts will say that holidays must be taken within the year or may be forfeited so check your contract and make sure you take your full allocation. You need to adopt the habit of planning ahead when it comes to holidays, because the member of staff producing the rota will have to plan for each vet to take their holiday entitlement while also ensuring the practice is adequately staffed throughout the year. It is not always possible to let someone take time off at the last minute as cover needs to be arranged and there cannot be too many

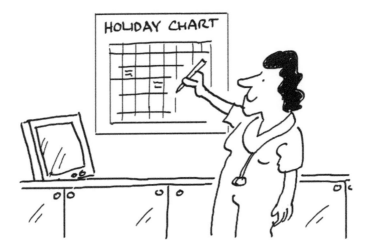

vets in the practice off work at the same time. Check with the practice manager to find out how the holiday system works and book yours into the diary well in advance or you may end up with whatever days off are left after everyone else has made their choice. Members of staff with small children will be constrained by school holiday times so they will rush to book those times well in advance. It is far more expensive to go away then anyway, but if you want to book a specific week off during school holidays to go to a wedding, for example, then you might need to be quick off the mark and book early.

Most practices are reluctant to allow more than two weeks to be taken at a time, simply because accommodating all the holidays can be quite a challenge and client care and continuity can be better served without overly long holiday periods.

Do not wait until you have been working for nearly ten months and are mentally and physically exhausted, and have to cram all your remaining annual leave into a short space of time.

Holidays of a full week or preferably two will give you the chance to completely unwind and it is not unusual to feel lethargic or go down with a cold in the first few days of a holiday. Your body seems to 'decide' it can afford to be ill once you relax the pace and the effects of the stress of work wear off. If you take several short holidays and long weekends you may not relax sufficiently or completely unwind for long enough for it to be of benefit, so I would recommend that you try to go for at least one decent holiday a year.

Check your progress and increase your experience

When you first started work in practice there was so much to think about and you were fully occupied like a manic hamster on a wheel dealing with a hundred new experiences a day and working hard to do the best you could with the work presented. As more and more of the day-to-day tasks become familiar and easier to perform, it is now worth taking stock of how far you have come and the areas in which you still have to improve and refine your skills.

Is there an area which you still feel worried about and which you may be avoiding at work? It is very tempting to avoid the things that you find more difficult and in some smaller practices, it will be more obvious both to you and to others that this is what you are doing. That challenge of the hefty Labrador bitch spay becomes the size of a hippo in your mind and there is always someone else in the practice who you think could do it better than you. In a smaller practice, you will probably just have to get on and do one, and will indeed be encouraged to do so by your mentor who has faith in your capabilities and is going to be there in the background supporting you. In bigger practices, it may be much easier for you to continue to walk round those things which challenge you and to waive the opportunity to do something difficult, but the more you avoid them, the more intimidating they become and the harder it gets. The months and years go by and that buxom bitch spay becomes a bigger and bigger obstacle in your mind and you worry about it and tell yourself that someone else would be better at it than you. Take on the chance to operate on Fatty McFatdog now while you have help and support available and the sense of achievement from mastering and over-coming that challenge will be all the greater. It will become easier every time you perform it and though it can still be a difficult operation, you have the confidence and the reassurance of knowing you can do it, and if the worst happens and you are faced with a bleeder then you can stay calm, get exposure and sort it out. There will probably be times even after you have been qualified for 20 years, when some surgery will still make you sweat and get the adrenaline circulating, but the more you do, the more confident you will become.

Increasingly, you need to be able to use the equipment which is present in most practices, such as the X-ray machine, ultrasound machine and the endoscope competently, and not continue to rely on someone else.

Every experience of operating the scanner and looking at scans will improve your skills and you need to see a lot of normality to be able to navigate an abdomen and to have the abnormal jump out at you on a screen. Take any opportunity that arises when other people are performing scans or endoscopy to gain experience and on a quiet day, use that spare time to learn how to operate the blood analysis machine or other equipment.

I was speaking to a young vet recently who was being praised by the nurses as 'king of the ultrasound machine'. Though he was a relatively recent graduate, he was now becoming the one who the other vets frequently deferred to in his expertise in ultrasound scanning and I asked him how he had become so proficient. He told me it was because when seeing practice, he heard the nurses say how boring it was holding animals for ultrasonography and so, as a student, he volunteered to hold all the animals to allow the nurses to carry on with other tasks. This gave him the opportunity to see a large number of scans and to be given guided tours of the normal abdomen and chest, as well as seeing various pathologies identified.

You are well aware that you are a working vet now and not a student, and so the income-generating work in the practice does have to take priority over learning experiences and opportunities. You may have to be proactive and use your own time to gain more experience if you want to improve in confidence and competence. You have to seize opportunities to learn during quiet times of the day, during evenings on call and sometimes even be prepared to come in in your own time when something really interesting is happening. The practice will undoubtedly benefit from your enthusiasm and increased knowledge but, primarily, it will be your gain as you become a better vet.

Learning from routine consulting

The art and science of being a good veterinary surgeon is in recognising the abnormal in our patients and to do this you need to be completely familiar with that which is normal. Running your hands over an animal's body and performing manual palpation of every abdomen presented to you in a consultation, even in the course of a health check for a booster, gives you the ability to identify an abnormal abdomen in an ill animal. Everyone starts off as a vet student palpating an abdomen and nodding sagely when asked if they can feel the kidney whereas, in reality, they cannot distinguish anything at all and it is only with continued practice that you reach a stage where an enlarged spleen jumps out at you on palpation. X-rays and ultrasound scanners are widely used but palpation is still an invaluable and undervalued skill especially in an apparently healthy animal. You can use imaging to confirm your suspicions, but it is not feasible to scan every animal which comes in and a gentle, skilful palpation can be really effective in detection of abnormality when no symptoms are evident. I have frequently identified abdominal masses during a booster examination of an otherwise healthy dog or cat and clients regularly assume that their pet is just slowing down in their old age when actually something more insidious is going on. It is so satisfying to diagnose a mass before it bleeds and presents as an emergency, and your abdominal palpation can save a dog's life.

Continue to use the ophthalmoscope and auroscope whenever you can so that you become adept at using the instrument and increase your expertise. Use your stethoscope and listen to every heart you can so that when you put your stethoscope on the puppy and there is the unusual sound of a machinery murmur, it will immediately register as an abnormality and you will not miss that patent ductus arteriosus. Any diagnostic instrument is only as good as the ability of the person listening and practice really does make perfect. An added benefit of the use of a stethoscope during a consultation is that the client usually stops talking to allow you to listen and it can give you valuable time to think.

If you are in a hurry and want to make up time in a busy surgery, it is tempting to skip the full health check for booster examinations but if you do, you will inevitably miss something that becomes apparent a couple of weeks later. You are doing that animal a disservice if you do not perform a full examination, so check heart sounds and for lumps and bumps, bad teeth and smelly ears, even if the client has not mentioned them.

Review your PDP

Your personal RCVS PDP record is there to assist you and for logging the expected competences and experiences as you approach the end of the first year as a qualified vet. It needs reviewing now so that you can make sure you are on track compared to your peer group.

You should seek out opportunities in the areas where you have not been able to gain experience and discuss your progress with your employer, using the PDP as an aid to ask them to help you review your progress and help you to broaden your experience. Your employer or mentor should meet regularly with you, but this commitment might well have slipped their mind as the days go by. They have to sign to confirm that you have taken part and also that they themselves have engaged with the process, and it is recommended that you allocate an hour every four to six weeks to update your PDP record. The record is for your benefit and needs signing off by your allocated Postgraduate Dean; you can choose whether to allow full access for your mentor or employer or just share specific pages. There is a BVA guide to PDP and the RCVS has a booklet and information on their website.

Reviews and appraisals

Most good employers will have regular, structured reviews or appraisals with their vets and may have an organised and official appraisal system in place. In smaller practices, this may be less formal and more a discussion over a coffee with your employer if there are just two or three of you in the practice.

If you feel the need for a more in-depth discussion, then do ask your employer for a properly scheduled meeting to talk about things more thoroughly. Your employer or manager should be more than happy to sit down with you at a suitable time and discuss your progress but it may not have occurred to them to actually suggest it, especially if you have been performing well. A busy employer tends to focus on dealing with matters which are the most pressing and if you are apparently doing well and not seeking their attention, then time may just pass by. It is often the good assistant who gets overlooked while the one who is a problem to the employer receives all the attention, but you need feedback too so if it is not forthcoming, go and ask for it.

Remember the BVA young graduates' support network and find out where the nearest group meets and attend if you possibly can. These are reported to be very helpful and often have very interesting content in addition to giving you the chance to meet other young vets experiencing the same triumphs and disasters that you are meeting. There is nothing quite so cheering as hearing another vet's survival stories and there is always someone who has been in the same boat as you and has lived to tell the tale. If you can get to the young graduate reunions organised by the VDS and supported by other organisations such as SPVS and the BVA, then do go as it is a wonderful opportunity to catch up with friends and also to share experiences and help one another.

Keep up your contacts with your friends but do not be intimidated by the one smug mate who says they have performed three GDVs and a cruciate op single-handed as they are either singularly talented or more likely being economical with the truth. These are the same people who go on social media and give the impression that their working life is as perfect as their hectic social life when, in reality, they are usually in bed by nine, all the nurses hate them and they are still panic-stricken over doing a cat spay.

Is the grass greener on the other side?

It may seem to you that during your first six months you have been putting a great deal of effort into working hard and hence you may assume that you must have been extremely productive and earned pots of money for the practice. Indeed, you should have been putting a huge amount of effort in to your work, but the reality is that you are unlikely to have even covered the costs of your employment. You have to take into account the amount of support you have needed from other people and your reduced caseload and complexity level of work compared to your more experienced colleagues. Employers accept this and expect that most new graduates are unlikely to be productive in their first six months at work and they look on the development of a new graduate as an investment for the future. Once you start to increase the speed at which you can spay a cat and gain the confidence to manage a more complex case, which may need investigations and surgery, and which you become able to perform yourself, then your productivity will increase markedly.

It may be tempting to look round at other jobs after six months, especially if you feel that your initial choices as a new graduate were very limited; if the job market is very buoyant, you will see some tempting terms on offer. You might start looking at the possibility of handing in your notice and getting another job, but I would urge you to think very carefully before you opt to move so soon and to weigh up the pros and cons.

Moving now would mean that you will be the new person in the practice all over again, needing to find out where everything is and getting used to different people and a different system of working. Every practice has its own style and culture and ways of doing things and although the practice you are in may have its drawbacks, it is familiar to you and that does makes life easier while you increase your experience.

It also looks better on a CV if you have demonstrated that you have a certain amount of staying power and can hold down one job for a reasonable length of time. A good track record of employment and good references are a significant advantage in a relatively small profession such as ours, and a history of short job placements may set alarm bells ringing when an employer is recruiting. Employers will understand that a first job and even a second may not have worked out, but if there are three or more short periods of employment then they will wonder what that says about you as a potential employee.

Staying in a practice you are happy in for a reasonable length of time, at least, say, 18 months to 3 years, will give you a good grounding in practice and you will be a very employable person at the end of that time. This may not be the job of your dreams but if you are reasonably happy and advancing your knowledge and becoming a good competent vet, then there is a lot to be said for staying where you are.

It might be that you are attracted to the offer of a higher salary and, as mentioned previously, it is not unreasonable to ask about a pay rise after six months if things are going well. Your employer may be about to offer you an increase, so do not move solely for a position offering a higher salary which might be available where you are now.

Good reasons to stay in the same practice at this stage:

- Knowing you have the support and encouragement of your employer or immediate supervisor and any criticism is given in a way that is constructive not destructive. You know who your supervisor or mentor is and what they expect from you and they know what you are capable of and where you need support.
- You feel confident that you have the opportunity to discuss any problems you may be having.
- You feel that you are enjoying your day despite being challenged by learning new skills and extending your experience.
- You are familiar with the structure and routine of the practice and you know where everything is and how the practice works.
- You have hopefully formed good working relationships with your colleagues and you feel appreciated and part of the veterinary team.
- You know some of the regular clients and are gaining job satisfaction by seeing cases through.
- You feel well in yourself and are sleeping and eating well.

Some employers may have reservations if they see a pattern of relatively short terms of employment without a good explanation. The reader of a CV may wonder if you have a problem with committing to work, or struggle to get on with colleagues or have some health issues which have made you move on. Eighteen months on a CV in one position looks much better than ten months or less, and you have proved you have the ability to hold down a job for a reasonable length of time and have given it a fair shot.

Recruitment is expensive for a practice when the advertising costs and the time and effort spent interviewing is taken into account. There is always some reduced productivity as a new vet settles in and some demands on the time of the existing staff as they introduce them to the way the practice works. Clients love continuity and frequent changes of staff can lead to a reduction in turnover for the practice, so employers prefer vets who will stay for a reasonable length of time. If they are choosing between two equally employable candidates and one has a track record of short terms of employment in several practices, then they may prefer to choose a vet with a track record of longer periods in the same job.

If you are having a rough time

You may be reading this after six months in your first job and feeling that you are really desperately unhappy and not enjoying being a vet at all. If this is the case, then do not immediately think that it is you who are not cut out to be a vet or that you are a failure. It is far more likely that the practice you are in is simply not the right one for you and another practice would be far better suited. Do not despair and blame yourself or assume it is a failing on your part, but logically and rationally identify what is wrong and why you are feeling the way you do.

There are still practices where young graduates are not treated at all well and there are practices which take advantage of the desire of those new graduates to get a foot in the door. The worst practices overwork their new graduates by expecting them to work long consulting sessions with little or no support and may underpay them and not support their further development. This can shatter their confidence and this lack of support and the neglect of the needs of a new graduate can drive them out of the profession altogether. These conveyor belt practices fully expect their young vets to leave after a relatively short time and indeed they do not want them to stay for long because once they are more experienced they can command a higher salary. This is completely irresponsible and shortsighted and it is all too easy to damage the confidence of a new graduate and make them regret their choice of career, even making some young vets leave the profession forever. If you think this is the sort of practice you are in, then extricate yourself as soon as you can and do not wait for six months or more to pass because you can find a more suitable place to follow your chosen career and there are good practices out there.

There are also those difficult employment situations where no one is at fault but that particular practice is just not the right fit for you. Every individual is different and a practice in which one vet may thrive may simply not be suited to another new graduate who has different needs. Innate self-confidence, character and personality make a great deal of difference to where individuals thrive in practice and some new graduate vets hit the ground running and love being under pressure in a busy practice where they relish the challenge. Other new graduates take a little longer to settle in and adapt to employment in general practice and need to grow at a slower pace with help and encouragement. Eventually, over the years, both vets can become equally competent and able and it is just a question of finding the right environment in which each vet can flourish.

Reasons to seriously consider leaving a practice after six months:

- If there is a distinct lack of encouragement and support for you and you feel that you are being asked to work beyond your current abilities.
- If you have been asked to do an unreasonable amount of extra work which was not specified in the job offer or contract.
- If there is a severe restriction of opportunities to increase your experience and you are being asked to perform all the basic tasks without any foreseeable opportunity to gain experience.
- If reasonable requests to address a problem you have at work are refused by those in charge.
- If you feel that there is no one at all who you can relate to within the practice team and no one who cares about your well-being.
- If bullying by other members of the veterinary team has been tolerated and not addressed by management.

- ☙ If you feel that you do not have the backing of your employer and that criticism of you to the clients by other members of the team is being permitted.
- ☙ If you feel that you hate being a vet and are feeling depressed and unhappy most of the time, and not sleeping and eating well.

Do discuss your problems with a third party and see if there are ways in which these problems could reasonably be resolved. The most charitable view could be that you might be the first new graduate the practice has ever employed and they may not realise what you have been experiencing and wish to rectify it. There are still practices where the person managing the practice has not had any training in managing people and being an excellent vet does not necessarily make you a good employer. Some independent practices owned by one or two vets may never have employed anyone before and may have unrealistic expectations of a new graduate and have forgotten what it is like to be newly qualified and needing support. They may have no comprehension that an employee is rarely going to be able to work at the same rate as they are willing to work.

You may be reasonably happy with the practice but want to leave because of personal circumstances. It may be that an opportunity to work in a particular field that you aspire to has become available or because you now realise that the type of practice you are in is definitely not for you. Some vets have a dream that they will be really happy in mixed practice only to find that once they are actually doing the job, large animal work is not for them after all.

As long as the decision to leave is made because of the type of the work and not because of the shortcomings of that particular practice, then it may be completely reasonable to move into a completely different sphere of veterinary work. However, do not let one bad employer put you off a particular area of practice, as you may be able to find a much better practice because you now know what to look for.

In my opinion, moving to get more money is not a very good reason to move after six months in a practice where you are reasonably happy. If another practice is offering a markedly higher salary, then it is probably going to be because they are desperate to fill a position that has some drawback or because they are going to be expecting a great deal of work from you. Once you have been qualified for a year or two, the opportunities will be plentiful and being in a practice where you are able to increase your knowledge and capabilities in a supportive working environment is far more important than money at this stage.

If you know of a vet who is a friend and who is in what sounds like a truly hideous job, then do support them emotionally and encourage them to look after their health, even if it does mean encouraging them to move on. It can be very hard to find the energy to make a decision to move when you are miserable and depressed and your confidence is at rock bottom. In your first job, you have no parameters to compare it to and you may need the help and advice of someone else to show you that you are in a bad situation and that there are alternatives available. Remember to offer them the links to the Vetlife support line and to other organisations which can help, especially if you feel that someone's mental health is at risk.

www.vetlife.org.uk
telephone 0303 040 2551

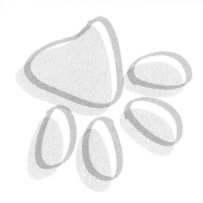

CHAPTER 20

Itchy feet and greener grass

After 18 months in practice, you are likely to be a really valuable asset to the team wherever you are working and have transformed from a bright-eyed but relatively inexperienced new graduate to a really capable veterinary surgeon. The first 18 months in practice are not easy at all and however well-prepared you are, it is a long journey with many ups and downs, but you have survived and become a good vet. You have come such a long way from that first day when you didn't even know the name of the head nurse or where they kept the ear drops.

You will have seen a wide range of different animals and their owners and done many of the routine procedures expected of a veterinary surgeon and you now know every quirk of the practice that you are working in. You can follow the numerous protocols without thinking twice and know where everything is to be found in the midst of an emergency. Basic tasks will have become second nature to you and you can relax much more now when doing the routine work and enjoy it. Your confidence will have grown considerably and you will be enjoying using your mental energies to expand your knowledge and experience and welcome new challenges.

You will, by now, have developed your own unique style of consulting and when you start an evening surgery you can effortlessly orchestrate a good consultation and case work-up and can concentrate on the most important aspects of veterinary care for your patients. You will be seeing all sorts of medical cases, however complex they might be and you will be enjoying the satisfaction of diagnosing diseases and treating them effectively, and will have performed a wide variety of different surgical procedures. You have probably done enough routine procedures such as neutering to feel very confident with them now and you have developed basic surgical skills which hold you in good stead even with more complex procedures which may arise.

Some clients will ask for you by name and some may show their appreciation when you go the extra mile for them and their pet during a difficult time. We are fortunate to be in a job where people often do appreciate us and thank us for doing our job and if they write a card to you or send an email or post a positive comment about you on Facebook or other social media, savour it and keep it or screenshot it to save it. Remember those clients who think you are great and read those positive comments when you next have a bad experience with a case or an ungrateful client. Despite your increased confidence and ability, that will still happen from time to time because this is the nature of being in veterinary practice. You might do a really good job in difficult circumstances and yet receive a complaint, or you might receive a bottle of wine for a straightforward euthanasia when you were just doing your job with kindness.

There probably will be occasions when you do still need to ask for help and this is likely to continue to happen as long as there is someone working with you who is more experienced than you are. However long you have been in practice, never be reluctant to ask the opinion of another vet because sometimes just another perspective is all that is needed. A wise vet never allows pride to stand in the way of what is best for their patient and there are times when your thought processes channel you along one line of thinking about a case and you can feel you are up a blind alley. Another vet's assessment without any preconceptions can shed new light on a case and my partner and I often used to refer cases to each other for an in-house second opinion if we felt we might be missing something or were flummoxed about a case. Talking a case through with a colleague really helps to focus your mind, whilst forums and clinical discussion groups online can be a very valuable source of advice.

You will still be learning new things all the time and this will be a constant state through-out your life as a vet. No vet has ever seen it all, however long they have been in practice and this exposure to new surprises is one of the bonuses of being in this profession and what makes going to work each day interesting and rewarding. Hopefully, you will have enjoyed the past 18 months and been well looked after in your first practice, with plenty of support and opportunity, and have received excellent mentorship. Most vets remember their first practice all their lives and hopefully you will too, and for all the right reasons.

Review where you are in your life

You are most likely leading a very busy life but take time now to take stock of where you are in your life as a whole, both personally and in your career as a vet.

You now know the aspects of the job that you look forward to the most and you may have found that you really enjoy feline medicine or soft tissue surgery or dermatology, even though you did not anticipate doing so. A colleague may have inspired you with an enthusiasm for ophthalmology and it is not too soon to consider which way you want your career to go as you continue on the path of lifelong learning.

You should be having regular appraisals or reviews with your manager or employer and can discuss the opportunities within the practice or the company which are available to you for continuing professional development.

If you are in a mixed practice, you may enjoy working with one particular species, such as horses, so much that you wish to move to a practice or a branch of the practice dedicated to that species. On the other hand, after 18 months of being in practice, you may have decided that large animal or mixed practice is not right for you after all and you wish to focus on small animal work. Do make sure that you really have given it enough time before you decide to concentrate on one particular species or type of practice, because the first few years really are a roller coaster ride of highs and lows of confidence and job satisfaction, and you might need a year or two more to be absolutely certain.

Consider your life outside work and how happy you are with your social life and about where you are living and where you would like to live in the future. You may have been so busy just getting your first job and becoming proficient that this may not have been a high priority for you, but you should not just live to work, even at this stage of your career. You might be living in an area which you do not like, such as in a city when you would prefer to be in the countryside, near the sea or closer to family.

Look at your life as a whole and if you are not getting to do the things which make you happy then consider making some changes. Think of yourself as a case study and examine what your life is like inside and outside of work so that you can make a differential diagnosis and come up with some treatment plans to improve your quality of life.

If you are happy in your current job, then make an honest appraisal of where you are in terms of your career and look and plan towards where you want to be in the next two to three years. Most veterinary practices are in a continuous state of change in relation to staffing as people's life circumstances change, and it may be that you can see a different opportunity that exists within your practice. If you can see that an opportunity for you is in the offing, perhaps working for a different branch or developing an interest in a particular area of practice, then do point this out to your employer or clinical director as it may simply not have occurred to them. You don't have to be pushy, but it really helps if you let them know that you are interested and, to put it bluntly, if you do not ask, you will not get!

There may be opportunities which could exist for the practice which you as a more recently qualified graduate can see and could propose. You may be able to suggest introducing a new service, such as senior pet care or laser therapy, and your employer may be happy to invest in it if they feel you would take ownership of the proposal and drive it forward. I used to really appreciate a vet coming to an appraisal with ideas of what they wanted to do in the future or with a proposal for increasing their level of knowledge, and I was more than willing to help them achieve their goals. It is usually well received if you come forward with a proposal or business plan having done some background work and perhaps give a presentation for what you are suggesting, mapping out the benefits for the practice.

At this stage of your career, you may already be thinking about following a particular area of practice such as orthopaedics, cardiology or ophthalmology, and be looking for a career path to allow you to follow that specific interest. Interested and motivated vets benefit the practice overall and if someone decides to undertake a certificate, for example, then everyone in the practice learns from them and gains by it. It is worth pointing out that an interest in the less glamorous and trendy disciplines such as dermatology or dentistry could stand you in good stead too, as they comprise such a relatively large proportion of first opinion practice cases.

You may have really enjoyed your 18 months in your first practice and be happy to stay on and increase your experience and expertise where you are currently employed, but you will no longer be 'the new graduate' and your role may have changed. You might now be the one offering advice and support to a new vet just starting out in practice.

I am sure you will remember just how you felt 18 months ago and I am sure you will extend the hand of friendship and support and be an excellent mentor. You can make such a difference to that person's life and you will also find that teaching and mentoring is an excellent way of consolidating your own knowledge. Vets find themselves teaching other vets and nurses throughout their careers and education of clients happens every day, so look on it as a learning experience as well as a kindness. The ability to teach is a skill that is very useful in a veterinary career in practice and one for which it is unlikely that you have had any significant amount of training, but in some cases a vet finds that they enjoy teaching so much that they make it their career path and return to academia.

Moving on

You might decide after careful consideration that it is definitely time to move on; because of your experience, you are now in a position to be much more aware of what you want. You are no longer a new graduate, so you are far more employable and attractive a proposition for practices who are recruiting and your range of opportunities will be greater. You can change tack very easily at this stage of your career and, if you prefer large animal work and had settled on a position in a small animal practice because that was the only one available when you qualified, you are now in a much better position to look for a job in mixed practice or equine. You have a proven employment record and general experience of being in practice, with many transferable skills and capabilities.

An employer's point of view when you leave your first job

If you are a reliable employee and a good vet, then your employer will be understandably disappointed if you move on now because they will have invested time and effort in supporting you as a new graduate and they may have been hoping that they would have the benefit of your increasing efficiency for longer. They may well be motivated to encourage you to stay and assist you with developing your career, so it is worth listening to any proposals they come up with to make you want to stay.

If you do decide to look for another job now, then compose a list of the essential factors, then the desirable but not absolutely vital factors, and then those things that would be the icing on the cake and go and look for the job that gives you the best fit. When you have perused all the adverts, just make sure you are definitely going to move to something better than you already have and that you are not leaving a good job that your current practice could improve by making minor adjustments, if you just approached them and asked.

The novelty has worn off a little and you get that restless feeling that makes you want to kick your heels up and look for pastures new. The grass really may be greener on the other side and it is human nature to wonder if there is a massive salary increase awaiting you elsewhere. Just look carefully before you gambol off into the sunset and make sure this is the time to make a move.

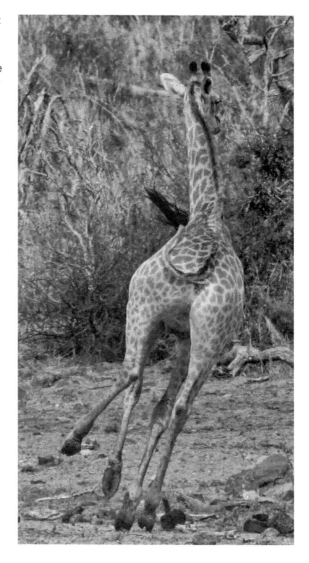

The possible benefits of moving:

- ❧ You might get a significant pay increase, especially if the current job market is very competitive.
- ❧ You might have more choice of practices and be able to move to an area of the country which you like.
- ❧ You might be able to find work in the type of practice you always aspired to, such as an equine practice or a bigger practice with referral vets working under the same roof.
- ❧ You might feel the practice you are in at the moment is not supporting you well enough or is restricting your potential and that a different practice is what you need.

A few words to the wise when you are thinking of leaving but have not yet discussed it with your employer:

❧ Do not talk about the fact that you are thinking of leaving with your work colleagues. If you do discuss it at work, it is highly likely that word of it will reach your employer and even if you decide you want to stay, it will always be in the back of their minds if they are considering internal promotions. It is also quite unsettling for everyone else in the practice who would be left behind when you leave, because they do not like change and they may feel that you are pulling away from the team. Just make sure you have completely made your mind up before you tell anyone and have the courtesy to tell your employer first.

❧ Do not announce on social media that you hate your practice and everyone in it and are off to look for another job! Definitely do not do this after a drinking and complaining session down the pub.

❧ When you apply and go for interview, do not criticise your current practice and employer to your potential future employer because this really sets alarm bells ringing with your prospective employer. Even if it is all fact, you will sound indiscreet and a difficult person to please and there is also the possibility that they know your current employer socially.

❧ Of course, I know you would never take a sick day to go for an interview! That would be dishonest.

❧ Be aware of exactly what financial package you are on at the moment, including subscriptions, perks such as transport and accommodation and CPD allowances, and so on, so that you can compare like with like accurately.

❧ Have some idea in your mind of the salary you hope to command in your next job, as they are quite likely to ask you what you are hoping to earn.

❧ Make sure you are comparing working conditions and rotas on a like for like basis as regards total hours worked and the out of hours commitment, holiday allowances, and so on.

❧ Ask about the opportunities for further study, such as financing for certificates and about CPD generally and if it is in-house or an allowance.

Leaving like a professional

❧ Behave professionally if you do leave and work out your notice diligently and honourably unless the circumstances are really exceptional. It is unfair to walk out and leave a practice in the lurch when you chose to accept the position there in the first place and they have fulfilled their obligations to you. It is far better to leave on good terms if you can; do remember that you may need good references in the future and that the profession is relatively small with many employers knowing one another and it is better not to be perceived to be unreliable.

- When you hand in your notice, do it politely, courteously and professionally and express appreciation of your boss and colleagues. This is not the time for petty comments, even if you feel a little hard done by, because that feeling of victory at having spoken your mind will most likely fade very quickly and you may need some goodwill from them some time in the future.

- Work out your notice diligently and cause as little problem as possible for everyone who is still in the practice by writing everything up and not leaving any loose ends. It is also better for your patients if you can make sure you have left comprehensive clinical notes for ongoing cases and you have some responsibility to the other members of staff too.

- Be aware that some employers will not require you to work out your notice but may put you on 'gardening leave' because they do not wish you to remain in the workplace for various reasons. This can include a ban on entering the practice premises and a ban on any contact with clients and this might be in your contract. This is more common when you have been a longstanding member of a practice, or are setting up or moving to a practice in competition, where the departure of a long-established and popular vet can cause potential damage to the practice. If you move to a neighbouring practice, it is discourteous and unprofessional to encourage clients to follow you and this may well be expressly forbidden under the terms of your contract.

I have experienced all sorts of ways in which vets have chosen to leave their jobs and move on and some have behaved beautifully: we have thrown a farewell party and the practice as a whole has been disappointed to see them go.

Most vets are very honourable and do their job conscientiously right up to the last minute before they leave and their colleagues are really sad to see them go, but they understand that they need to move on. The boss is sorry to see them go too but wishes them well and is likely to go above and beyond expectation when it comes to any references in the future. The most telling and frequently occurring question in a reference is 'would you employ this person again in the future?'

The other end of the spectrum is the obnoxious vet who continually tells everyone how they can't wait to leave and that the practice and the poor suckers who are still having to work there are fools because it is the worst practice in the world. They lose interest in their patients and put little or no effort into consultations because they won't be seeing that client again and do not have the perspicacity and professionalism to see that they are letting those animals down. They are often mysteriously ill in the last few days and ring in sick, necessitating other veterinary colleagues to cover for their shifts. They still expect an amazing farewell party and give constant reminders of how terrible life will be when they have gone and generally behave really badly so that everyone breathes a sigh of relief when they finally depart.

I have had some vets behave so badly that I have asked them to leave without working out their notice because, even though their absence may cause a staffing problem, they are so disruptive that the practice is better off without their negative influence in the weeks before they move on. Some vets with little self-awareness behave very badly by telling everyone that they cannot wait to leave the practice and then a few months later, they ask for references because they are moving on a second time. I have known vets and nurses ask to come back to work at the practice because they have found that they regretted leaving, but you will be unlikely to be welcomed back if you have spent your last days at work telling all and sundry how glad you are to be going to a better place.

Drowning not waving

I am sure that there will be some vets reading this and thinking, hang on a minute, I don't feel confident and collected and experienced at all. Negative thoughts may be overwhelming you and your dreams of being an accomplished vet, loving your work, look further and further away.

You might have been reading this and thinking: 'I don't really feel at all confident in my work or my progress in this practice and I am not sure I like being a vet at all. I worry about coming to work every day and I feel as if I am flying by the seat of my pants all the time, narrowly escaping disaster and hating every moment. Everyone is bad-tempered with me all the time and it is not at all what I was expecting or hoping for and I feel isolated and miserable. I am a failure as a vet and I do not know what to do.'

If you do feel like this and you are sure that you have tried your best but to no avail, then please do not assume it is the whole of veterinary practice that does not suit you and that you are a failure because you have not settled into this particular practice. This may just not be the practice for you or the area of veterinary work for you or perhaps the career path for you.

The most likely explanation is that you are not receiving the correct support in the appropriate way for you as an individual and it may be that you would flourish in another practice with a different structure and a good mentor and different support. Some practices do expect far too much of their new graduates and think that because the last one or two thrived on minimal support and positively jumped in at the deep end without a life jacket, then all graduates will survive.

I have known some excellent vets who took considerably longer to become happy in their own skins and they became confident working in practice and became excellent vets. It was a matter of finding what worked for them and treating them as individuals and not battery chickens.

You might need to change practices altogether or you might possibly be able to remedy the situation in the practice you are in if you talk to the management and explain how you feel. If they do not want to listen or cannot help, then look for a practice who can give you what you need to be able to function and grow and, most of all, to enjoy being a vet.

There are practices who do not treat their vets well and it can be a little bit like being in an abusive relationship as you can feel so downtrodden and self-critical that you stay where you are because you do not feel you have what it takes to move. Rest assured that there will be a place for you because you have proved your worth already by graduating with a veterinary degree and you have scaled all those hurdles and you are an achiever.

Working in practice is not the be all and end all and you are a highly qualified, intelligent individual who is capable of many things. Every vet has the odd crisis of confidence and vets have to work hard but the only reason for continuing to work as a vet is if fundamentally you are enjoying it and finding the work rewarding and, most importantly, that you feel happy in yourself. If not, then maybe it is time to move practices or even look for a career in another line of veterinary work. Talk to someone about it, but do not suffer in silence and stay where you are because it appears the easiest option. It is not an admission of failure to move on and, in fact, may be the best career decision you ever make, opening new possibilities which could impact on the rest of your life.

The British Veterinary Association in the UK provides a career coaching service at a discounted cost and offers one-to-one coaching by email or in person. They may help if you want to discuss your options confidentially with someone who has the knowledge of what career paths are available.

If you really have not enjoyed your time in first opinion general practice, then there are other options available to you with your degree and your time in practice will not have been wasted but will be valued even if you change career path now. All the different options which existed when you first qualified are still possible and you are likely to be more employable in these areas now because of your experience. You will have many transferable skills and many companies would be glad to employ you and offer you the career that suits you.

Some vets who experience a life-changing health problem or injury and are forced to look for work outside practice, find that life takes them down a new career path that they were not aware of and they find fulfilment in other employment despite having had to change their plans. Some achieve far more than they would have if they had stayed in practice, so do not settle for being unhappy because there will be the right opportunity out there somewhere for you too.

CHAPTER 21

So now you know it all

The first two to three years in practice are the bedrock of your future as a vet. Every day you will have been increasing your knowledge and skills and these intense and hardworking years are the basis for your future as a vet, whichever career path you decide you wish to pursue.

You will most likely have worked extremely hard and the demands on you will have been great in terms of time and mental and emotional challenge. You will probably have had much less free time than some of your friends who are not vets to enjoy a good, hectic social life and this can be hard when you are young and wanting to participate in everything that is going on in life.

The benefit of these intensive years of work are that you will become familiar and skilled at many routine procedures and they will become progressively easier as you grow in experience and confidence. These first intense and challenging years are an investment in your future and every 'first', whether it be a caesarian or stabilising a diabetic, means less fear and apprehension when the next one comes along.

Every year consider the following:

a) Are you happy with your current job?
b) Do you have the opportunity within this practice to improve and progress?
c) What are you good at?
d) What do you really enjoy doing?
e) Where do you want to be in your career in five years' time?
f) Are there opportunities for advancement where you are?
g) Are there future opportunities for ownership or management?

It might be worth looking beyond the next five years, especially if you are fairly sure of your future goals and aspirations. Plan ahead and aim high but avoid reducing your options if you

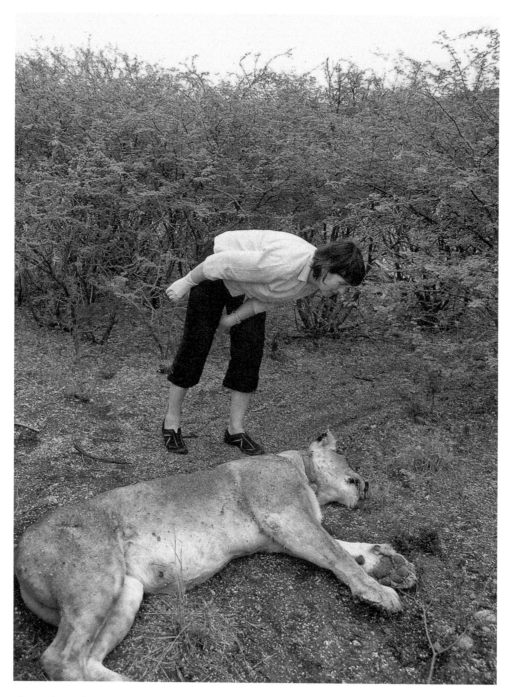

This is the author in South Africa, showing a great deal of confidence in the dose of anaesthetic administered by the ecologist with the dart gun. Many veterinary graduates would like to work in conservation with wild animals such as lions and elephants. If that is your dream, then work towards it but always keep your mind open to change in direction and new opportunity and be the best you can be in whatever career path you choose.

are not exactly sure of what you want to do, because there are many diverse opportunities out there for a vet. There is really nothing to stop you doing anything you want to do if you set your mind to it.

Think about what you need to do to achieve your ambitions and try not to let any feelings of insecurity or fear of the unknown prevent you from following your preferred path. You have so much potential and the only person who is likely to prevent you from fulfilling your potential is you.

The future becomes more complicated when we form relationships and put down roots, such as buying a property and starting a family. Moving home and changing jobs inevitably becomes more complicated when other people are involved and I would urge you to follow your dreams while you are young and can be flexible and responsive to opportunity when it arises.

When you look at the number of job advertisements asking for experienced veterinary surgeons, you should be in no doubt that you have a very good chance of being able to choose the type of practice and the area of the country you want to work in. You will have far more choice now than when you were a new graduate or 18 months qualified and the opportunities abound. If you have outside interests which would be better served by living near the sea or in good cycling country, then this may attract you to certain areas of the country and this might be a good time to move on so that you live your life where you choose to be, rather than letting circumstances dictate. Think carefully and do your research and be choosy, because you should now be a highly employable veterinary surgeon and have much more choice about your next post than when you were a new graduate.

If you do decide to look for another practice to work for, look very carefully at what is on offer and have some idea of what work pattern and salary package you are looking for. Always compare like with like so make sure you take every factor into consideration. Do not underestimate your value if you have several years of experience and have much to offer a potential employer. There is a tendency to underestimate how much is reasonable to ask for, especially if you have worked for a practice as a new graduate and have been underpaid and undervalued.

When I decided to move practices at five years qualified, I went for three different job interviews. One practice offered me a position which I refused for various reasons and they were very affronted by this and made me feel that I had offended them and wasted their time. I went for another interview at a practice and soon after arriving, I realised that there was no way I was going to work for them so, when they asked me what salary I was looking for, I thought that I would ask for a ridiculously large amount which would prevent them offering me a job. I named a figure way above my wildest dreams which I thought they would be deterred by, but to my surprise they still offered me the job. This taught me a valuable lesson not to underestimate my own worth and when negotiating a salary to make sure I had done my homework and not to be too modest because of a misplaced lack of confidence.

Some jobs can sound very appealing with no out of hours work, or a rota involving a week on and two weeks off, but do also consider how you can ensure that you maintain and preferably advance and improve your skills, because with another few years of experience you will be an even better vet and this opens doors to opportunity. I believe that the more experience you gain in the first five years in practice, the easier and less stressful the rest of your working career will be because you will have seen and done most procedures and you will be experienced enough to handle most new challenges. Your clinical and surgical experience will have given you the ability to be more than capable of managing just about anything that practice can throw at you. If you have been qualified for six years without having performed a caesarian on your own or a GDV, then the prospect of doing one for the first time still hangs over you. Some vets do prefer to opt for no out of hours work and may actively avoid surgery, opting for routine work and consulting, but this should be a career choice rather than something you drift into through lack of opportunity. Your first five years in practice can set you on a certain career path almost by default, but it is better to keep your options open and make sure that it is your choice rather than just chance and circumstance dictating where you go with your professional career.

Ours is a relatively small profession and there is a lot of goodwill out there for younger members of the profession, so make the most of speaking to older colleagues at meetings and on forums and find out what is available out there.

Some career options which you might consider after your first few years in general practice include:

- Working towards a further qualification such as a certificate enabling you to work in a referral centre
- Working for a dedicated emergency services provider
- Locum work
- Working in the charity sector
- Teaching and academia
- Careers in research and development
- Careers in industry
- The Royal Army Veterinary Corps
- Government positions
- Food hygiene and meat inspection work
- Laboratory work
- Global health
- Animal welfare
- Management services.

Emergency work

The provision of dedicated emergency services is a rapidly expanding sector as more practices outsource their work which arises out of regular opening hours. Further training in emergency work is widely available by expanding companies such as VetsNow and the work is exciting and varied, requiring good decision-making skills and an ability to work under pressure within a small team where you may be the only vet on the premises.

You are likely to be dealing with complex cases and performing interesting and challenging surgery, but you will also see the usual routine out of hours cases such as vomiting animals, cut paws and anything else which worries a client enough to seek help from a vet out of hours.

The facilities and equipment are usually excellent and there is opportunity to use advanced diagnostic and surgical equipment.

Emergency care companies can offer a career path which may appeal to you if you wish to pursue other interests, such as competitive sport. At this stage of your career, you are likely to have the experience to cope with the pressure that emergency work brings although you should be under no illusion that you will be faced with several complex cases requiring decisive actions and the work can be challenging and unpredictable. You may have several emergencies at once and you will be speaking to clients you have never met before under very stressful circumstances and be working with different people rather than a familiar team. Some vets thrive on the variety of cases they see and enjoy the adrenaline buzz, but it is not for everyone and your success may depend on how confident you are in your own abilities at this stage of your career.

Out of hours work usually commands a higher rate of pay and fewer hours, which can allow daytime free to do other things. The work is well paid to compensate for the antisocial hours and the rota often offers blocks of time off which may appeal to you if you have other outside interests, such as a sport or study. Some vets find it easier to organise childcare and spend more time with their children with this working format, preferring to work intensively for a block of time to maintain a reasonable income, but with good time off in between. It can be a very practical means of bringing in a decent income for a vet with a family who may find it a more attractive option than employing a child minder or can be a way to build up a reasonable sum of money over a relatively short time.

To equip their vets with the necessary skills for this type of work, intensive training courses are often provided comprising several weeks with lectures and practical sessions. This may be followed by a period in a clinic with a mentor to guide and advise you until you are able to work unassisted when necessary in an emergency clinic. They usually require you to have had some previous experience of general first opinion practice and there is likely to be an obligation to work for them for a specified length of time to make it worth their while to invest in your training.

I would advise you to think carefully about the demands of this work at an early stage of your career and give careful consideration as to whether you have the confidence and experience and if it will suit your personality. Ongoing support is provided, and it does offer the opportunity for continuing professional development, but you will inevitably be working nights and weekends and so there will be occasions when you will be under quite some pressure. Some vets enjoy this work while others struggle with working at night and changing sleep patterns and prefer the environment of a close-knit practice team and regular daytime hours.

Working in academia

If you enjoyed your research projects at vet school, there are opportunities for vets to work in research and in teaching positions at vet schools and this can provide interesting and exciting opportunities to gain further qualifications which could lead to future career pathways. Experience of having worked in practice for a time can be an advantage when applying for such positions and many of the skills learned in practice will be extremely useful to you.

You will need good communication skills and attention to detail and to be able to demonstrate problem-solving ability, all of which you will have been using in practice on a daily basis. Many vet schools need vets who can combine work in practice with teaching, and this is particularly valued by vet schools who teach their final year out in practice in the distributed models of veterinary education. Working in research does not always involve working in a lab environment and is often diverse in interest, intellectually challenging and can offer the opportunity to meet interesting and highly educated people. It may offer opportunities to travel, for example to international conferences, and the satisfaction of feeling you are contributing to a bigger picture in health generally. You might enjoy the opportunity to work with young, like-minded, highly intelligent and enthusiastic people in an academic setting, although you will of course meet such individuals in practice too.

The downside can be that much of the work may be desk-bound and that you will find that contracts in research tend to be time-limited so the job security and continuity of employment that you find in general practice may not be there. You may need to move location to follow the work available with all the upheaval and uncertainty that can bring.

There are opportunities to become a resident or an intern in referral practices, where you can advance your knowledge and experience in a particular area that you are interested in such as orthopaedics. These positions tend to attract an initial low remuneration and the hours can be long and the work arduous, but if this is a means to acquiring a further qualification and you have an inspiring mentor, then you may love the work. It might be the means to open the door to your ambition to progress in that field and will be time and effort well invested.

Working for a charity

Charities such as the PDSA and Blue Cross are large and well-organised bodies and the quality of the work they do is comparable with most first opinion practices. There may be some financial constraints, for example they will be unlikely to prescribe costly chemotherapy drugs, and each charity will have its own ethos and protocols to deliver the maximum benefit from the money that is donated to them.

You are likely to meet clients whose values and behaviours you may find quite challenging and you may find the condition in which your patients are presented to you distressing because of their home lives. You would frequently be making a big difference to the quality of life of your patients, which you would find rewarding, but be faced with some emotionally harrowing experiences. You do not have to ask owners for payment for treatment and you will have clear guidelines as to what you can and cannot do for your patients, so there will be limits to the options you can provide. Compliance by owners in acting on your advice may be poor and there may be a lack of appreciation from owners, although as we know only too well, this occurs in private practice too.

You are likely to be able to have good access to complex cases in which you can gain surgical experience and you will be able to perform complicated procedures which may not have been possible in private practice. You are likely to see many interesting medical cases which are rewarding to treat and the work offers a good opportunity to gain experience generally which will stand you in good stead for any future work in practice of any type.

Other positives which may appeal in working for a charity are good rates of pay, a pension scheme, generous sick pay schemes and funding for continuing professional development, plus opportunities for upward progression and advancement in the organisation.

Locum work

A career as a locum vet may attract you because of the flexibility it can offer and the freedom to choose where, when and for whom you work. It offers the opportunity to travel to many different areas of the country and indeed different areas of the world, and enables you to choose the dates on which you wish to be available and when you are not. The different ways of approaching cases in different practices gives you the chance to learn a great deal from the vets you work with and also to observe good and bad practice. This may be very helpful in the future if you have to make decisions about where you wish to settle down, in what sort of practice you will enjoy working and what you would avoid. If you want to own your own practice eventually, you can incorporate the best aspects of the different practices you have worked in and learn from having seen the worst and so avoid the same pitfalls.

The daily rate is relatively good and working as a locum may give you the opportunity to accumulate some capital by working harder for a length of time than you normally would if you were employed by someone else. When you compare the potential income for locum work to an annual salary as an employed vet, you do need to take into account the fact that there is no holiday or sick pay entitlement and that you will be paying your own national insurance, subscriptions and CPD and other costs.

Locum work can offer opportunities overseas, such as in vaccination schemes, and for those who prefer to have variety in their careers at this stage, it has the potential to take you in many and varied directions. You have a high degree of control about where and when you wish to work and so you can choose to work long hours or antisocial hours which pay a premium rate, thus accumulating enough money to take a block of time off to travel, if that appeals at this stage of your life.

You will learn a great deal from other vets in the practices but they will also expect a good day's work from you and the mentoring and support of working within a familiar team in a permanent position is unlikely to be present. Practices benefit from investing their time and effort in assisting their permanent employees but not necessarily their locums, and it is possible that you may be worked quite intensively and have little support. As a locum, you are there to provide a service and the practice wants to ensure they receive value for money from you.

The best and most popular locums for a practice are positive, friendly, reliable and hard-working individuals who do not criticise the host practice, the protocols, the staff or the equipment. They do the best job they can with what is available and are true to their word, turn up on time, are friendly and smile at the clients, do not cause trouble with the permanent staff, work to a good standard and charge correctly. A good locum is appreciated and will never be short of offers of work, always welcomed back with open arms and can build a close relationship with a practice and the people working there.

The downsides of locum work:

- As a locum, you may find yourself working in practices you do not like, with people you do not like and with equipment that you are unfamiliar with which may not be up to the standards you are used to.
- You may be given the most unpopular and most mundane work to do, although often the workload may be lighter than usual because some clients will wait for their regular vet to return from holiday.
- You will have no influence on how the practice functions or the protocols which are in place.
- You will never know where anything is until the day before you are about to leave.
- You will need to be able to use several different practice management systems and every practice has their own peculiar little ways of doing things.
- You will be living out of a suitcase in a variety of lodgings, some good, some not so good and some shockingly bad, by all accounts.

Some individuals can find the constant change and uncertainty quite stressful and it can pall after a while, so it does not suit everyone. You may enjoy the work in a practice and move on and never return, though some locums will return several times to do sessions in a practice where there has been mutual appreciation and may even take a permanent job there if one should arise.

It is always advisable to maintain a good reputation for reliability, even if you hate an individual practice and vow never to go back, because the veterinary profession is relatively small and word will get around if you let people down. Never agree to take a locum position and then drop out at the last minute because you will most likely have ruined a family holiday for someone and this will not be forgotten or forgiven. This may ruin your reputation for reliability and you should never underestimate the speed of communication within the veterinary community, where bad news travels fast and far.

Joining a company or group with opportunities for running your own practice

You may plan to run your own practice eventually and may want to join a practice as an assistant now, where there may be a future option of ownership, or you may wish to work for a company with a view to becoming a clinical director.

Corporate practices are frequently looking for clinical directors and currently constitute 40 percent of practices in the UK, as whole, and 50 percent in Scotland, although this has probably changed even more since the time of writing. You can run a practice yourself and command a higher salary commensurate with the amount of responsibility you have and the profitability of the practice you are in charge of.

Joint venture partnerships can offer you the chance of having your own practice to manage and give you the opportunity to benefit financially for the work you do without the level of investment needed when setting up on your own. Look carefully at what is on offer and the small print of the contracts. There are positives and negatives about every business relationship and joint venture investors understandably expect a return on their money.

The practice will be provided for you ready and fully equipped, taking away a great deal of the pressures of setting up your own practice. You will have management support, which can be very useful if you have no experience of business, although you will quickly learn, especially when it is your own money you are dealing with.

You may be working alone or with one or two other vets and have a variable amount of autonomy and clinical freedom. You need to know just how much clinical freedom you will have, especially if this is important to you. The buying power of corporate practice is huge and so you will most likely be using drugs and pet foods from an agreed list to make the best savings, but you can check the fine detail of this and other factors when looking at what is offered in the agreement.

These practices are often set up with access to an out of hours emergency centre, which means that you do not have to work at night or at weekends and this may be very appealing to you and provide an attractive work–life balance. Some vets still wish to reap the rewards of doing much of the lucrative work at weekends during the day and in the early evenings, and they may opt to transfer calls just at night as, of course, it makes a difference to their profitability.

Do not be carried away by the thrill and anticipation of being your own boss and sign up without being sure exactly what terms you are agreeing to. Take care to look at the small print and get someone else to check it over too; employ a lawyer to ensure you are aware of exactly what happens should you wish to leave the practice if your circumstances change and you want to walk away. I know of vets who have thought that there was no question of them not wanting to continue to be a joint venture partner but when they found that in fact it was not working out for them, they found the conditions of leaving very difficult. It was all there in black and white in the contract and the parent company had been completely open about their procedures, but the vet had not read it through carefully enough or thought about every possible eventuality. We often make better vets than we do business people and it is important to seek professional advice if you do not possess the necessary skills and knowledge. Good financial and legal advice are a wise investment.

In the past, vets who have been qualified for less than five years have set up or bought their own practices and been very successful, though it is important to be aware of the commitment involved in running a practice and the time and effort needed for it to be a success. Setting up your plate requires in-depth research of what is involved, careful planning and full awareness of the demands on a practice owner, but with good employees, effective delegation and outsourcing it is possible and has been done in the past, though times are changing as ever, and ownership of small independent practices is becoming less common.

It is easier in fact now, since the advent of emergency service providers and referral centres, to set up a single-handed practice which may ultimately expand in the long term or stay as a one-vet practice should you choose. I often see premises in great locations that would make excellent small animal practices but you need to take advice and do your homework about the local competition and resources. Working for yourself is very motivating and, of course, you reap the rewards of your own endeavour, so your commitment to client service and your engagement with your clients tends to be far greater than when you work for someone else. You may be able to build a very successful practice which can provide a good source of income and which you can sell to fund your future.

There are still opportunities to buy into partnerships and limited companies, though as is often said, it is rather like entering into a marriage but without the romance. Far easier to get in than to get out and it is vital that you have a fair and comprehensive partnership agreement and seek legal advice before you sign on the dotted line.

After due consideration, you may decide that you are very happy working in first opinion practice and content to be an employed vet and that you like working in your current practice. In our practice, we had new graduates arrive 20 years ago and never leave. I became a partner in a practice and stayed there for 30 years and have never regretted my decision.

It may be that opportunities exist in the practice for you to progress and follow your interests and you may be in a good, supportive practice with an employer who values its vets and treats them really well, giving them the chance to grow and have autonomy. There is no reason to move just for the sake of it, as long as you have considered all the options and made a conscious decision to stay.

You can study for a certificate in general practice or other further education options and remember to ask the practice owners or managers about further training. Some practices are proactive in encouraging their vets to train but a busy practice owner may just not have thought about offering you the chance to study for a certificate or to involve you in management or offer a change in role and responsibilities.

Do not stay in the same practice simply because you are nervous of moving and because you are reluctant to experience change. The longer you have been in a practice, the more comfortable you are because you know the other vets, the clients and the nursing staff and if you move on you would be entering the unknown. This is all true, and perhaps this practice gives you everything you could desire and still nurtures and supports you to grow, and staying might be the right decision for you, just as long as you are not denying your ambitions and stifling your chances of career advancement for the sake of familiarity.

I have talked with vets who have stayed in the same practice for years when they really wanted to do something else with their working lives; they just stayed put because they became too comfortable or life became too complicated. Although they have been content and had a good life, as they get older some regret not following their wish to own their own practice or become an orthopaedic surgeon or even to live by the sea. Some people stay because they have to, because of their partner's or spouse's career situation or because they have other responsibilities. If you have to stay in a geographical area, then do look at other options in the area or how you may be able to develop within the practice you are in and try to have a plan in mind rather than just going with the flow.

Salaries for employed vets are at a level driven by supply and demand, so if there are not enough experienced vets around, practices will compete to recruit the best vets by offering the best pay and conditions and they should also be willing to pay well to keep good vets. It is always essential that you look at the entire package and take into account extra benefits such as health care, opportunities for further qualifications and fine detail such as holiday allowance and expected working hours. If you are in long-term employment and are an asset to a practice, then do not be hesitant in asking about a pay increase and do your research by looking at the SPVS salary survey so that you know what you should be earning.

Royal Army Veterinary Corps (RAVC)

You can access a career in the RAVC by applying for and attending an 11-week professionally qualified officers course at Sandhurst in the company of medical and dentistry graduates and become a lieutenant in the First Military Working Dog Regiment. There are further opportunities for career advancement and the work can evolve beyond veterinary work. There are also opportunities in the Territorial Army for reserve vets while continuing to work in practice which offer travel, training and a tax-free bonus.

Zoo and conservation work

Opportunities are not as widespread as demand appears to be but if you are very attracted to this sector, then gaining some experience in large animal work is advisable as you are likely to need to have acquired some transferable skills and experience. There are internships and residencies but these are oversubscribed and few and far between.

Working in this field is more accessible when you are young and without family ties such as children at school, so if you have ambitions then do not wait until you have a mortgage and four children.

There are many providers of career advice and it is worthwhile investing in some excellent advice such as that provided by the BVA careers advice provision. I would urge you to choose what you really want to do with your life and to work towards it even if it is a little nerve-wracking. You are young and highly qualified and in a new and exciting, developing veterinary world and have so much opportunity at your fingertips. Talk to other vets who are working in the areas you are attracted to and it is highly likely that you will find that there is help and advice available for you if you seek it out. There is a wealth of experience out there from older vets who have great generosity of spirit towards younger vets in practice and who would be only too happy to help.

Leaving veterinary work altogether and exploring pastures new

If you are sure, after several years as a vet, that veterinary work is not for you, then perhaps it is time for a complete career change. If you are convinced that you are in the wrong career and have exhausted all options, do not continue working in a job that you are not enjoying. Remember that as a veterinary graduate you have an excellent science degree and this means that you are not confined to working in the veterinary field but well qualified to apply for a myriad of other opportunities available in the world of employment. You can choose to make a complete change of career and follow in the footsteps of many other vets who found that it was just not the right job for them.

Keep an open mind and look for opportunities where you can and use all those excellent transferable skills that you have acquired in practice, such as communicating effectively with the general public. You now have well-developed and proven organisational and decision-making skills, and you have demonstrated your ability to work within a team and in providing leadership to the nursing staff. You may have educational experience of teaching student vets and nurses and all these skills, together with the excellent science degree you have attained, make you eminently employable in many fields.

I do sincerely hope, however, that you are still enjoying being a vet and that you feel optimistic about your future in the profession. I know that I have found it to be an amazing vocation which has brought me intangible benefits of job satisfaction, unfailingly interesting work and the mental stimulation of every day being different from the one before, so that I have rarely been bored in all my years as a vet and I still feel so lucky to be part of our unique profession.

I know that not every vet feels as I do and at the moment there are many factors affecting the way young vets feel about their chosen profession. The fear of litigation, consumer

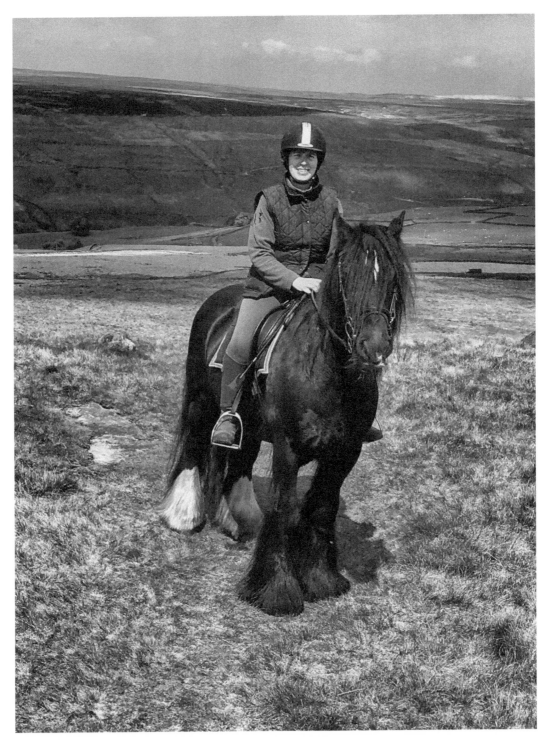

'There is something about the outside of a horse that is good for the inside of a man [or woman].'
(Winston Churchill)

expectations and the many changes in the way practice is structured, combined with dissatisfaction with the relatively low pay and conditions compared with other qualified professionals, can create feelings of discontent and uncertainty about the future.

I think that our fee structure in first opinion practice is currently being driven down by excessive competition for market share without sufficient foresight to the future and is a reflection on how we undervalue ourselves as a profession. The fees charged in first opinion practice should produce sufficient profit to pay a sufficient number of staff to provide the service effectively and to pay those people at a level commensurate with their ability and their investment in their education. Practices need to be profitable enough to reinvest in the practice premises and equipment and to move forward with new technology and the services that the public want for their animals.

You may not become as wealthy as a doctor or a dentist, but you should be able to earn a decent salary and have a really good life working in a job you enjoy the majority of the time. Every occupation has its downside but, although there will be times when things go wrong and clients are unreasonable or your patients try to injure you, there will also be those days when you will think it is the best job in the world.

This is a time of great change, but animals will always need veterinary care and we must make sure that we are there as the gatekeepers and providers for animal health and well-being as vets have always been. We should keep hold of the passion that drove us to choose this profession and the intangible personal and immeasurable benefits of being a vet which, for me, have outweighed all other considerations.

If you are still enjoying being a veterinary surgeon in practice, then I am so delighted for you because nothing makes me happier than to see a young vet embark on the same rewarding life of a veterinary surgeon in general practice that I have experienced. There are many further qualifications you can obtain but, for me, being a really good vet in first opinion practice is a wonderful thing to be. I hope you never lose that great feeling you get when a new puppy comes in or when you have successfully treated a family pet or performed a caesarian and you know that you achieved that outcome and that you have saved that precious life.

I wish you all the best, whatever your future holds and I hope you always remember that your life as a vet can be whatever you want it to be. Hold fast to your aspirations and your principles and practice the art of veterinary medicine as effectively as you can, facing each new day that comes without dwelling on those that are in the past. Most of all, be kind to yourself and remember that every day you will have made a positive difference, however small, to the well-being of animals in the course of your work, and that is what really matters.

Notes for employers and mentors

Our new graduates today are the future of the veterinary profession and they are not the same as those of us who have gone before, not the same but much more knowledgeable in fact. In many ways, they are much better veterinary graduates than we were ever were and they have been trained to use more complex equipment than we ever had to master. They have had the benefit of learning in a digital age with all the resources that offers and with tuition from lecturers with all the current knowledge of learning styles that a modern university can offer. They may not have had the opportunity we had as students to practice our skills in practice but with the right support in their first job they excel.

The curriculum at vet schools today is packed full of subject matter that was not even mentioned twenty years ago such as business skills but it is simply impossible to include everything within the curriculum that would be advantageous for a new vet in general practice to know. This is where you as employer and mentor come in and the weight of that responsibility and the potential benefit of it should be recognized by both you and the graduate.

Mentoring is hard work and demanding of your time, patience and your willingness to give of yourself in order to enable a young vet to become proficient and confident and thus content in their chosen career. It should not be undertaken lightly, and you should not be tempted to cut corners or be ungenerous with your time or dedication to this important task, because the future career satisfaction and possible happiness of a new vet is likely to be heavily influenced by this first year in practice.

Protected regular booked time should be allocated to this task and every new graduate should have a named mentor who is easily accessible to him or her even before they start work. Practices should recognise the importance of the work of the mentor and afford the necessary resources to do the job well and give structure to support the relationship and reward the role. This is in the interests of the practice and not just the new vet as employers have a duty of care to their new graduates and should look after their interests and wellbeing.

There are many more available resources for practices to draw on than previously and courses are available for mentors. The mentoring programme should be approached in an organised manner with regular reviews which are documented in such a way that progress can be assessed and areas for attention highlighted.

A good mentor should consider the following.

- Make contact before the new graduate starts work. Ensure they have all your contact details but also other essential contact details for practice personnel.
- All mentor meetings should be given due importance and not cancelled for trivial reasons and both parties must make time for them and approach them with enthusiasm.
- Progress and achievement should be documented on a regular basis using the PDP where appropriate.
- Include monitoring wellbeing as this is a stressful time for a new vet and a mentor is in a position to seek help and assistance from elsewhere for situations which are beyond their capabilities.
- When the mentor is away from the practice on holiday another member of staff should be organized to cover and help out.
- The mentor should praise achievement and progress however small and not focus solely on areas that could be improved.
- The mentor should listen to the new graduate as they will have the latest knowledge from vet school that may well be useful for the practice.
- The mentor should listen with an open mind to suggestions the new vet may have for improvements in the practice as they have arrived with a fresh eye and new perspective.
- If the mentor and the new vet are not working well together for whatever reason, or it is not possible for the mentor to find the necessary time, then do not continue regardless. Organise a new mentor without delay as a priority as mentoring of new graduates is essential and not just an added bonus.

I have the utmost respect for new graduates today who are dealing with things that previous generations never had to face such as student debt, pressures of social media and a rapidly changing structure in general practice. Perhaps we older vets envy the opportunity they may have, and which we did not, to enjoy a working life that still allows them to spend time with their friends and families and to follow other interests. Our role as older vets and mentors should be to support the next generation of vets positively and generously, and we should be rightly proud of our excellent young vets.

Employers have a responsibility to protect the wellbeing of vets working for them and there is no excuse for damaging their confidence or their mental health in asking too much from them in the first phase of their working lives. Young vets should be given a reasonable workload that allows time to learn the practical application of their professional skills and still have time to live lives as young and sociable adults. No vet employed in practice today should suffer from burn out due to unreasonable pressures of work and it should be an embarrassment for the employer who allows this to happen.

Wellbeing

Here is a brief wellbeing checklist for vets.

- Do not be a martyr to the job. There is more to you as a whole person than being a vet and it is just a part of who you are, an important part, but still just a part.
- You cannot make everyone happy whether it is in your personal life or in your working life. The happiness of other people is not your sole responsibility but you should make your own wellbeing a number one priority.
- If something is not going well in your professional life or in your private life, then you can take steps to change it. Changing direction is not an admission of failure but of strength.
- Be honest with yourself and kind and do not set higher standards for yourself than you would for other people. Do not dwell on the one negative experience but on the multitude of small positive achievements.
- Vets are often caring people and have a tendency to care for everything and everybody but themselves. Allow yourself a fair amount of time for doing what makes you happy such as a sport or interest, give it due priority and make it an essential part of your life.
- Spend time with people who lift your spirits and not with those who drain the joy out of your life. See friends in person and not just online and do things together which you enjoy and which make you smile.
- Do something in the fresh air every day, get some sun on your face and look around you. Spend some time with healthy animals. Feel the wind in your face and listen to sounds that are not related to humans. Empty your mind of minor worries; allow good thoughts in.
- Do not deprive yourself of sleep, good food, and good company. They usually make you feel much better whatever you are up against.
- Avoid excess alcohol, rubbish food, and negative people.
- You are a medically trained person so if you are not well mentally or physically go and get some help from an expert. You deserve help when you need it, you are important and your health and wellbeing is important so make that call just as you would advise an animal owner to ring the vet. You can and will improve with the right help.

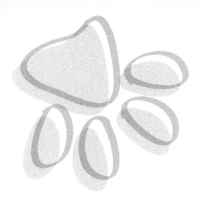

Acronyms

BSAVA	British Small Animal Veterinary Association
BVA	British Veterinary Association
CPD	continuing professional development
EMS	Extramural Studies
PDP	Professional Development Phase
PDR	Professional Development Record
RCVS	Royal College of Veterinary Surgeons
SPVS	Society of Practising Veterinary Surgeons
VDS	Veterinary Defence society

Common acronyms in clinical records

With thanks to contributors on the Veterinary Voices Facebook page.

BAR	bright alert responsive	EUGA	examine under general anaesthetic
BB	bring back		
BIOP	been in owners possession	FI	further investigation
BS	blood sample	HBC	hit by car
CCF	congestive cardiac failure	HR	heart rate
COA	calved on arrival	HX	history
C+	cough	INI	if not improved
DUDE	defecating drinking urinating eating	INVMB	if not very much better
		IVFT	intravenous fluid therapy
D+	diarrhoea (D++ even more diarrhoea, etc.)	LAPM	left a phone message
		MYF	mind your fingers
DNA	did not arrive	NAD	no abnormality detectable/ diagnosed
DOA	dead on arrival		
EAG	empty anal glands	NBM	nil by mouth

NFT	no further treatment		STOOP	spoke to owner on phone
NWB	non-weight bearing		Sx	surgery
O	owner		TGH	to go home
OA	osteoarthritis		TGHW	to go home with
OR	owner reports		TPR	temperature pulse respiration
POC	post op check		UA	urine analysis
PTS	put to sleep		US	ultrasound
RTA	road traffic accident		UTI	urinary tract infection
RV	revisit		V+	vomiting
SHIG	see how it goes		VMB	very much better
SO	stitches out		VMI	very much improved
STO	spoke to owner		WYF	watch your fingers

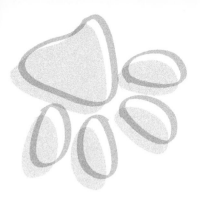

Index